AF838596

INHUMAN RESEARCH
Medical Experiments in German Concentration Camps

Alfred Pasternak, M.D. F.A.C.O.G.

INHUMAN RESEARCH

Medical Experiments in German Concentration Camps

In memory of all those
who perished in the Holocaust,
Alfr Pasternak

AKADÉMIAI KIADÓ, BUDAPEST

This book has been published with the financial assistance
of the Hungarian Academy of Sciences

Cover design:
Krisztina Kállai Nagy

ISBN 963 05 8382 8

Published by Akadémiai Kiadó
Member of Wolters Kluwer Group
P.O. Box 245, H-1519 Budapest, Hungary
www.akkrt.hu

© Pasternak, A. 2006

All rights reserved. No part of this book may be reproduced by any
means, or transmitted or translated into machine language without the
written permission of the publisher.

Printed in Hungary

In memory of my parents,
Simon and Anna Pasternak

CONTENTS

"The Holocaust is the burden of the twentieth century."

Hannah Arendt

Preface

Irma Liebman was seventy-one years old when she was taken to Auschwitz. She was the widow of Aaron Liebman, a great Talmudic scholar, a deeply religious, well-to-do, respected man. She was small, and had beautiful snow-white hair. She was a gentle, kind, quiet, fragile little lady. She always walked with a silver-handled cane.

Dr. Josef Mengele, who conducted the selections of the newly arrived prisoners at Auschwitz, immediately waved her to the right side. A few hours later, her frail little body was reduced to a few ounces of ash.

Irma Liebman was my grandmother. She was killed in Auschwitz, along with ninety-six other members of my family, according to the marble memorial we erected on Mount Zion in Jerusalem. Also killed were every one of my childhood friends, leaving me the only child survivor of our little Hungarian community.

■

The psychological effect of the Holocaust upon survivors has been extensively studied. Some of these studies have examined how survivors respond to the portraying of the Holocaust. Researchers have found that survivors can be divided into two categories: a large group of people who try to avoid everything related to the Holocaust because they fear nightmares and depression; and a small minority who compulsively seek out everything that presents, in any form, any part of the Holocaust history.

I most definitely belong to the second group. I read every available book, attend every lecture, see every movie, every exhibit about the Holocaust.

This predilection has led me to realize that the subject of the medical experiments conducted by Nazi physicians in various concentration camps is a relatively neglected part of Holocaust historiography. People, from all walks of life, have only heard of Mengele and his experiments on twins. The true extent and content of the camp experiments, doubtless one of the most shameful chapters in the history of medicine, is unfamiliar except to some historians specializing in Holocaust history.

Without having a specific goal or purpose in mind, quite some years ago I began to collect documents on these experiments. After awhile, prompted by friends, I presented a lecture at the History of Medicine Society. This presentation led to invitations from local medical associations, the Maimonides Society, and hospital annual general staff meetings, all across the United States. Eventually, some fellow survivors encouraged me to compile a book from my materials. The result is the volume you are holding in your hands.

I have created this book only with a great deal of reluctance, on many accounts. I knew from the beginning that I would have to retire from my very active medical practice, in order to free up the time required for such an undertaking. I also knew that no part of my book could ever be exhaustive. Besides the materials in major archives, libraries and museums, which I have read, many additional sources must lie waiting in Germany, the former Soviet Union, and other places; these data I will never find. Similarly I knew that I might actually fail to select the most informative and therefore the most important documents, or even the most significant part of a certain document. Eventually, I still decided to do it, no matter how incomplete the result of my work.

I was urged by a self-imposed feeling of moral obligation. Why? Even though about 80% of my large family perished in the Holocaust, my parents and two older sisters survived. Among the Jews of Hungary, outside of Budapest, this was almost as astonishing as the fact that I, a skinny 13 $^1/_2$ year old when I arrived at Auschwitz, survived. And I survived, in my own judgment, without any physical disability or major emotional scarring.

However, probably because of the above experiences, the Holocaust was and will always remain the primary determining and influential experience of my life. I simply must make whatever little or insignificant contribution I can to the telling of the complete "story," to prove the "Holocaust denyers" false and evil. As a physician, I feel this imperative especially strongly.

None of my childhood friends survived Auschwitz. While working on this book, I have always had them in mind; as was also my very special friend, my fellow camp mate in Dornhau, my partner *"Putzer"* in cleaning the guards' barrack for a few months, the late John Saunders (Jeno Schwartz).

I wish to thank Mr. Nathan Shapell, Mr. Jonah Goldrich, Mr. Max Webb and Terrace Tower USA for their financial assistance in the research of this book; Dr. Robert Levy for his valuable help in the actual research; and Ellen Wilson for her tireless editorial guidance. Finally, I wish to express my gratitude to my wife Elizabeth for letting me postpone the plans we had made for our retirement.

CHAPTER 1

The Nazification of German Medicine

From his prison cell in the Bavarian town of Landsberg, Adolf Hitler penned these words on the troubles roiling German civilization of the 1920s: "Anyone who wants to cure this era, which is inwardly sick and rotten, must first of all summon up the courage to make clear the causes of the disease."[1] The medical metaphor is unmistakable; Hitler viewed his era as one of decay and German society as a sick organism afflicted with a dangerous malady that was threatening its integrity and continued viability.

Traditional social and economic structures in Germany were indeed being challenged by ambivalent forces, which were simultaneously destroying traditional relations and ways of being, and creating complex, confusing new ones. The population was growing rapidly, as agricultural innovations increased the

1 Adolf Hitler, *Mein Kampf* (Boston: Houghton Mifflin, 1943), p. 435; cited in Robert Jay Lifton, *The Nazi Doctors: Medical Killing and the Psychology of Genocide* (New York: Basic Books, 1986), p. 16. The survey material in this chapter is especially indebted to Lifton's excellent study. In addition, it draws from Robert N. Proctor's *Racial Hygiene: Medicine under the Nazis* (Cambridge, Mass: Harvard University Press, 1988). Lifton introduces two important concepts, "medicalized killing" and "the killing/healing paradox", to describe the process of rationalization that allowed physicians to participate in the Nazi experiments and exterminations in the camps. Proctor provides a nuanced analysis of the intellectual arguments and resulting policies that transformed concepts from eugenics and racial hygiene into full-blown racist ideologies and practices.

The following secondary works have also proved invaluable: Götz Aly, Peter Chroust and Christian Pross, *Cleansing the Fatherland* (Baltimore and London, 1994); Michael H. Kater, "The Burden of the Past: Problems of a Modern Historiography of Physicians and Medicine in Nazi Germany", *German Studies Review,* 10: 1 (February 1987) and *Doctors under Hitler* (Chapel Hill and London: University of North Carolina Press, 1989); Robert N. Proctor, "Nazi Biomedical Policies", in *When Medicine went Mad: Bioethics and the Holocaust,* ed. Arthur L. Caplan (Towota, New Jersey: Humana Press, 1992); Barren H. Lerner and David J. Rothman, "Medicine and the Holocaust: Learning More of the Lessons", *Annals of Internal Medicine,* 122: 10 (1995); Ernst Edzard, "Killing in the Name of Healing: The Active Role of the German Medical Profession during the Third Reich", *American Journal of Medicine,* 100 (May 1996); *Medizin ohne Menschlichkeit: Dokumente des Nürnberger Prozesses,* ed. Alexander Mitscherlich and Fred Mielke (Frankfurt am Main: Fischer Taschenbuch Verlag, 1960), first published in English as *Doctors of Infamy, The Story of Nazi Medical Crimes* (New York: Henry Schuman, 1949).

food supply and medical advances joined with better nutrition to extend human longevity and decrease mortality rates. In response to industrialization, people were relocating to burgeoning cities, following jobs and seeking new opportunities. In congested, filthy urban areas, old human afflictions – crime, poverty, squalor and communicable diseases – acquired disturbing visibility and terrifying new dimensions. Faced with these circumstances, the Germans resorted to fighting with their European neighbors, in an effort to relieve the pressure. But war failed to resolve the problems, bringing tragic consequences in its wake. The search for answers to the ills of industrialization and urbanization had to begin anew.

In turning to medical metaphors and models for his solutions to these problems, Hitler was drawing on a long-established philosophical tradition that conceptualized human societies in biological terms, as living organisms constructed of interrelated, mutually dependent parts and locked in a natural struggle against other such organisms for survival. Germany, from this point of view, was a sick body. The solution to her ills lay in finding the causes of the malady and disabling or eliminating them, much as a doctor would attack an illness by removing its causes.

Nazism stands out from other fascist philosophies of the late nineteenth and twentieth centuries in its harnessing of biological theories – specifically population genetics – to a totalitarian nationalist-socialist program rooted in racism. The key to restored social and economic vigor was believed to lie not only in structural economic changes but also in medically strengthening the specifically "German" elements of society at the expense of "non-German" ones. The concept "race" justified the division of humankind into the categories of "German" and "non-German", while the discipline of eugenics (*Rassenhygiene* in German) inspired the idea of strengthening the population through genetic manipulations. The discipline of medicine provided the disease model, which prescribed cutting out, or otherwise removing "cancerous", "parasitic" racial elements.

Throughout the period of Nazi rule, the German medical profession acted as an extension of the regime. The reasons for this sad spectacle are many and complicated, far beyond the scope of this volume. What is relevant here is that a perversely skillful manipulation of the German medical profession, coupled with a co-optation of scientific practices, population genetics theories, disease models and the language of hygiene, allowed the Nazi program of racial cleansing to advance to unheard of extremes, with assistance from doctors. Never before has medicine been used to such murderous ends!

Rassenhygiene (the term was coined in 1895 by Alfred Ploetz) was the unruly late nineteenth-century offspring of Mendelian genetics. The latter discipline had turned the farmer's act of creating healthier, more productive livestock or crops into a recognized natural science, rooted in positive laws. *Rassenhygiene* simply applied the laws of genetic inheritance and natural selection to humankind, all in the name of bettering, maybe even perfecting, the human lot.

The problem with this approach lay not so much in its idealistic goals, but in the devilish ethical-philosophical questions associated with the goal: Who was going to control the processes by which human traits were classified as good or bad? What criteria were going to inform the classification? Who was going to take charge of selecting the genes to be passed along? How were the decisions to be legitimized? How were they to be implemented and by whom?

The answers in the early twentieth century did not require the division of humankind into races, some superior, others inferior; nor did they require brutal medical experiments with human subjects, forced sterilizations, "medicalized killing", or genocide. In other words, the horrors of the Nazi racial policies did not grow inevitably from these intellectual roots. Despite the connotation of racial cleansing conjured by the German term *Rassenhygiene,* Hitler and his fellow racists had to distort the discipline, or privilege one of its intellectual streams of thought – the racist Nordic supremacist idea – over others equally strong, in order to bend the broader discipline to their will. Once this distortion had occurred, the discipline lent inspiration and an aura of scientific legitimacy to acts of state-sponsored racial cleansing. Nazism, in the words of Rudolf Hess, was simply *applied* biology![2]

But the transformation of *Rassenhygiene* into a set of validated racist practices depended on more than this skillful intellectual hijacking; someone had to carry out the Nazi decrees, and the evidence suggests that many professional medical people were willing to do so. In fact, had German biologists, geneticists and physicians rejected a specific set of assumptions *not* essential to *Rassenhygiene* but critical to legitimizing Nazi policies, they might have resisted nazification more actively and even prevented some of the horrors associated with the later years of war. But many, too many, subscribed to these assumptions: Humankind can be divided according to objective, verifiable criteria into genetically distinct races, unequal in quality. The pure and superior "German" population in Germany is declining in numerical proportion to inferior racial groups, such as Slavs, Gypsies and Jews. It is also undergoing a qualitative decline with implications for the very survival of German culture and civilization. Given this dire situation, radical measures to purify, strengthen and preserve the population must be implemented, and the interests of the individual can and indeed must be sacrificed to the interests of the collective.

2 Lifton, *The Nazi Doctors,* p. 31, 129.

Once Hitler brought the Nazis to power, on 30 January 1933, he moved quickly to begin implementing his program of "racial hygiene". In keeping with his obsession that an "illness" afflicted Germany, he focused first on the medical profession: "You, you National Socialist doctors, I cannot do without you for a single day, for a single hour. If you fail me, then all is lost. For what good are our struggles, if the health of our people is in danger?"[3] In practice, his words meant that the medical profession was subjected to the process known as *Gleichschaltung;* that is, the restructuring of the profession according to the *Führerprinzip* to ensure that medical practice would conform with and reflect Nazi racial ideology and goals. The first targets were various professional medical associations, such as the Union of German Medical Associations (Deutsche Ärtzevereinsbund) and the Hartmann Association (Hartmannbund), which were placed under the control of a Reichärtzeführer [Reich Medical Leader]. The newly appointed Reichärtzeführer was Gerhard Wagner, who was already head of the Reich Physicians' Chamber, the Association of German Health Insurance Physicians, the Office for Public Health, the National Socialist Physicians' League, the Office of Racial Policy, the Expert Committee for Public Health, and the Office for Genealogical Research (Amt für Sippenforschung). Henceforth German physicians would be centrally controlled and required to assist in implementing Nazi racial hygiene programs.

The anti-Semitic implications of *Gleichschaltung* soon became evident. Jews in 1933 are estimated to have comprised 13% of the medical profession (though they may have represented more than 80% of the physicians in Berlin's hospitals). After *Gleichschaltung,* the new German Medical Association immediately passed a resolution calling for the removal of Jews from positions of influence throughout the Reich. No longer would they be permitted to join medical school faculties or to participate in professional medical organizations. As a sign of what was to come, Issue No. 1 of the *Deutsches Ärzteblatt,* the principal professional medical journal of the reorganized profession, carried a giant swastika on its cover, as if to advertise the arrival of a new era in German medicine. In the fall of 1933, Dr. Kurt Klare, head of the Association of the German Medical Press, announced that only "German" doctors would be permitted to edit and write for the medical journals. Publications and medical schools quickly embraced eugenics and racial theory. Textbooks written by Jewish physicians and scientists were banned. Meanwhile Jews were maligned as "anti-healers" and abortionists, corrupt with commercialism, bolshevism, and degenerate notions such as Freudian "sexology".

3 This speech by Hitler at one of the early meetings of The National Socialist Physicians' League is cited in Proctor, *Racial Hygiene,* p. 64. The National Socialist Physicians' League was founded at the Nuremberg Nazi Party Congress in 1929.

The three statutes of 1935 collectively known as the Nuremberg Laws made clear that the Nazi state would be dedicated to protecting its German Aryans from "infection" or "pollution" through contact with non-Aryans, especially Jews.[4] The first two laws, the Reichbürgergesetz (Reich Citizenship Law) and the Gesetz zum Schutze des deutschen Blutes und der deutschen Ehre (Law for the Protection of German Blood and German Honor; or the "Blood Law"), were promulgated on 15 September 1935. The first narrowly defined Reich citizenship to exclude Jews while the second proscribed intermarriage, and even casual sexual relations, between Jews and Aryan Germans. So-called "racial heritage", categorized according to the degree of "Jewishness", determined individual rights under this law. On 18 October 1935 came the third law, the Gesetz zum Schutze der Erbgesundheit des deutschen Volkes (Law for the Genetic Health of the German People), requiring couples to submit to a medical examination before marrying and prohibiting the marriage of people with specified "genetic defects". The transformation of racial hygienics into full-blown racism was now enshrined in a set of laws, and German medical journals applauded the development. The message was loud and clear: Jews should not be allowed to propagate. In fact, Jews were already being marked for extinction.

Following the promulgation of the Nuremberg Laws, hundreds of ordinances were passed to further separate Jews from the rest of German society. One of their targets was the continued presence of Jews in the medical profession. On 25 July 1938, a new law specifically excluded Jews from the practice of medicine, and on 6 October, all Jewish physicians were removed from the official registry of physicians. Henceforth Jewish doctors were restricted to treating other Jews, and then only *after* obtaining official permission. An article by Dr. H. H. Meier advertised the triumph of the Aryans in its very title "Das Ende des jüdischen Arzttums" (The End of Jewish Medicine).[5]

German physicians were eager and willing participants in these events. They joined the Nazi Party in record numbers (an estimated 45% of the profession, proportionately more than any other profession) and reaped distinct economic benefits as their Jewish competitors from medical school faculties, insurance boards and clinics were removed from the profession. Individual physicians acquired greater numbers of paying patients, while faculty positions and promotions became more readily available. In their failure to protest these early

4 A note on orthography: I have elected to preserve the German umlaut in all spellings, except for the cities Nuremberg and Munich. In accord with this principle, variant spellings in documents (Fuhrer or Fuehrer for Führer, for example) have been converted to the umlauted form.

5 Meier's article appeared in *Ziel und Weg* (Objective and Method), 9 (1939).

acts, indeed in their willingness to sacrifice their Jewish colleagues on the altar of personal greed and ambition, German physicians became accessories of Nazism, even before they began assisting in the criminal and unethical acts associated with the camp experiments and exterminations.

From the early days of their power, the Nazis also set in motion their program of medical interventions on behalf of greater racial purity. Compulsive sterilization, then prohibited, even on eugenic grounds, was made legal through the 14 July 1933 "Law for the Prevention of Genetically Diseased Offspring" (Gesetz für Verhütung Erbkranken Nachwusches). Under this statute, an individual could be sterilized against his or her will, if a genetic health court (Erbgesundheitsgericht) determined that the person suffered from a so-called genetic illness, such as schizophrenia, manic depressive illness, syphilis or alcoholism. The law specified the establishment of a network of genetic health courts and appellate courts to handle these cases. On 1 May 1934, the former Aufklärungsamt für Bevölkerunspolitik und Rassenpflege (Bureau of Education for Population Policy and Racial Hygiene) became the Office of Racial Policy (Rassenpolitisches Amt), charged with bringing all education and training on population and race matters into line with Nazi ideology. This bureau played a critical role in the design of both the sterilization program and the Nuremberg Laws. Through its training programs, it imbued physicians with the precepts and practices of racial hygiene. It also conducted important public propaganda campaigns to ensure that the new laws and policies would be endorsed and implemented.

In 1934, 181 genetic health courts and appellate courts were established throughout Germany. Operating as part of the civil justice administration, each court consisted of a panel composed of one lawyer and two doctors. Every German doctor was now a "genetic doctor" responsible for incorporating racial hygiene into his medical judgments. The duty to report genetic information now took precedence over the confidentiality of the doctor-patient relationship. Just as physicians routinely reported births and deaths to the authorities, they would now report the presence of genetic defects; it was a matter of public health and hygiene, of keeping population statistics and records. But the implications of the change were far greater: thenceforth, patients were no longer going to be treated as individuals but as members of the *Volk;* the doctor's primary allegiance would be transferred from his patient to the State.

The results of the sterilization program reveal the degree to which physicians participated from the very beginning in Nazi programs. An estimated 400,000 persons were sterilized, ninety-five percent before the outbreak of World War II. The majority of these sterilizations were done by surgical means, vasectomies for men and tubal ligations for women. In some instances experimental means such as chemical injections or radiation were used. Persons chosen for sterilization had the right to appeal but almost all appeals were rejected. The so-called feebleminded were most frequently targeted (42.5% of the total number of procedures). Many of these individuals protested. The program required a bureaucracy to generate and screen applications, and physicians and hospital staff to perform the surgeries and provide post-operative care. All such personnel were participants in and accessories to these crimes. Imagine the time and costs involved in these sterilizations and you have some idea of the complicity of the German medical establishment, even at this early stage.

There was no great public outcry against the Sterilization Law (the Catholic Church opposed the law in principle but made no concerted effort to challenge it), but there were internal disagreements among Nazi officials over the scope of the law. One faction headed by Arthur Gutt of the Reich Ministry of the Interior disputed with another headed by Gerhard Wagner and the Physicians' League about the intent of the law. Gutt argued that the law needed stricter standards for determining genetic defects. Wagner felt that the law was more political than medical and that the need to purify the Aryan race and rid it of defective elements justified a loose, flexible standard. This power struggle between two individuals and their respective institutions culminated in a 1938 amendment to the law, mandating the appointment of two German lay persons – loyal party members of course – to each panel in the genetic court system. These new appointees were intended to counterbalance the occasionally reluctant medical members of the board. But no matter, after 1939, for several reasons, among them a shifting of resources and priorities, the sterilization effort slowed down.

One of the new priorities, and one that would further entwine the German medical profession with Nazi policy, was the euthanasia program. The cleansing of the German race, by euthanizing or simply murdering anyone who did not fit the Aryan ideal, was part of the Nazi agenda for the Reich from the outset. Doctors and other leaders simply had to have the "courage", as Hitler put it in *Mein Kampf,* to do the job, however distasteful or immoral it might seem. In effect, with the euthanasia program, the Nazis were beginning to demand that doctors violate their fundamental commitment to preserve individual lives, to act instead as murderers rather than healers.

The Nazis grounded their arguments for euthanasia on two assumptions: first, that human beings are not biologically equal; and second, that this inequality relieves the State of the duty to protect all its citizens: the weak can be sacrificed. Euthanasia was simply one way of putting these assumptions into practice. These ideas had been spelled out in 1920 in the book *Die Freigabe der Vernichtung lebensunwerten Lebens* [The Permission to Destroy Life Unworthy of Life], by two eminent German professors, Karl Binding, a legal authority and Alfred Hoche, a professor of psychiatry. Binding and Hoche demonstrated that "assisted death" could be justified on medical and legal grounds. Their argument was primarily utilitarian in nature: putting people to death can be a "useful act" because it relieves individuals and the State of the tremendous economic burdens associated with caring for the incurably ill, the mentally ill, the feebleminded, the retarded, and the deformed. The phrase "lebensunwerten Lebens" [life unworthy of life] passed into the German lexicon as a respectable concept, which Hitler embraced and which, under the Nazis, acted as a euphemism signifying all people who did not meet the Nazi's criteria for membership in the master race.

Unlike the sterilization program, the euthanasia program was implemented extra-legally; that is, in the absence of specific authorizing statutes. The practice of euthanasia was too controversial, too politically sensitive for open embrace, so it was instituted instead through a series of executive actions accompanied by an extensive propaganda campaign. The propaganda used two sorts of argument: the first, an economic one that appealed to human "reason"; the second an emotional one that appealed to the German sense of the heroic. The intent was to transform murder into an act of mercy for the affected individuals, necessary for their own good and for the health of the community. Reichärtzführer Wagner outlined these principles at the notorious 1935 Nuremberg Nazi Party Conference: The State should place a greater value on the healthy than on the sick. The care of the sick is a drain on the regime, at the expense of the healthy; the notion that all people deserve equal care is insane and the Nazi regime must tackle this problem. Government bureaucrats, SS and SA officials, party leaders, police and members of the press, meanwhile, were exposed to the worst cases in German mental hospitals in order to underscore these points. Certain hospital budgets were cut so that the patients would suffer and either die or become less worthy of life. Meanwhile Nazi propaganda films contrasted healthy Germans with Jewish mental patients and appealed to the German love of the heroic. The film of Helmut Unger's 1936 novel *Sendung und Gewissen* (Mission and Conscience), for example, told the story of a physician-husband who honors his beloved wife's request for euthanasia in order to spare her from the ravages of end-stage multiple sclerosis. He is accused of murder but exonerated. The film *(Ich klage an!)* was a success, a cultural event of great psychological impact.

In testimony after the war, Wagner revealed that Hitler had actually decided early on to eliminate the mentally ill, indeed that even in 1933 euthanasia was being practiced clandestinely in certain mental hospitals. But the program did not really take off until 1939, when the order was given to set up the Committee for the Scientific Treatment of Severe, Genetically Determined Illness. Under the direction of Karl Brandt, the committee was to formulate a plan for the killing of all deformed and retarded children in Germany. Hitler had already personally authorized one such killing in what was to become a model case: a child born blind, retarded, and without an arm and leg, allegedly in response to a written request from the child's father. (No doubt this story has been mythologized; the specifics of how this particular letter and request got to Hitler, and how many other such requests he reviewed are not discussed in sources.)

Although the euthanasia program was to be clandestine, its implementation required extensive cooperation from the medical establishment. Doctors and midwives delivering children with any deformities were asked to report the births to the state government. Similarly doctors were asked to report to local health authorities the names of any children in their care less than three years of age with any such infirmities. The doctors were obliged to fill out elaborate health questionnaires. Conditions to be reported were listed in medical journals, and the regulation of these diseases was treated as a public health issue, much like the reporting of venereal disease.

The questionnaires were returned to the office of Hans Hefelmann, who was charged with overseeing the business of the committee. With the help of three physicians, Hefelmann marked the questionnaires with a plus (death) or minus (allowed to live). Individuals slated to die (the euphemism was "selected") were sent to one of twenty-eight hospitals where the deaths were brought about by a variety of techniques including pills, injections and gassing. Death certificates were carefully filled out and always listed a natural cause of death, in a conscious falsification designed to deceive the Red Cross and to prevent criticism from foreign nations, the press or health organizations. Parents received a standardized letter informing them of a child's death, listing a false cause of death, and containing the misleading explanation that, for health reasons, their child's body had been cremated.

Robert Jay Lifton, in *The Nazi Doctors,* introduces the concept of "medicalized killing" to describe the complex of ideas and actions that allowed medical personnel to be party to such crimes. The creation of an elaborate web of lies by the participants at each step of the euthanasia process allowed them to deceive themselves about what they were doing. Lifton calls this web "the healing/killing paradox", and argues that it forms the foundation for a new way of thinking in which killing and healing were interchanged. The result was a significant psychological shift within the German medical community as a whole. Physicians deceived themselves into believing that they were saving or healing the German Nation, even as the result was that individuals were being "selected", "treated", or "eliminated", the preferred euphemisms for what were really acts of medical murder.

At his post-war trial Karl Brandt was asked about whether euthanasia was cruel. He explained that the underlying motive was the desire to help individuals who could not help themselves, for whom the prolonging of life would mean torment. He went on to say: "This reflection is certainly not anything inhuman. Nor did I ever feel it to be in any degree unethical or immoral..." Asked if he felt any blame for the euthanasia, he answered: "No. I do not feel myself to blame. I have a perfectly clear conscience... I was actuated by purely humane sensibility..."[6]

The program slowly expanded beyond its original scope. In December 1940 Hefelmann decided that children older than three could be "treated", and by the autumn of 1941 children as old as seventeen were being screened. Jewish children, originally excluded from the program on the grounds that were unworthy of "mercy" killings (as we well know, the Nazis had other plans for them), were swept into its purview in 1943 when the killing of healthy children of non-German races was authorized; the psychiatric hospital at Hadamar began executing Jewish children in May of that year.

The aforementioned Committee for the Scientific Treatment of Severe, Genetically Determined Illness also began administering an adult euthanasia program in the summer of 1939. The orders for this program were passed along through several intermediaries (Gerhard Wagner to Helmut Unger to Hans Hefelmann to Viktor Brack, who was told that Hitler had authorized Wagner's successor Leonardo Conti to set up the program), all sworn to strictest secrecy. Hans Lammers, head of the Reich Chancellery, later recalled that "[Hitler] considered it proper that the 'life unworthy of life' of severely mentally ill persons be eliminated by actions *(Eingriffe)* that bring about death."[7] Conti, with assistance from Philipp Bouhler, the party chancellery leader, and Herbert Linden, one of the authors of the Blood Law, obediently created a plan to murder all of Germany's handicapped and mental patients.

The adult program was initiated officially by an October 1939 decree from Hitler, backdated to September 1, to coincide with the start of the war: "Reich

6 For Karl Brandt's testimony, see Mitscherlich and Mielke, eds., *Medizin ohne Menschlichkeit*, pp. 206–208; here p. 208.

"F.: Wenn Sie das Ganze betrachten, fühlen Sie sich selbst heute irgendwie belastet durch die Ausübung der Euthanasie?"

"A.: Nein Ich fühle mich dadurch nicht belastet. Ich habe die Vorstellung und Überzeugung, dass ich das, was ich in diesem Zusammenhang getan habe, vor mir selbst verantworten kann. Es war getragen von einem absolut menschlichen Empfindung..."

7 Lifton, *The Nazi Doctors*, p. 62.

Leader Bouhler and Dr. Brandt are charged with the responsibility for expanding the authority of physicians, to be designated by name, to the end that patients considered incurable according to the best available human judgment *(menschlihen Ermessen)* of their state of health, can be granted a mercy death *(Gnadentod)*."[8] At the 1935 Nuremberg Congress, Hitler had remarked privately to Wagner that the outbreak of war would provide a smokescreen behind which the elimination of the mentally ill could take place with little protest from the people. Thus it should not surprise us to learn that the euthanasia program began in earnest after the September 1939 invasion of Poland.

As Lifton points out, the war provided not only a smokescreen behind which the murders could take place, but also several other rationales for the questionable program: to the German people it could be said that if the best of Aryan youth were headed to the front where they might lose their lives for the Reich, it was not to protect those "unworthy of life"; and it could also be pointed out that the "mercy-killings" would free up hospital beds for military purposes. The disappearance of the weak, the infirm, and the disabled from the boundaries of the Reich was taking on ever increasing urgency in the twisted minds of Nazi officials. Their mission of murder assumed heroic proportions.

"Operation Euthanasia", along with the bureaucratic apparatus that supported it, came to be known as "T4" because its administration, which included more than fifty volunteer physicians, was headquartered in Berlin at Tiergartenstrasse 4. Reporting to the T4 operation were three separate organizations, "dummy corporations" set up to camouflage the operations, each a party to the murders in its own way. The Working Committee for Hospital Care was the name that appeared on letterhead for official correspondence; The Charitable Foundation for Institutional Care, or Central Clearinghouse for Mental Hospitals, handled fiscal affairs; and The Non-Profit Transport Corporation, or The Common Welfare Ambulance Service, Limited, moved patients from their care facilities to extermination centers.

The program involved most of the German psychiatric establishment as well as other doctors and hospital employees throughout the Reich. As in the child murder program, questionnaires asking for information about the presence of "genetic disease" (Down's syndrome, schizophrenia, Huntington's chorea, among others) were drafted and sent to hospitals and homes for the chronically ill. For the adult program, however, the T4 leadership also sought to identify individuals who had been continuously hospitalized for five years or more, or

8 Ibid., p. 63; citing, Trial of Werner Heyde, Gerhard Bohne, and Hans Hefelmann, Generalstaatsanwalt Frankfurt, Js 17/59 (GstA), 4 VU 3/61, Strafkammer des Landgerichts Limburg/Lahn, p. 203.

who were criminally insane and in custody, as well as patients who were "not of German blood". These questionnaires gave the impression of being some sort of statistical survey, but they signaled their diabolic intent in the weight given to questions about the ability of an individual to work. The fine print specified "no vague answers" and asked for a specific evaluation of "productivity": how much the person works (full or part-time), how skilled he or she is, and how hard he or she works.[9] Anyone unable or unwilling to work was slated for elimination. The first murders were carried out in Poland in January 1940, of 4,400 incurable mentally ill patients – they were shot.

Originally, as Dr. Viktor Brack's famous dictum, "the syringe belongs in the hand of a physician", makes clear, injection was envisioned as the preferred means for administering euthanasia; but death by injection was quickly rejected in favor of carbon monoxide. The superiority of the latter was demonstrated in January 1940 when Conti, Brandt and others met in a hospital in Brandenburg, a former prison, for a full-scale test of adult euthanasia. The demonstration began with the euthanizing of six patients by injection. Conti and Brandt pushed the syringe on the first two to show the commitment of the leadership to Hitler's order. But the patients died too slowly. So it was decided to try carbon monoxide.

Christian Wirth of the SS Criminal Police, who had been assigned to the T4 staff (he would later be involved in the extermination camps), supervised the construction of a special tiled gas chamber designed to resemble a shower room. A "water pipe", situated a few inches above the ground, emitted carbon monoxide. The hospital had two crematoria ovens for burning the bodies. In the test, approximately eighteen to twenty persons were made to undress in an adjacent room and then to enter the shower room where they were gassed. The observers included Dr. Imfried Eberl, who was soon to become head of the T4 killing center at Brandenburg, would later assume that role at the Bernberg facility, and eventually be appointed the first commandant of the Treblinka extermination camp.

The results satisfied the observers. The shower room setup disguised the fact that people were being murdered, to both the killers and their victims. A "humane and efficient" way had been found to euthanize. Karl Brandt judged the technique "a major advance" in medical history.[10] Subsequently, six hospitals were chosen and outfitted with the special gas chambers and crematoria. T4 directives mandated that the procedure was to be carried out by doctors within the first twenty-four hours after patients arrived. The plan was to euth-

9 Lifton, *The Nazi Doctors*, pp. 68–69, reproduces the questionnaires.
10 Ibid., p. 73.

anize 65,000-70,000 persons out of a population of 65-70 million. By August 1941 not only had the Nazis accomplished their goals, they had also generated detailed records of the murders.

These records reveal that by August 1941, a total of 70,273 individuals had been murdered according to an established pattern. Once patients were selected, they were transported to the designated hospital killing centers. Lists identifying the patients accompanied them, along with detailed instructions concerning the collection of their case histories and valuables. SS men, often dressed in white coats to impersonate medical personnel, manned the transport buses. The bus windows were blacked out lest the population observe anyone inside becoming upset. The doctors at the delivering institutions were not informed of the location to which their patients were being sent. Sometimes the patients were actually taken to one destination "for observation" before actually being sent to the killing centers.

The T4 program operated at a profit. German historian Götz Aly has noted that the program made money by sequestering its victims' assets and the gold from their teeth, thus foreshadowing the treatment accorded Jewish concentration camp inmates. The most important source of income for the program, however, was the service fee charged for each patient assigned to the program, up to the moment of death, and sometimes beyond, as the death certificates carried falsified dates.

Residents of the towns near the killing centers were not meant to know what was happening in their communities. Most of the killing centers were set up in former mental hospitals, nursing homes, castles, or, in one instance, a former prison. Walls were built to surround the facilities so that no sounds from within – patients' screams for example – could be heard outside the walls.

But such large-scale murders could not have been accomplished without the knowledge and complicity of great numbers of people at many different institutions and from many walks of life. Consider the bureaucracy involved: the Nazi officials who planned and authorized the program, the persons who prepared the forms, who mailed them and retrieved and compiled them; the doctors, midwives and nurses who reported on those marked for death, the ones who enforced the decision, the drivers who transported the patients, the workers who built the gas chambers and crematoria, the hospital workers, and the populace surrounding the killing centers disguised as health facilities.

Then there was the matter of the death certificates. Professor Werner Heyde of Würzburg, a prominent psychiatrist, initially oversaw the program and was directly involved in issuing the death certificates. Given the circumstances, filling out the death certificates required inventing possible causes of death. Thus, in yet another perversion of medicine, doctors were asked to put their medical knowledge to use not to save people but rather to come up with credible explanations for the murders. This practice added another layer of deception and treachery to the operation. Deception did not even end with death. The victims' ashes were sent to each family, but these were not the individual's ashes, as the corpses were cremated in groups.

At a post-war trial, Helge Grabitz, a German war crimes prosecutor, was asked about how the T4 workers could accomplish their task. Based on the testimonies in post-war trials, she answered:

"Those who were immune, looked on day in and day out and helped to gas the children and infants; those who had to participate against their will, they would have preferred to do something else, nevertheless they participated. And finally there were those who did not know how to bring this into balance with their conscience, but they did not have the courage to refuse... According to my own knowledge, I would say the greatest group was those who did it as a matter of course. Those who did with enthusiasm, that is the second largest, and the least large group is that group that had qualms of conscience."

Proctor notes, "It is important to note the banality of the operation. In 1941 the psychiatric institution at Hadamar celebrated the cremation of its ten thousandth patient in a special ceremony, where everyone in attendance – secretaries, nurses and psychiatrists – received a bottle of beer for the occasion."[11]

In August 1941, Hitler told Karl Brandt that the euthanasia program was to be "stalled". There is some testimony that Hitler was reacting to negative publicity and complaints received about the program. Brandt claimed to have telephoned Bouhler to relay the order, but no written documents confirm this. Whatever the reason, the euthanasia operation was transferred from the control of Hitler's Chancellery back to the individual hospitals, and in the fall of 1941, the gas chambers were shipped from the mental hospitals east to Belzec, Majdanek, Auschwitz, Sobibor and Treblinka. But that is to step ahead of the unfolding events.

The T4 program thus came to an official halt, but German Nazi medical professionals had become so inured to the culture of medical murder that physicians continued the practice until the very last minutes of the war. This was the period of so-called "wild euthanasia", during which doctors who no longer had access to gas chambers euthanized selected patients by whatever other means were available. Patients also died by virtue of neglect – from starvation, dehydration, and the withholding of basic care – as well as from the effects of punishments.

11 Proctor, *Racial Hygiene*, p. 191, citing Fredric Wertham, *A Sign for Cain: An Exploration of Human Violence* (New York, 1966), p. 157.

Despite its official halt, the T4 operation had been a success. The Nazis had met their goal of euthanizing 1% of the German population. More importantly, T4 had laid the groundwork for the next phase of the Nazi agenda: the extermination of the Jews.

After Germany invaded Poland, Polish Jews were forced into ghettos in a move portrayed as a quarantine of sorts, a public health measure: "a hygienic necessity", as the Nazis called it. As a result of overcrowding and malnutrition, the ghettos would indeed become disease-ridden places, thereby making it possible for the Nazis to claim that cleaning them out was necessary for the public health, thus reducing opposition from urban residents. Self-serving as well as self-fulfilling, these arguments provided a circular medical rationale for the isolation and murder of the Jews. The high rate of disease had the desirable coincidental effects of causing Jewish deaths and weakening overall Jewish morale and resistance. This, too, was part of the Nazi plan.

However, the ghettoization of Jews created another quite real danger, that the diseases being allowed to ravage the ghettos might spread outside their walls. Thus German officials pondered: what should become of the Jews? Some argued for keeping them as a class of slave laborers, particularly during the war, as so many of Germany's finest sons were being sacrificed at the front. Brack suggested a variation on this theme: keep the healthy Jews as workers but sterilize them to prevent them from propagating their "race". This idea was rejected. Others proposed removing the Jews to another land, perhaps Madagascar. Still others argued that the Jews might prove useful as pawns in negotiations with the French and the English: the Allies just might agree to the removal of the Jews from German-controlled areas in exchange for peace. Yet another proposal was to create a Jewish preserve in Eastern Europe, so that Jews could be studied in a "natural habitat". However, these solutions were merely academic discussions among the lower rungs of Nazi leadership. In retrospect, it is clear that at the highest levels, Hitler and his henchmen were moving inexorably towards a more radical solution; programs of racial hygiene and euthanasia, applied to the Jews, would soon metamorphose into cold-blooded murder.

The Jewish extermination program began well disguised, in the same institutions that were charged with administering the general euthanasia program, with an April 1940 order from the Reich Ministry of the Interior that all Jewish patients be identified in three weeks time. In June two hundred of these patients – men, women and children – were gassed at the Brandenburg center. The gassings continued through July at Brandenburg as well as other euthanasia centers. In August, however, a new directive ordered the removal of Jewish patients to different facilities. Apparently, employees of the killing centers and families of the patients marked for euthanasia were complaining about being housed in a facility with Jews. In the fall of 1940 the first Jewish patients were sent to the East, to Poland, as part of the policy of removing all Jews from Germany. Others were moved in December to Neuwied in the Rhineland. There they were incarcerated in the Bendorf facility, which, in a touch of malevolent irony, had been founded in 1869 as a private Jewish owned institution, later transformed into a state facility for mentally impaired children. In 1941, the Reich Ministry of the Interior ordered the killing of all hospitalized Jews for no other reason than their Jewishness. The Bendorf patients ended up in Poland, transported in sealed railroad cars, sixty-to-seventy patients per car, allegedly destined for Lublin. It is assumed that they were murdered at the extermination camps in the Lublin area: Belzec, Sobibor and Treblinka. To conceal this reality, death notices and condolence letters were written on fictitious "Chelm Insane Asylum" stationary. The T4 staff even had the letters taken to the town of Chelm in Poland, there to be properly postmarked.

The extermination camps, of course, were simply the end point in a graduated series of institutions designed to serve the goals of the Nazi program of racial hygiene. The system of prison camps, which included forced-labor camps, prisoner-of-war camps, transit camps, and concentration camps, as well as extermination camps, thus complemented and completed the work begun in the ghettos and mental institutions: persons deemed undesirable or dangerous to the State were to be separated from the general population. One of the first concentration camps was Dachau, opened in 1933, just outside Munich. At first Dachau held only political opponents, such as Communists and Social Democrats, or those who had been sentenced in a court of law. But its population soon expanded to include Jews, homosexuals, Jehovah's Witnesses, Gypsies, clergy and others who were denounced for making negative comments about the regime. The other concentration camps filled quickly as well. Meanwhile the conquest of the East was bringing ever greater numbers of Jews and other "undesirables" into the boundaries of an expanding Reich.

The killing in concentration camps originally began as an attempt to address the problem of overcrowding. Himmler asked Bouhler, the leader of T4, for the use of T4 personnel to rid the camps of "excess" prisoners. In April a new program was instituted to murder concentration camp inmates, including Jews, who were incapable of working – "14 f 13" is the reference number of the operation in Concentration Camp Inspectorate lists. The action was also referred to as "prisoner euthanasia" or "Operation Invalid".

In December 1941 several concentration camps were notified that a commission of psychiatrists would be arriving to select prisoners with mental and/or physical infirmities for "special treatment". Jews were to be included in the group, regardless of their health. For these Nazi doctors there was no distinction between the physically inferior and the racially inferior.[12] The physicians conducted superficial examinations, when they conducted any at all. As in the T4 operation, forms were filled out with diagnoses fabricated to justify execution. But no real justification was necessary for the murder of Jews. The term "special treatment" was recognized as a Gestapo term justifying extra-legal execution.

The first murders of Jews as part of the "special treatment" program took place at either Dachau or Buchenwald, but the policy was also instituted at other work camps such as Ravensbrück, Sachsenhausen, and Mauthausen. As the war dragged on and the camps became overcrowded, Operation 14 f 13 provided a way to eliminate undesirables, including those who were less productive, thereby reducing the overcrowding that was believed to be inhibiting production efforts. In effect the policy allowed those camps that were not purely killing centers to establish an extermination component.

As the notion of medicalized killing was accepted and extended, the Nazi Reich faced new strains. The plans for the invasion of the Soviet Union meant growing numbers of Soviet prisoners. After the June 1941 invasion, orders were given to four SS Einsatzgruppen to murder the Jews in conquered Soviet regions. The Nazis also encouraged pogroms against Jews by the local populations and made sure that Jewish prisoners-of-war were selected for "special treatment". Early in the campaign, the infamous mass shootings into ditches were used, but this method was deemed too wasteful of ammunition and too difficult emotionally for the soldiers. Next, under the supervision of Christian Wirth, the Nazis tried "killing vans"; Jews were sealed into trucks and, as the trucks drove, carbon monoxide was re-circulated inside to asphyxiate the occupants. The trucks' destinations were giant ditches where the bodies were dumped and buried. But this method too, was deemed inefficient.

On 31 July 1941 Reich Marshall Goering wrote of going ahead with preparations for a *Gesamtlösung* or comprehensive solution of the Jewish problem. In January 1942, Nazi officials met just outside Berlin at the Wannsee Conference to discuss an *Endlösung,* a "final solution". The green light was given to building extermination camps in Poland where mass killings could occur without arousing protests from neighboring communities.

Six extermination camps were constructed in Poland: Auschwitz-Birkenau, Treblinka, Belzec, Sobibor, Majdanek, and Chelmno. These camps had as their main purpose the murder of millions of innocent men, women and children. The first, Chelmno, began operating in late 1941, the others, in 1942.

12 Proctor, *Racial Hygiene,* p. 208, states, "Operation 14 f 13 represents the transition from the systematic destruction of the handicapped and the mentally ill to the systematic destruction of the ethnically and culturally marginal."

Christian Wirth was made chief extermination specialist and first commander of the Belzec camp. Based on his experiences at T4 and with the mobile killing vans, Wirth decided that carbon monoxide would be used and that gas diesel engines would be installed adjacent to the gas chambers to produce the poisonous fumes. Dr. Irmfried Eberl, who had already been directing the T4 killing centers, was made first commander of Treblinka. Eberl would turn out to be unsuited for the logistical challenges presented by mass murder. Nevertheless, during his brief tenure at Treblinka, he represented, in the words of Robert Jay Lifton, "the ultimate healer turned killer".[13]

At Auschwitz, doctors participated in every step of the systematic extermination of millions of Jewish men, women and children. Upon arrival doctors conducted the selections on the ramps; later, in the camps, they oversaw the selection of those no longer able to work who were to be sent to the gas chambers; and finally, they even dropped the poisonous Zyklon B pellets into the gas chambers. This was medicalized killing taken to an extreme.

In conclusion, the writings of certain German physicians inspired Hitler, and Hitler placed their medical theories at the core of his murderous laws and programs. The German medical establishment accepted the pseudo-science of eugenics and racial hygiene and embraced the racist laws and statutes that followed from these theories. They benefited from the misery, exclusion, expulsion and deaths of their Jewish colleagues. They violated their Hippocratic oaths and the confidentiality of the patient-doctor relationship. Doctors played major roles in the Nazi government and in the sterilization, euthanasia and extermination programs. Medical and health care workers participated willingly in the medicalized murder of their fellow citizens of all faiths. Regarding the Jews, in effect, doctors took an active role in the Nazi regime that systematically took away first the dignity, then the human rights, then the possessions, and finally the lives of millions of Jews.

The argument that Lifton makes so forcefully in *The Nazi Doctors* is that "the medicalization of killing – the imagery of killing in the name of healing" – was crucial to the Nazi "final solution"; that by couching murder in biomedical terms and by using physicians and health professionals to participate at every stage of the process genocide was made psychologically possible and even permissible.[14] Thus Fritz Klein, one of the camp physicians in Auschwitz, when asked how he could reconcile his Hippocratic Oath with the death camp crematoria, could answer: "Of course I am a doctor and I want to preserve life. And

13 Lifton, *The Nazi Doctors*, pp. 123–124 offers a thumbnail sketch of Eberl.
14 For the Lifton quotation, see Ibid., p. 14.

out of respect for human life, I would remove a gangrenous appendix from a diseased body. The Jew is the gangrenous appendix in the body of mankind."[15]

Writing in the *Annals of Internal Medicine* in 1995, Drs. Rothman and Lerner wrote, "It is no exaggeration to declare that the greatest blot on the record of medicine in the 20th Century is the role played by German physicians in the Nazi era."[16] I must concur!

15 Ibid., pp. 15–16; paraphrasing prisoner-physician Ella Lingens-Reiner, *Prisoners of Fear* (London: Gollancz, 1948), pp. 1–2, who is reporting a conversation with Klein, in the camp.

16 Barren H. Lerner and David J. Rothman, "Medicine and the Holocaust".

CHAPTER 2

The Experiments

INTRODUCTION

I present the following chapter to provide evidence of the experiments Nazi doctors performed on prisoners in different concentration camps. The chapter consists of brief descriptions of the various experiments, with supporting evidence in the form of reprinted materials collected from primary and secondary sources.

This chapter is the most important part of the book. As I mentioned in the preface, the fact that most people have heard only of Josef Mengele and his experiments with twins, is one of the major reasons for my decision to tell about the other doctors and the many other experiments. We must not make the mistake of thinking that the horrors of the Nazi era were a matter of a handful of evil men doing terrible things. Many people were involved, and they could do the things they did, in part because they had accepted a specific intellectual framework as valid.

At the Nuremberg Trial, held in the years 1945–46 by the International Military Tribunal, the Prosecutor argued in his closing statement that "the SS was able to obtain an allocation of government funds for research [on prisoners in the camps] on the grounds that they had access to human material not available to other agencies". The materials I present in this chapter bring the implications of this statement clearly to the fore. The concentration camp experiments were carried out methodically, on human beings whom the researchers treated as if they were simply objects, not individuals with hopes, fears, loved ones and lives. The dehumanization of the experimental subjects, which is so evident in the documents, adds a chilling note to the well-known stories of concentration camp gas chambers and mass graves.

The experiments fell into three categories: those designed to solve medical problems for the military; those intended to prove the superiority of the "Aryan race"; and those carried out to satisfy the curiosity of certain powerful individuals. The hypothermia, high altitude, and seawater experiments, for example, addressed naval and air force combat and rescue problems. Experiments with sulfa drugs, with treatments for mustard gas and phosphorus burns, with various approaches to wound healing, and with medications for blood coagulation, aimed at minimizing the effects of common wartime injuries. Experiments with typhus, malaria and infectious hepatitis aimed to discover preventive vaccines and the most effective therapy. Hirt's skeleton collection and Mengele's anthropological studies sought to provide experimental evidence of Aryan superiority claims, while the various sterilization experiments aimed at preventing the "inferior races" from propagating. Finally experiments, for example, with the treatment of homosexuality, with sun exposure, and with lethal doses of anesthetics simply satisfied the curiosity or whims of individuals; the camp experiments provided a unique opportunity to use human beings as guinea pigs. Where else could medical professionals have experimented on human beings without concern for possible consequences?

I wish to finish this introduction to the experiments by stating that I am aware of the fact that the documentary that follows is incomplete. It is my sincere hope that other scholars working on this subject will make up for its shortcomings.

TYPHUS EXPERIMENTS

Typhus is a serious viral infectious disease. It can be prevented by fighting the lice that can spread the disease and by using protective vaccines made from either killed or live typhus virus. The killed virus vaccine does not provide absolute protection and may actually cause a mild form of the disease. The live virus vaccine is more effective. It is usually first attenuated so that it is no longer pathogenic to human beings but retains its ability to stimulate production of antibodies, thus protecting the recipient from contracting the disease. Vaccines always have to be tested for effectiveness (immunizing qualities) and tolerance. In the German concentration camps, prisoners rather than animals were used as test subjects for the first time in history.

In the fall of 1941, there was a real threat of a typhus epidemic in Germany. Paul Hoedeman's book *Hitler or Hippocrates,* describes the urgency of the situation:

> A few weeks after Hitler had declared war on Russia, serious problems came to light. At least 10,000 German soldiers were suffering from typhus. This illness was turning out to be deadlier than the Russian barrages. Consequently, there was considerable uneasiness amongst the troops, and some regimens refused to advance but there was insufficient

> protective vaccination. The military staff was in serious difficulties; such disobedience was at odds with their idea of rigid discipline.[1]

The Army Chief of Staff, General Franz Halder, noted in his diary in February 1942: "Ten thousand cases of typhus and thirteen hundred deaths!" Dr. Eugen Haagen, one of the doctors actively involved in typhus research in the camps, testified at Nuremberg:

> The development of typhus throughout the war was such that typhus no longer became purely a war epidemic, but because of the many refugee camps, prisoner of war transports and military transports, typhus was brought into Germany itself. In the overcrowded camps especially, with lack of sanitary installations, there was considerable danger from typhus, particularly where people assembled who came from the East. In the Auschwitz camp, for example, there had always been extensive epidemics. Typhus pressed further and further into Germany. In every close community such as the camps itself, there was a great source of typhus, not only the danger of an epidemic within the camp, but also an epidemic that spread to the surrounding civilian population. Most of the concentration camp inmates worked outside the camp in factories, and they came into close contact with the civilian population, so you can easily see the danger of contagion.[2]

The highest level of the German government was seriously concerned. Dr. Leonardo Conti, Secretary of State for Health in the Reich's Ministry of the Interior, appointed Chief of the Medical Corps of the Waffen SS, Dr. Grawitz, to be in charge of a solution. Dr. Grawitz, in turn, instructed the Head of the SS Institute of Hygiene, SS Standartenführer Dr. Mrugowsky, to start research on typhus and work out a vaccine that would effectively protect from the disease. According to Hoedeman:

> The existing typhus vaccine, the Weigl's vaccine, was effective but was so expensive and time-consuming to prepare that not enough was available. Only physicians and officers were being vaccinated with it. The newly developed vaccines by Cox, Gildermeister and Haagen, produced from egg-yolk cultures, could be produced in large quantities, but their actual effectiveness had yet to be satisfactorily demonstrated. The results of the experiments upon animals were too inconsistent for the vaccines to be designated efficient.[3]

1 Hoedeman, *Hitler or Hippocrates*, p. 125.
2 Extract from the Testimony of S. E. Haagen, in *Trials NMT*, vol. 1, pp. 555–531.
3 Hoedeman, *Hitler or Hippocrates*, p. 125.

Mrugowsky's research program progressed very slowly. Therefore, Grawitz recommended something up to this time unimaginable in the history of medical science: The testing of experimental vaccines on human subjects before animal testing had been completed.

On 29 December 1941 Grawitz held a conference on the subject in the Ministry of the Interior, with Army Sanitation Inspector General, Chief Surgeon Professor Dr. Handloser; State Secretary for the Department of Health of the Reich, SS Gruppenführer Conti; President of the Robert Koch Institute (Reich Institute to Combat Contagious Diseases), Professor Gildemeister; and SS Standartenführer Mrugowsky of the Institute of Hygiene, Waffen SS, Berlin, among the participants. The conference concluded, "Since tests on animals are not of sufficient value, tests on human beings have to be carried out."[4] Reichsführer Heinrich Himmler approved the recommendation.

Professor Gildemeister recommended his own discovery, a vaccine he had developed with Drs. Koch and Haagen. Keeping in mind the economic interests of I. G. Farbenindustrie, Dr. Demnitz recommended a vaccine worked out by Dr. Lautenschlager, an employee of the company. At the end of the conference participants selected several vaccines for testing. On 2 January 1942, Buchenwald and Natzweiler concentration camps were selected as experimental sites – with Dr. Ding in charge at Buchenwald and Dr. Haagen, at Natzweiler. (As an irony of fate, shortly after the beginning of the experiments, Ding accidentally infected himself with the virus, became ill and had to be treated in a Berlin hospital. His case was written up in the *Zeitschrift für Hygiene und Infectionkrankheiten,* vol. 124, 1943.)

At Buchenwald, one of the camp physicians, Dr. Waldemar Hoven, acted as Ding's assistant. The two doctors transformed Block 46 into a research center officially called the "Experimentation Center, Department for Typhoid and Virus Research". On 9 December 1946, in his opening statement at Nuremberg, Chief Prosecutor Brigadier General Alfred Taylor described the general pattern of the typhus experiments:

> A group of concentration camp inmates, selected from the healthier ones who had some resistance to disease, were injected with an ant typhus vaccine, the efficacy of which was to be tested. Thereafter, all the persons in the group would be infected with typhus. At the same time, other inmates who had not been vaccinated were also infected for the purpose of comparison – these unvaccinated victims served as the "control" group. Perhaps the most wicked and murderous circumstance in this whole case is that still other inmates were deliberately infected with

4 Ibid.

> typhus for the sole purpose of keeping the typhus virus alive and generally available in the blood stream of the inmates.[5]

The "researchers" started by giving a dose of Rickettsia-prowazeki, the virus that causes typhus, supplied by the Koch Institute, to a few prisoners, in order to create a supply of infected blood for the actual vaccine experiments. The virus was delivered by various methods. Sometimes the researchers used lancets to cut the skin and infect it with typhus culture; they also occasionally used contagious lice. But mainly they used intramuscular or intravenous injections of fresh, virus-infected blood. Each subsequent month, new men were infected, in order to ensure a continuous supply of virus-tainted blood. These "passage persons" all died.

The doctors selected four different vaccines for the tests: the one made by Behring Factories; another based on Cox's egg yolk process; the Weigl vaccine, prepared from lice intestines; and the one manufactured from rabbit lung, developed in Paris at the Pasteur Institute by Durand-Giroud.

A total of twenty-four series of consecutive experiments were completed. In each a certain number of prisoners were vaccinated and all were later artificially infected. Unvaccinated subjects served as controls for comparing the progress of the disease and evaluating the efficacy of the vaccines. A total of 729 prisoners were used in the experiments, and 154 of them died. The 120 "passage persons" also died.

A second set of experiments at Buchenwald aimed at identifying more effective treatments for clinical typhus, among them I. G. Farbenindustrie drugs in various stages of development. The firm had requested permission and received authorization to test the drugs on human subjects.

Dr. Waldemar Hoven, one of the physicians who participated in the typhus research at Buchenwald, testified at the Nuremberg Trial.

Translation of Document No-429, Prosecution Exhibit 281[6]

> Extract from the Affidavit of Defendant Hoven, 24 October 1946, re: Typhus and Virus Experiments
>
> I, Waldemar Hoven, being duly sworn, depose and state:
>
> In the latter part of 1941 an experimental station was established in the Buchenwald concentration camp in order to determine the effectiveness of various typhus vaccines. This section was called the "Typhus

5 General Alfred Taylor (9 December 1946), "Opening Statement of the Prosecution", in *Trials NMT*, vol. 1, pp. 27–74.

6 Affidavit of Defendant Hoven, 24 October 1946, Document No-429, in *Trials NMT*, vol. 1, pp. 555–556.

> Experimental Station–Division for Typhus and Virus Research" and was under the direct supervision of Dr. Ding, alias Schuler. This experimental station was set up in Block 46 of the camp. The Hygiene Institute of the Waffen SS in Berlin, under the command of Dr. Joachim Mrugowsky, received all the reports of these activities and Dr. Ding took orders from Mrugowsky. In the early days, that is, between 1941 and the summer of 1943, Dr. Ding had many meetings in Berlin with Dr. Karl Genzken concerning his work at Buchenwald in connection with the typhus experiments. Dr. Ding told me that Dr. Genzken had a special interest in these matters and that he sent him reports at various times. Dr. Karl Genzken was one of his superiors. I understood that the chain of command in the supervision of the typhus experimental station was as follows: Reichsarzt SS Grawitz, Genzken, Mrugowsky, and Ding.
>
> I can recollect that Dr. Genzken gave orders to Dr. Ding in January 1943 to enlarge the experimental station. At this time Block 50 was cleaned out and made into a station for the production of the various vaccines to be used in the experiments at Block 46. From this time on the experimental station was known as the "Division for Typhus and Virus Research of the Hygiene Institute of the Waffen SS".
>
> The experiments in Block 46 in the Buchenwald concentration camp were conducted as follows: One group of victims was first vaccinated with the typhus vaccine and then infected with the typhus virus. In order to contrast the effectiveness of the vaccine, another group of inmates was merely infected with the typhus virus without previous vaccination. Between the autumn of 1942 and the summer of 1943 about 500 inmates of the Buchenwald concentration camp were used in these experiments. During my time about 10 percent of the total number of the inmates used, died as a result. I heard that a larger number of the victims died after my time, that is, about 20 percent.

Dr. Ding, who also signed himself as Ding-Schuler, Ding von Schuler and Schuler, kept a ward journal that was taken from Buchenwald by one of his assistants, Dr. Eugen Kogon. Kogon later delivered it to the Office of the Chief Counsel for War Crimes and testified as to the authenticity of the document and its signatures. The diary and Kogon's testimony provided valuable evidence for the prosecution at the Nuremberg Medical Trial. Kogon later published an account of his experiences.[7]

7 "Ding Diary", Document No-265, in Ibid., pp. 557–572. Testimony of Prosecution Witness Eugen Kogon, in Ibid., pp. 583–586. Kogon's memoir is *Der SS-Staat, das System der deutschen Konzentrationslager.*

Translation of the Ding Diary

5 Jan 42:
Preliminary test A

Preliminary test to determine the surest and most practical way of infecting human beings artificially. Five experimental subjects received intramuscular and subcutaneous injections of vitelline membrane diluted 1:25 with an emulsified Rickettsia-prowazeki strain from the Robert Koch Institute in doses of 1 cc. Infection was not possible.

Dr. Ding
SS Hauptsturmführer

■

10 Jan 42:
Preliminary test B

Preliminary test to establish a sure means of infection: Much as in smallpox vaccination, five persons were infected with vitelline membrane culture virus (strain Rickettsia-prowazeki, Robert Koch Institute) through two superficial and two deeper cuts in the upper arm.

All experimental subjects used for this test fell ill with genuine typhus. Incubation period two to six days.

20 Feb 42:

Case history and charts of the preliminary tests to establish a sure means of infection sent to Berlin.

One death out of five sick.

Dr. Ding
SS Hauptsturmführer

■

Feb 42:
Typhus Vaccine, Research Series I

Vaccination for immunization against typhus using the following vaccines:

1. 31 persons with Weigl vaccine from the intestines of lice from the Institute for Typhus and Virus Research of the Army High Command, Krakow.
2. 35 persons with vaccine from vitelline membrane cultures made by the Cox, Gildemeister, and Haagen process.
3. 35 persons with vaccine "Behring Normal" (1 egg in an emulsion of 450 cc. vaccine. Mixture of 70 percent Rickettsia-mooseri and 30 percent Rickettsia-prowazeki).

4. 34 persons with "Behring Normal" "Behring Strong" (1 egg emulsified in 250 cc. solvent).
5. 10 persons for control.

3 Mar 42:

All persons vaccinated for immunization between 6 Jan 42 and 1 Feb 42, and the 10 control persons were infected with a virus culture of Rickettsia-prowazeki in the presence of Professor Gildemeister. SS Hauptsturmführer Dr. Ding infected himself in the process (laboratory accident).

17 Mar 42:

Visit of Professor Gildemeister and Professor Rose (Head of the Department for Tropical Medicine in the Robert Koch Institute) to the experimental station. All persons experimented on fell sick with typhus except two who, as was established later, had already had typhus during an epidemic at the police prison in Berlin.

19 Apr 42:

Final report on the first typhus vaccine research series: five deaths (three control persons, one "Behring Normal", and one "Behring Strong").

Dr. Ding
SS Hauptsturmführer

■

4 Sep 42:

Typhus Vaccine, Research Series II

Vaccination for immunization against typhus using the following vaccines:

1. 20 persons with vaccines made by the Durand and Giroud process (Pasteur Institute, Paris) from rabbit lungs.
2. 20 persons with vaccine made by the process of Combiescu, Zotta, and collaborators from dog lungs. (Producer: Cantacuzino, Bucharest.) This vaccine was made available by Professor Rose, who received it from Naval Doctor Professor Ruge from Bucharest.

5 Oct 42:

Artificial infection of all persons vaccinated for immunization between 19 September 1942 and 4 October 1942, and 19 persons for control with vitelline membrane virus (Rickettsia-prowazeki).

25 Oct 42:

Infection has started with all persons experimented on.

20 Nov 42:

Charts and case history sent to Berlin.
Four deaths of control persons.

Dr. DING
SS Hauptsturmführer

■

5 Nov 42:

Typhus Vaccine, Research Series III

Vaccination for immunization against typhus of 20 persons with vaccine made according to the process of Giroud, Paris. (This vaccine was brought from Paris by SS Hauptsturmführer Dr. Ding immediately after production.)

30 Nov 42:

Artificial infection with vitelline membrane material from the Robert Koch Institute of the 20 persons vaccinated for immunization and of six control persons. This research series was observed for six weeks and then abandoned without results, as no sickness broke out in the control group.

Dr. DING
SS Hauptsturmführer

■

8 Nov 42:

Typhus Vaccine, Research Series IV

Vaccination for immunization of 20 persons with a vaccine from intestines of lice made by the Weigl process (sent by lecturer Dr. Haas of the typhus institute "Emil v. Behring" in Lvov).

30 Nov 42:

To test the effect of the immunization, the infection is to be carried out with lice suffering from typhus. The lice and their cages must be burnt immediately, as the latter became leaky during transport, and therefore represent a danger of epidemic in Buchenwald camp.

Dec 42:

Newly sent lice applied to 15 persons (five immunized and 10 persons for control). The lice must again be destroyed, as the cages are not tight.

Report made that infection with live typhus lice is not possible because the danger to the camp inmates is too great.

4 Jan 43:

Due to infection by lice on 3 December 1942, five persons show short nontypical illness.

The research series is concluded.

Dr. Ding
SS Hauptsturmführer

■

20 Dec 42:

Typhus Vaccine, Research Series V

To determine the immunization effect, 20 persons are being actively vaccinated for immunization with "EM" vaccine of the Behring Works-Dr. Demnitz-(vaccine in which vitelline membrane as well as chicken embryos were used).

26 Jan 43:

Artificial infection with vitelline membrane virus OP No. 223 and 226 (Rickettsia-prowazeki–strain from Robert Koch Institute).

Dr. Ding
SS Hauptsturmführer

■

28 Feb 43:

Typhus Vaccine, Research Series VI

To determine the immunization effect, the following were actively vaccinated for immunization:

20 persons with vaccine "Zürich" from the hygiene institute of the University of Zürich (lungs of mice), and 20 persons with vaccine "Riga" from the serum institute of the University of Riga (Professor Darsin, from vitelline membrane cultures).

31 Mar 43:

Artificial infection with egg Rickettsia (Rickettsia-prowazeki) of the Robert Koch Institute, Berlin.

11 Apr 43:

The infection of 31 March 1943 has not resulted in any sickness so far.

28 Apr 43:

Experimental series abandoned.

Dr. DING
SS Hauptsturmführer

■

11 Apr 43:

Preliminary test C

To determine a sure means of infection, experiments with fresh blood from persons stricken with typhus were made. Infection took place as follows:

3 persons – 2 cc. each of fresh blood intravenously.
2 persons – 2 cc. each of fresh blood intramuscularly.
2 persons – 2 cc. each of fresh blood subcutaneously.
2 persons – after scarification.
2 persons – with a vaccinating scalpel cutaneously.

Those infected intravenously contracted typical, serious typhus and died from failure of the circulatory system. The other experimental subjects complained only of minor discomfort, without becoming hospital cases.

Dr. DING
SS Hauptsturmführer

■

13 Apr 43:

Preliminary test D

The following were infected:

6 persons with 2 cc. each of fresh blood intravenously.
6 persons with 2 cc. each of fresh blood intramuscularly.
6 persons with 2 cc. each of fresh blood subcutaneously.
6 persons by scarification.
6 persons by means of vaccinating scalpel cutaneously.

The six intravenously infected persons again contracted very serious typhus; five died.

Of the six infected intramuscularly, one person contracted medium typhus. The others had no serious complications, and were not hospital cases.

The surest means of infection to produce typhus in humans is, therefore, the intravenous injection of 2 cc. fresh typhus-infected blood.

Dr. DING
SS Hauptsturmführer

■

18 Jun 43:
Typhus Vaccine, Research Series VII

Carrying out of typhus vaccination for immunization with the following vaccine:

1. 20 persons with vaccine "Asid".
2. 20 persons with vaccine "Asid Adsorbat" of the Anhaltinischen Serumwerke G. m. b. H., Berlin 7.
3. 20 persons with vaccine: "Weigl" of the Institute for Typhus and Virus Research of the Army High Command, Army (OKH) Krakow (Eyer).

27 Aug 43:

Infection of –
20 persons in the series "Asid".
20 persons in the series "Asid Adsorbat".
20 persons in the series "Weigl".
10 persons for control by intravenous injection of 1/4 cc. each of fresh typhus-infected blood, strain Bu II, Passage I.
All experimental persons got very serious typhus.

7 Sep 43:

Chart and case history completed. The experimental series was concluded –

53 deaths (18 with "Asid", 18 with "Acid Adsorbat", nine with "Weigl" eight control).

9 Sep 43:

Charts and case histories delivered to Berlin.

Dr. Ding
SS Hauptsturmführer

■

17 Jan 44:
High Immunization Experiment with Fraenkel Vaccines

According to an immunization plan of the Fraenkel high immunization for humans, the compatibility of Fraenkel-Formol-Toxoid (Formol-Toxin of bacterium perfringens) of humans was tested.

At first 15 experimental subjects were vaccinated three times at intervals of 14 days with 1 cc. Fraenkel-A1. F. T. (Fraenkel-Toxoid absorbed in aluminum hydroxide).

After an interval of 14 days, vaccinations with Fraenkel-Formol (Formol-Toxin of bacterium perfringens) as follows:

20 Dec 43 – 1 cc. subcutaneously – left upper arm.
26 Dec 43 – 2 cc. subcutaneously – right upper arm.

31 Dec 43 – 4 cc. subcutaneously – left upper arm.
3 Jan 43 – 6 cc. subcutaneously – right upper arm.
6 Jan 44 – 9 cc. subcutaneously – right and left chest.
10 Jan 44 – 12 cc. subcutaneously – both upper arms.
14 Jan 44 – 15 cc. subcutaneously – right and left chest.

17 Jan 44:
Observation of vaccination reactions completed and sent away.

Dr. DING
SS Hauptsturmführer

■

31 Jan 44:
Vaccine Preliminary Experimental Series "Weimar"

To test compatibility and the immunization effect, five persons were immunized by three vaccinations with typhus vaccine "Weimar" (producer: Hygiene Institute of the Waffen SS, Division for Typhus and Virus Research). On 22 Jan 44, 0.5 cc., on 27 Jan 44, 1.0 cc., on 31 Jan 44, 1.0 cc. were injected subcutaneously in the left or right upper arm.

For comparison, five persons were immunized on the above-mentioned dates with 0.5 cc., 0.5 cc., and 1 cc. of typhus egg-culture vaccine "Asid" (Anhaltinische Serumwerke, Berlin) and five persons were immunized with typhus vaccine "Giroud" (produced by the Pasteur Institute, Paris, from rabbit lungs), 1 cc. each.

25 Feb 44:

Twenty persons (15 immunized and five for control) were infected by subcutaneous injection of 1/20 cc. fresh typhus-infected blood.

Donor: G * * * Nr 713, 36 years old (6th day of sickness) Strain Bu IV/Passage 13.

All those infected fell sick with slight to serious typhus.

5 Apr 44:
Chart and case history completed.

25 Apr 44:
The experimental series was concluded –
Five deaths (one Asid, one Weimar, three Control).

Dr. DING

■

18 Mar 44:
Typhus Vaccine, Research Series VIII

Suggested by Colonel M. C. of the Air Corps, Oberstarzt Professor Rose the vaccine "Kopenhagen" (Ipsen-Murine vaccine), produced from mouse liver by the National Serum Institute in Kopenhagen, was tested for its compatibility on humans.

20 persons were vaccinated for immunization by intramuscular injection into the musculus glutaeus max. on the following dates: 8 Mar 44, 0.5 cc.; 13 Mar 44, 0.5 cc.; 18 Mar 44, 1.0 cc.

10 persons were contemplated for control and comparison.

Four of the 30 persons were eliminated before the start of the artificial injection, because of intermittent sickness.

16 Apr 44:

The remaining experimental persons were infected on 16 Apr 44 by subcutaneous injection of 1/20 cc. typhus sick fresh blood. Donor. W *** No. 763, 27 years old (6th day of sickness) Strain Bu VII/Passage 1.

The following fell sick

a) 17 persons immunized; nine medium, eight seriously.

b) Nine control persons; two medium, seven seriously.

2 Jun 44:

The experimental series was concluded.

13 Jun 44:

Chart and case history completed and sent to Berlin.

Six deaths (three Kopenhagen, three Control).

Dr. DING

■

27 Jul 44:
Typhus Vaccine, Research Series IX

The typhus vaccine "Weimar", produced by the Division for Typhus and Virus Research of the Hygiene Institute of the Waffen SS, Weimar-Buchenwald, was tested according to orders for its efficacy on humans.

This vaccine was produced from rabbit lungs according to the process Durand-Giroud. It contains virus (Rickettsia-prowazeki) of self-isolating types deadened and suspended in 2/00 Formol.

20 persons were immunized on the following dates with 1 cc. each: 17, 22, 27 July 1944.

The vaccinations were made subcutaneously on the right or left upper arm.

For comparison 20 persons were immunized at the same time with "Weigl" vaccine, produced from lice by the Army High Command in Krakow according to regulations.

Furthermore, 20 persons were provided for control purposes.

6 Sep 44:

The 60 experimental persons were infected by subcutaneous injection of 1/10 cc. fresh typhus-infected blood each into the right upper arm.

All persons fell sick as follows

a) "Weimar" – nine slightly, seven slightly to medium, four medium.

b) "Weigl" – six slightly to medium, eight medium, six seriously.

c) Control – one medium, 19 seriously.

17 Oct 44:

The experimental series was concluded.

4 Nov 44:

Chart and case history completed.

24 deaths (5 "Weigl," 19 Control)

Dr. SCHULER

■

31 Oct 44:

Taking of Blood to Produce Typhus Convalescent Serum (FFRS)

To produce FFRS, 20.8 liters of blood were taken from 44 typhus convalescents between the 14th and 21st day after the fever had subsided, and sent by courier to the SS Main Operational Headquarters, Office Group D, Office XVI (blood conservation) SS Sturmbannführer Dr. Ellenbeck, Berlin-Lichterfelde.

Dr. SCHULER

■

13 Nov 44:

Therapeutic Experiment with Typhus Vaccine

By order of the senior hygienist of the Waffen SS of 12 August 44, it is to be determined whether the course of typhus can be tempered by the intravenous or intramuscular injection of typhus vaccine.

For the experimental series 20 persons were considered, of these, 10 for intravenous injection (Series A), 10 for intramuscular injection (Series B) and, in addition, five persons for control.

On 13 Nov 44, the 25 experimental persons were infected by subcutaneous injection of 1/10 cc. each fresh typhus-infected blood.

All persons fell sick as follows

Series A	10 serious
Series B	1 medium
	9 serious
Control 1 serious	

22 Dec 44:

The experimental series was concluded.

2 Jan 45:

Chart and case history completed.

19 deaths (9 Series A, 6 Series B, 4 Control).

DR. SCHULER

The following document from the Nuremberg Medical Trial offers further testimony about the typhus experiments.

Extracts from the Testimony of Prosecution Witness Eugen Kogon[8]

Direct Examination

Mr. McHaney: Now, will you please explain to the Tribunal in your own words exactly how these typhus experiments were carried out.

Witness Kogon: After 40 to 60 people, sometimes up to 120, had been detailed for a series of experiments, one-third of them were separated, and the other two-thirds were either vaccinated with a protective treatment, or it was otherwise administered to them, if it was a chemical therapeutical treatment. Those people who were protected against typhus remained in Block 46 for several weeks until their infection with Rocketries prowazeki, the typhus agent. The first selection, that is to say, the first third, was also infected together with them. They served as so-called control persons, with the help of whom it was possible to ascertain whether the infection took and what course the disease took in their cases, so that this course could be compared with that of those who had been vaccinated and then infected.

8 Testimony of Prosecution Witness Eugen Kogon, in Ibid., pp. 583–586.

A category of the experimental persons was used to maintain the typhus cultures. Those were the so-called passage persons, amounting to three to five persons per month. They were merely infected for the purpose of ensuring a constant supply of fresh blood containing typhus. Very nearly all those persons died. I do not think I am exaggerating if I say that 95 percent of these cases were fatal.

Q. Witness, do you mean to say that they deliberately infected three to five persons a month with typhus just to have the viruses alive and available in blood?

A. Just for that particular purpose.

Q. Can you tell the Tribunal whether these experimental subjects suffered to any appreciable extent during the course of these typhus experiments?

A. After a certain period, when the actual illness had set in after the infection, ordinary symptoms of typhus would appear, which, as is well known, is one of the most serious illnesses. The infection, as I have already described to you, became so powerful during the last two and a half years that the typhus almost always appeared in its most horrible form. There were cases of raving madness, delirium, people would refuse to eat, and a large percentage of them would die. Those who experienced the disease in a milder form, perhaps because their constitutions were stronger or because the vaccine was effective, were forced continuously to observe the death struggles of the others.

The following letter to Dr. Rose of the Robert Koch Institute demonstrates that physicians of the German Reich did indeed know what was going on in the concentration camps in the name of scientific research.

Extracts from the Testimony of Defendant Rose, Cross-Examination[9]

Rose: (Reading):
29 November 1943-Registered
To Oberstarzt Professor Dr. Rose
Inspectorate of the Medical Service of the Luftwaffe
Saalow (Post Office Zossen-Land)

9 Testimony of Defendant Rose, in Ibid., p. 587.

> Dear Herr Rose:
>
> Enclosed I am sending you the report about our experiments with dehydrated typhus vaccine which I promised you several days ago. As I intend to publish the findings, I have already written the report in manuscript form. After it has been reviewed, I would like it to be submitted to the competent authorities for their approval, of its publication in the *Zentralblatt für Bakteriologie* (Central Periodical for Bacteriology).

In the spring of 1943 Prof. Dr. Eugen Haagen resumed active military duty as a consultant to the Air Fleet Reich Physician, and he also received a research commission from the Luftwaffe for typhus experiments at Natzweiler and Schirmeck concentration camps. He developed a murine (rat) typhus vaccine, which contained an attenuated virulent (live) virus.

Extracts from the Testimony of Defense Witness Dr. Eugen Haagen[10]

> Experiments in Schirmeck (Subcamp) of Natzweiler
>
> Witness Haagen: Vaccinations were performed on 28 persons altogether, in several groups. The first vaccination was of eight persons. They were given one injection of 0.5 cc. of the vaccine into the breast muscle in the customary manner. The second group consisted of 20 persons, divided into two subgroups of ten each. The first group – let's call this group A – was also given 0.5 cc. of the vaccine intramuscularly. Subgroup B, the last ten persons, were first given a vaccination of 0.5 cc. of a dead typhus vaccine produced in the Robert Koch Institute. Then, eight days later, there was a second vaccination with a live vaccine, again 0.5 cc. intramuscularly. I should like to say that the first vaccination with the dead vaccine, which I have just mentioned, was performed for two reasons: First of all, in order to be able to see whether this preliminary examination produced more protective bodies; and, in the second place, to see whether this preliminary examination with (dead) vaccine might reduce the reactions of the living vaccine.
>
> At the same time, I carried out protective vaccinations on persons outside the camp, on volunteers. They were again performed in such a way that there were three injections this time: the first, 0.25 cc., the second, 0.25 cc., and the third injection 0.5 cc. of the live vaccine.

10 Testimony of Defense Witness Dr. Eugen Hagen, in Ibid., pp. 606–631.

Q. The Court will be especially interested, Witness, in the reactions of the persons after this vaccination. Can you tell us that?

A. In the first group of eight persons who were given 0.5 cc. of the living vaccine only once, three had a reaction consisting of a short fever of over 39 degrees. The rest of the persons, however, had no reaction.

In the second group, among the ten persons in group A, there were no noticeable reactions. In the other group there were very negligible symptoms, in some cases only a headache and depression. Typical symptoms of typhus, brain symptoms or vessel symptoms, and other symptoms, did not appear in any case.

The same was true of the third group. Here again there was no reaction. I must say in this connection that I used a vaccine produced from dead typhus virus. I must point that out because later, in Natzweiler, I used the classic epidemic or louse typhus virus vaccine.

■

Experiments in Natzweiler

Q. Now, Professor, we were talking about your letter to Professor Hirt of 15 [13] November 1943, in which you ask him to make other prisoners available. Was this request met later and were you able to carry out vaccinations in Natzweiler later with your new vaccine?

A. Yes. I received the persons I had requested, and in December of 1943 and January of 1944 we were able to carry out these vaccinations. I performed them in two groups of 40 persons each with my live attenuated virus which is no longer pathogenic to human beings, and this I want to state explicitly.

Q. Professor, please describe these vaccinations briefly to the Tribunal.

A. First, a group of 40 persons was vaccinated. The first vaccination was done with 1 cc. intramuscularly. One was a vaccine made of murine typhus virus vaccine. In no case did local reactions of temperature or other symptoms occur. The second vaccination took place a week later. This was again 1 cc. of vaccine introduced intramuscularly. This was no longer pathogenic to human beings. To complete the story I have to say that between the Schirmeck vaccinations in May and these vaccinations, I had turned to the production of a louse typhus vaccine; this vaccine contained live virus. Before it was used in Natzweiler as a vaccine, we tested it on ourselves, that is, with some collaborators, to ascertain the tolerability and effects. We were roughly ten persons, members of the institute and also students. Only then did we use the vaccine on the prisoners in Natzweiler. Four weeks after the last vaccination there were the usual serological examinations. The Weil-Felix reaction was used. The average titer value, let me say, was better than in the vaccinations with the rat virus. It was, namely 2,000. I need not go into these details. The general reactions were normal reactions to inoculation, temperature, and headaches; but there were no manifestations of actual typhus as a result of inoculations.

Q. You are speaking of a first group, so I assume there must have been a second group. How did you carry out the vaccination of the second group?

A. It occurred to me that instead of injecting the vaccine, the vaccination could be performed by scarifying the skin in the same way as you scrape the skin to make a smallpox vaccination. Therefore, as with the first group, with the same living virus vaccine, I vaccinated 40 additional persons with scarification of the skin. Let me point out that the experiments on myself and on my assistants were carried out in the same way, with scarification of the skin. The reactions were comparatively mild, corresponding roughly to the reactions to vascular typhus vaccine, so that we had no misgivings about undertaking this kind of vaccination.

Q. You described the reactions of yourself and the volunteers as very slight. Now, the reactions of the prisoners were stronger, were they not?

A. Yes. They were stronger again. And this can only be explained by believing that the general state of health among the prisoners was lower than among my associates; but there was no such thing as a natural manifestation of typhus or any fatalities.

The mentality of the Nazi leadership is revealed in a letter from Himmler's office to Wolfram Sievers, SS Standartenführer, which suggests that Himmler was proud of this program, whatever the consequences for experimental subjects. The letter was written on Himmler's orders, on 6 June 1944, the day the Allied Forces landed in Normandy. It stresses that the experiments at Natzweiler could never have taken place without his "patronage". Himmler thought, in fact, that "the S.S. Central Administrative Office and the Waffen S.S. War Institute of Economic Research should have been mentioned in Haagen's report. Moreover, he might also mention that the Reichsführer had made these experiments possible." Professor Hirt attempted to persuade Haagen to stress the cooperation of the S.S. in this letter of 10 July 1944:

The S.S Reichsführer asks that your report contain the following paragraph:

"This research has been carried out under orders from the Chief of the Luftwaffe Medical Corps, with the support of the Reich's Research

Council. It was likewise encouraged by the S.S. Reichsführer personally, by the S.S. Administrative Service and by the Waffen S.S. Institute of Scientific Military Research."[11]

The following testimonies, which describe the methods and results of the typhus experiments, reveal that it was well known that the procedures were causing deaths among the experimental subjects.

Translation of Document No-370,[12] Office of U.S. Chief of Counsel, PRV 292

Experiments with Spotted Fever Vaccines at the Natzweiler Concentration Camp

I, Rudolf Emil Hermann Brandt, being duly sworn, depose and state:

In the fall of 1943, Dr. Eugen Haagen, Oberstabsarzt, and consultant in hygiene for the Luftwaffe and Professor at the University of Strasbourg, requested through Wolfram Sievers of the "Ahnenerbe" that 100 concentration camp prisoners be made available to him for experimentation on the effectiveness of spotted fever vaccines. Obergruppenführer Oswald Pohl, Chief of the WVHA had requested this number of prisoners sent to the Natzweiler concentration camp and the experiments were conducted by Dr. Haagen there.

Again in the summer of 1944, Haagen obtained 200 additional prisoners for the spotted fever experiments. In each case it was specifically required that the experimental subjects be in a physical condition comparable to members of the Armed Forces. This was because the vaccines were being developed primarily for the Armed Forces. Haagen was working under the auspices of the Medical Service of the Luftwaffe.

I am not familiar with the technical details of the experiments but I know that they were carried out. Moreover, I am sure that some of the prisoners died as a result of the experiments. As a matter of fact, the experimental persons were at times not in good physical condition as requested and some of them even died before the experiments began.

11 Aziz, *Doctors of Death,* pp. 236–237.

12 Testimony of Emil Hermann Brandt Document No-370, Office of the U.S. Chief of Counsel, PRV 292.

Extract from a Paper by Professor Robert Waitz, Former Prisoner of Auschwitz (Camp No. 157261)[13]

Experimental Typhus in the Buchenwald Camp

In Buchenwald research was conducted on typhus fever, in one of the hospital buildings, located in the center of the large camp and strictly isolated by a double barbed wire.

There was a large number of hospital personnel, subjected to a strict discipline; they also had to keep everything an absolute secret.

The food in this block was better and of a greater variety than the regular camp rations. This block also had a supply of all the necessary medicines.

The big chief of block 46 was SS physician Sturmbannführer Schuler-Ding, Director of the Institute of Hygiene/Block 50. Schuler-Ding rarely came to Block 46. He only gave directives for the experiments. The permanent administrative and medical chief was a prisoner, not a doctor of medicine, Artur Dietz. He was the one who examined the sick and prescribed medicines.

How were the human guinea pigs or "Kaninchen" /rabbits/ as Dietz called them, selected?

1. From among criminal prisoners

2. Volunteers, i.e. prisoners, physically and morally exhausted. Though they actually were aware of the danger threatening them if they let themselves be inoculated with typhus, they knew, that should they survive the infection, they would stay for three months in block 46, get more and better food, without the need to do hard labour. Therefore they chose a kind of suicide that gave them a certain chance to survive.

3. The following problems were studied: the incubation period of the disease, its gravity and the course of the disease, depending on the dosage and place where the virus was injected, the rapidity with which the Weil-Felix test showed reaction, the agglutination curve in regard to Eberth's bacillus and paratyphoid bacteria, the effect of certain medicines and particularly the Bayer's sedatives against typhoid encephalitis.

Death was caused most frequently by encephalitis and cardiovascular collapse.

Death occurred between the 7th and the 13th day, as an average between the 8th and 9th day. Mortality was high, higher than, in the case

13 Robert Waitz, "Experimental Typhus in the Buchenwald Camp", in IAC, *Inhuman Medicine,* vol. 1, pt. 2, pp. 120–130.

of spontaneous typhus, even during the period of an epidemic. A sick person around 40 years old had very poor chances to survive.

For such insignificant results, obtained during experiments conducted without adhering to scientific principles, by an incompetent personnel, thousands of people suffered and their lives were taken. The same happened in other experimental centers. In concentration camps, in experimental centers, the characteristic feature of Nazism was clear: disregard and contempt for the human being and absolute negation of his rights.

Translation of Document No-3560[14] Office of the Chief of Counsel for War Crimes

Copy of Document No. 18 of the Military Tribunal of Strasbourg pertaining to the Legal Proceedings against HIRT, HIMMLER, BICKENBACH, and HAAGEN, indicted for Murder and Complicity.

"Scientific" Extermination
by Henri Chrétien
Prisoner No. 98.752, Dachau Camp.

Henri CHRÉTIEN, a young Parisian doctor, was arrested in January 1943 as medical officer in charge of the sanitary service of the F.T.P. in the Paris area. Deported without trial in July 1943 to the concentration camp Natzweiler, was later transferred to Allach near Dachau in September 1944. He was liberated on 30 April 1945 by the 45th American Division and it was from this concentration camp of Allach, that he forwarded to "Le Médicin[e] Français" the following testimony, inexorable indictment against Nazi-barbarism...

(Extract)
In January 1944 a party of Gypsies arrived at Natzweiler, during a violent snowstorm. We saw how the SS hurried living, dying and dead people from the lorries, throwing them in disorder on to the snow-covered ground. These gypsies were confined in the hospital.

Two groups of 40 Gypsies were distributed in two wards of Building 5, the second Hospital Building. On Saturday a professor in SS uniform

14 Henri Chrétien, "Scientific Extermination", *Le Médicine Français* (25 May 1945), quoted in Translation of Document No-3560, Office of the Chief of Counsel for War Crimes, Mimeo, p. 1.

came from Strasbourg with his female laboratory assistant and – by means of incisions – proceeded to inoculate the Gypsies with typhus, both the 40 previously vaccinated one and the 40 who had not been vaccinated.

A fortnight after the inoculation, at the time when the disease had just broken out among the 40 non-vaccinated patients, I was posted to an external unit at Oberne.

I was therefore unable to watch the final result of the experiment. I did not return to Natzweiler until six weeks later. I could obtain not the slightest information from anybody. The experiment was over... but a typhus epidemic had broken out in the camp and in certain external units.

It is necessary to know under what conditions these barbaric experiments took place. For the typhus experiments, the gypsies were crowded together, 40 of them, in a small room: three-tiered bunks, two men on each narrow straw mattress. They remained confined there, and only went out in order to go to the latrine in groups and with an escort. From time to time, they received some rations in addition to their meager camp diet.

HITLER's "Science" gave vent to its perverted imagination in the concentration camps. It produced, in most cases, a display of quack experimental methods with no preliminary scientific theory. Could HITLER's "Science" at least yield important results? Colleagues have assured me that these appeared to be very scanty.

Document No-434, Affidavit of Ferdinand Roemhild[15]

I, Ferdinand Roemhild,, being duly sworn, depose and state:

In 1934 I became associated with the German Communist Party (KBD).

On March 22, 1935, I was placed under arrest.

I was put into prison on 2 April 1938, then transferred to the Buchenwald Concentration Camp.

In the summer of 1939, I was assigned to the prisoners' hospital as a clerk.

In 1941, Dr. Waldemar Hoven became the first camp physician and from that time on, my knowledge of the activities in this sector of the camp and in the hospital was complete.

Due to the above positions as an inmate of the Buchenwald Concentration Camp for a period of seven years and as a clerk and private

15 Affidavit of Ferdinand Roemhild, Document No-434, in RG-30.001M.

secretary to the first camp physician, I am able to give the following information.

Block 46 was established as an experimental station for research on spotted fever and virus in December 1941.

Block 50 became a part of this department for spotted fever and virus research and was used for the purpose of manufacturing spotted fever vaccine.

After the experiments had been completed, the number of human guinea pigs killed in the course of these experiments was reported to us for the records.

In all cases, the inmates transferred to Block 46 for experimental purposes were healthy prisoners. They were forced to undergo the experiments, they were not volunteers. No prisoners, as far as I know, were ever released as a reward for having undergone experiments. From the reports received in our office, I can state that roughly 300 of the prisoners used in these experiments died.

Excerpt from the Testimony of Dr. Balachowksy, Former Prisoner of Buchenwald[16]

After the conclusion of the experiments, no survivors were allowed to live, according to the custom prevailing in Block 46. All the survivors of the experiments were "liquidated," murdered, in Block 46, by the customary methods, that is by means of intracardiac injections of phenol. Intracardiac injections of 10 cubic centimeters of pure phenol was the usual method of extermination in Buchenwald.

From the records and the charts – we could identify 12 different cultures of typhus germs, designated by the letter BU (meaning Buchenwald), and numbered Buchenwald 1 to Buchenwald 12. A constant supply of these cultures was kept in Block 46 by means of the infecting healthy individuals through sick ones; this was achieved by artificial inoculation of typhus germs by means of intravenous injections of 0.5 to 1 cubic centimeter of infected blood drawn from a patient at the height of the crisis. Now, it is well known that artificial inoculation of typhus by intravenous injection is invariably fatal. Therefore all these men who were used for bacterial culture during the whole time such cultures were required (from October 1942 to the liberation of the camp) died, and we counted 600 victims sacrificed for the sole purpose of supplying typhus germs.

16 Testimony of Alfred Balachowsky, in *Trials NMT*, vol. 6, pp. 308–309.

M. DUBOST: They were literally murdered to keep typhus germs alive?
BALACHOWSKY: They were literally murdered to keep typhus germs alive. Apart from these, other experiments were made as to the efficacy of vaccines.

M. DUBOST: What is this document?
BALACHOWSKY: This document contains a record of the typhus cultures.

M. DUBOST: This document was taken by you from the camp?
BALACHOWSKY: Yes, I took this document from the camp, and its contents were summarized by me in the experiment book of Block 46.

Excerpt from the Testimony of Dr. Fritz Menneke, Director of the Insane Asylum in Eishberg, 14 January 1947[17]

Q. Were any of the inmates used in the experiments volunteers?
A. You can hardly speak about volunteers in a case like that.

Q. Were any of these inmates used pardoned after successfully undergoing such experiments?
A. No. I can't remember any such case.

Q. Were the inmates used all healthy persons?
A. They had to be healthy. Otherwise they wouldn't have stood up to the experiments.

Q. After the inmates died, were records kept as to the cause of his death?
A. Yes, then a death report was made and the cause of death was always designated as something different.

Q. In other words, most of the death certificates stated that the inmate died of natural causes. Would that be a correct presumption?
A. Certainly.

17 Testimony of Dr. Fritz Menneke, 14 January 1947, Nuremberg Trial Transcript, pp. 1632–1634, reprinted in Mendelsohn, ed., *The Holocaust*, vol. 9, pp. 82–84.

The major German drug companies I. G. Farbenindustrie, Bayer and Behring-Werke, as well as the Robert Koch Institute, saw the concentration camp experiments as an opportunity to test their drugs directly on human beings, thereby significantly shortening the time required to bring new drugs to the market. Dr. Ding's diary serves as a primary source of information.[18] It records the unfolding of experiments at Buchenwald with I. G. Farben's drugs Rutenol and Acridine (trade name: Akridin). The tests had been suggested by Drs. Neumann and Bieling, the former a representative of I. G. Farben, the latter one of the developers of these particular preparations. Prof. Lautenschlager of I. G. Farben assisted with the planning. Noteworthy is the fact that, in order to approximate the health condition of army personnel, only people in good general condition were chosen as experimental subjects.

Excerpt from Dr. Ding's Diary, Read by the Chief Prosecutor in Opening Statements at Nuremberg[19]

13 and 14 Apr 43: Unit of SS Sturmbannführer Dr. Ding ordered to I. G. Farbenindustrie A.G., Hoechst. Conference with Prof. Lautenschlaeger, Dr. Weber and Dr. Fussgaenger about the experimental series "Acridine Granulate and Rutenol" in the concentration camp Buchenwald.

24 Apr 1943: Therapeutic experiments Acridine-Granulate (A-GR2) and Rutenol. To carry out the therapeutic experiments, 30 persons (15 each) and nine persons for control were infected by intravenous injection of 2 cc. each of fresh blood of a typhus sick person. All experimental persons got very serious typhus.

1 Jun 1943: Charts of case history completed. The experimental series was concluded with 21 deaths; of these, eight were in Buchenwald, eight with Rutenol and five control.

7 Sep 1943: Chart and case history completed. The experimental series was concluded with 53 deaths.

18 See also Stanislaw Klodzinski, "Inhuman Medicine", in IAC, *Inhuman Medicine*, p. 43.

19 Excerpt from Dr. Ding's diary, read by the chief prosecutor in opening statements at the Nuremberg Doctors' Trial, in *Trials NMT*, vol. 1, pp. 50–52.

Translation of Document No-265, Office of U.S. Chief of Counsel[20]

DIARY [of Dr. Ding] of the Division for Research of Spotted Fever and Virus at the Institute of Hygiene of the Waffen SS.

10 Jan 43:
Therapeutic Experiments Akridin and Methylene Blue

On suggestion of the I. G. Farbenindustrie AG, as spotted fever therapeuticum were tested:

a) Preparation 3582 "Akridin" of the chemical pharmaceutical and sero-bacteriological department in Frankfurt-on-the-Main-Hoechst – Prof. LAUTENSCHLAEGER.

A) Therapeutic Experiment A

b) Methylene blue, tested in an experiment on mice by Prof. KIEKUTH.

B) Therapeutic Experiment M

26 Jan 43:
Artificial infection with Ridotter-Virus Op No. 223 and 226:

20 persons for therapeutic experiment A: Akridin
20 persons for therapeutic experiment M: Methylene blue
7 persons for control

20 Feb 43:

From the spotted fever infections of 26 Jan 43 the persons for control show no typical spotted fever symptoms.

Vaccine "EM" of the Behring Works
Akridin
Methylene Blue
About 1/4 are without sickness, the remainder have medium spotted fever.

The research series was designated to the manufacturer as "negative" as the persons for control could not be infected clearly.

1 death in therapeutic experiment Akridin.

Dr. DING
SS Sturmbannführer

16 Jun 43:
Typhus – Therapeutic Experiment "Otrhomin"

On suggestion of the Robert Koch Institute, Berlin (Prof. Dr. LOCKEMANN) the effect of a new "Therapeutikum" of the Rhode series –

20 "Diary of Dr. Ding", Document No-265, Office of the U.S. Chief of Counsel, in RG-30.001M.

Otrhomin should be tested on humans. For this purpose, 20 persons of the series "Otrhomin" and 20 persons for control (10 immunized, 10 not immunized) were infected on 10 Jun 43 respectively on 15 June 43 with 2 cc each of typhus bacteria swelling in a physical salt solution, given in potato salad. Of the 40 persons, seven got sick slightly, 23 medium. Furthermore, there were six ambulatory cases.

23 July 43:
Charts of case history completed of the series "Otrhomin" and sent to Berlin.

26 May 44–12 June 44:
Withdrawal of blood to produce spotted fever convalescent serum (FFRS)

To produce FFRS, 6,500 cc blood were taken from 15 spotted fever convalescents between the 14th and 21st day after the fever had subsided, and sent by courier to the SS main headquarters (SS Führungshauptamp), departmental group (Amtsgruppe) D, department (Amt) XVI (blood conservation) attn. SS Hauptsturmführer (Capt) Dr. Ellenbeck – Berlin, Lichterfelde.

Ding

31 Oct 44:
Withdrawal of blood to produce spotted fever convalescent serum (FFRS)

To produce FFRS, 20.8 liters of blood were taken from 44 spotted fever convalescents between the 14th and 21st day after the fever had subsided, and sent by courier to the SS main headquarters (SS Führungshauptamp) Departmental group (Amtsgruppe) D, Department (Amt), XVI (blood conservation) – SS Sturmbannführer (Major) Dr. Ellenbeck, Berlin-Lichterfelde.

Kluber

13 Nov 44:
Therapeutic experiment with spotted fever vaccine

By order of the highest hygienist of the Waffen SS of 12 Aug 44, it is to be determined whether the course of spotted fever sickness can be tempered by the intravenous or intramuscular injection of spotted fever vaccine.

For the experimental series 20 persons were considered, of these 10 for intravenous injection (Series A), 10 for intramuscular injection (Series B) and in addition five persons for control.

On 13 Nov 44, the 25 experimental persons were infected by subcutaneous injection of 1/10 cc each spotted fever sick fresh blood.

All persons fell sick, as follows

Series A	10 serious
Series B	1 medium
	9 serious
Control 5 serious	

22 Dec 44:

The experimental series was concluded.

2 Jan 45:

Chart and case history completed.

19 deaths	(9 Series A)
	(6 Series B)
	(4 control)

Dr. Kluber

In the preceding document, the entries for 26 May and 13 October 1944 speak of withdrawing blood for use in the production of a typhus convalescent serum. The blood was withdrawn from inmates recovering from typhus.[21] The witness Kogon testified that this work was done by SS Hauptsturmführer Dr. Ellenbeck on orders from Dr. Joachim Mrugowsky. Ellenbeck obtained the blood from typhus convalescents in Block 46. Blood was taken regularly from these experimental subjects, usually in amounts between 250 and 350 cubic centimeters. A number of them, already weakened by disease and thus unable to tolerate the loss of blood, died. While the precise cause of death could not be definitely ascertained under the circumstances, there is no doubt that the withdrawal of blood was a contributing factor.

Another typhus remedy, produced from the urine of pregnant women, and administered as an enema, was also tested.

21 Aziz, *Doctors of Death*, vol. 3, pp. 109–114.

Translation of Document No-875[22]
Office of the Chief of Counsel for War Crimes

Experiment with Clysters (Enemas) of Pregnant Women's Urine
Deposition of MV Dr. Zdenka Nedvedova-Nejedla
6 September 1945

Dr. Treite put me in charge of the ward of those suffering from typhoid fever, where he experimented with clysters of urine of pregnant women as a new method of treatment. I treated by this method about 30 cases of typhoid fever. As this method was according to my expert opinion harmless, and I was able to apply normal treatment besides the method mentioned above, half of the above mentioned patients did not suffer, though neither did I observe having any favorable results from this method.

The following document actually disputes a report by Drs. Holler and Zajitschek, which had been sent by Dr. Ding to his immediate superior, Dr. Mrugowsky, Chief of the Hygiene Institute of the Waffen SS. The document summarizes the therapeutic experiments and provides an analysis of the results. It also gives a surprisingly frank conclusion.

Translation of Document No-582[23]
Office of the Chief of Counsel for War Crimes

From the Hygiene Institute of the Waffen SS – Berlin
Chief: SS Oberführer Dozent Dr.med., Dr.rer.nat. J. Mrugowsky
(Stamp:)

From the Medical Service Officially
No Objections
(Stamp:)

22 Deposition of MV Dr. Zdenka Nedvedova-Nejedla, 6 September 1945, Translation of Document No-875, in RG-30.001M.

23 "On Treatment of Typhus with Acridine Derivates", Document No-582, Office of Chief of Counsel for War Crimes, in RG-30.001M.

The Reich Physician SS and Police
Berlin, 29 September 1944
by order (signature:) A. Poppendick, SS Sturmbannführer

On Treatment of Typhus with Acridin[e] Derivates
By Dr.med. Erwin DING
Sturmbannführer
Waffen SS Officer

4 October 1944

Publication of HOLLER's and ZAJITSCHEK's "A very successful, strictly causal-pathogenetic therapy of Typhus" [1] induces us to make a report about therapeutic experiments which we made with the same drugs Rutenol and Nitroacridin 3582 on 30 persons, as long as half a year before the two authors did.

FUSSGAENGER and WEBER [2] had used those two drugs for the treatment of mice, which were infected with murine typhus. 70% of the animals thus treated survived in contrast to an optimum of 6% of the untreated controls. The result of these experiments was so encouraging that we considered ourselves justified in starting clinical tests of the two Acridin derivates on human beings afflicted with typhus. From April to May 1943, 39 persons, whose spotted fever disease had been ascertained serologically and clinically came to the clinical station attached to the "Department for Spotted Fever and Virus Research" of the "Hygienic Institute of the Waffen SS" for treatment. These were very serious cases, judged by the significant involvement of their central nervous system and cardiovascular system. Accordingly there was a lethal outcome in over 50% of the cases.

According to the instructions of the firm BAYER/Hoechet, Rutenol was administered in form of a granulate, of which a heaped teaspoon full roughly corresponds to a single dose of 0.4 g. The treatment included a normal series of six to ten single doses at intervals of six hours; in the case of Nitroacridin, sugar-coated, it was one to two tablets three times a day, possibly from the start of the disease. Patients, whose infection could be regarded as rather certain, were given Rutenol, resp. [or rather] Acridine already during the incubation time. If the patient could take it even only to some dosage, we continued the treatment beyond ten doses.

Treatment with Rutenol
The complications were bronchial pneumonia, nephritis, intestinal bleeding, and subcutaneous phlegmones below the larynx.
Eight of the 16 patients vomited after Rutenol up to seven times a day.

Mortality was extraordinarily high with 53.3%. No connection showed between tolerance and death rate: four patients responded well to Rutenol and regained their health, three responded well and died; no complications appeared in any of these cases.

Eight patients vomited after Rutenol, three of them regained their health, the five others died.

Treatment with Acridine

The complications were parotitis, nephritis, in one case, gangrene of the shank, furunculosis, bronchitis, and decubital sores.

The tolerance was by far less favorable than with Rutenol: 13 patients vomited after taking it (up to seven times a day).

Again, mortality was very high with 53.3%...

Mortality among the 3rd group of spotted fever patients, who during the same epidemic remained without Rutenol or Nitroacridin treatment, was only 2% higher, 56%. (Considering the small number of persons under observation, reference in % was only used on account of the better possibility of comparison; we are well aware of the medium error.) The complications – bronchitis and decubital sores – must not be held responsible for the lethal outcome of the cases. Death occurred either due to acute weakness of the heart or as a result of gradual failure of the circulation.

During the epidemic under observation, both drugs showed no alleviation or fever-shortening effect whatever. The death rate, compared to the controls not treated with these drugs, remains roughly the same.

Administered per os, the drugs cause a strong irritation of the stomach, which manifests itself by vomiting. Rutenol, however, showed a more favorable result than Acridin 3582 with roughly half the number of persons who vomited after taking it. Here, over 4/5 of the patients under observation reacted by vomiting.

In conclusion we want to point out, that on the basis of our own experiences with Rutenol and Acridin 3582 we do not believe that the "Magic Bullet" has been found which would kill the germ without damage to the organism. Although this could be expected from the title chosen by Holler and Zajitschek: "A Very Successful, Strictly Causal-Pathogenetic Therapy of Spotted Fever". For the time being we still deem that a warning against exaggerated hopes of success of the therapeutic method referred to is not altogether out of place.

Translation of Document No-484[24]
Office of the Chief of Counsel for War Crimes

Experiments and Research about Exanthematous Typhus at Buchenwald Camp.

The following statement was made by Alfred BALACHOWSKY, Doctor of Science, laboratory chief at the Paris Pasteur Institute, arrested 2 July 1943 by the Gestapo... Brought back to Buchenwald on 1 May 1944 in order to work in block 50 (Hygiene-Institut der Waffen SS), on the production of the vaccine against exanthematous typhus for the German army.

"In general, the internees serving as 'guinea pigs', if they survived an experiment, were put to death at its end by an injection of Prussic acid (1 cubic centimeter, intravenously or of 10 ccm concentrated Phenol solution (intracardiac)."

A list of publications, which was attached to Dr. Ding's diary, shows that some camp experiments were reported in German medical journals, evidence once again of the fact that German physicians were aware of the existence of the camps and of the medical experiments that were conducted there.

DING DIARY[25]

Literature

[1.] HOLLER G. and ZAJITSCHEK, R.: *Med. Klin.* 1944, No. 17/18, p. 247ff.
[2.] FUSSGAENGER and WEBER: Private Information, Spring 1943.
[3.] SCHULER (formerly DING): "Exceptional Incubation Periods with Spotted Fever", in print.
[4.] MRUGOWSKY, J.: *Med. Klin.* 1942, No. 9/10 p. 1ff.
[5.] WOHLRAB, R.: "Journals for the Combatting of Epidemics", Warsaw–Stuttgart 1944, Vol. 1 p. 42ff.
[6.] ASCHENBRENNER, R. and v. BAEYER, W. "Epidemic Spotted Fever", Stuttgart 1944.

24 Alfred Balachowsky, Statement on Typhus Experiments, Document No-484, Office of the Chief Counsel for War Crimes, in RG-30.001M.

25 Ding's list has been transcribed as he entered it, with one adaptation: his words "and following" have been converted to "ff".

[7.] SCHULZE: According to ASCHENBRENNER, R. and v. BAEYER, W., 1.c. 177.
[8.] Messrs. BAYER/Hoechst: Communication of 27 March 1943.
[9.] MIESCHER, G.: *Swiss Medical Weekly* 1944, No. 25, p. 684ff.
[10.] SCHULER (formerly DING, E.): "Blood, Serum and Spinal Fluid in the Treatment of Spotted Fever" Annex of Intern Medicine, Vo[l]. 65 (1944).

This is an exact copy of a list Compiled by Schuler, including e.g. lack of some first initials.

MALARIA EXPERIMENTS

Malaria can be an acute or chronic disease, often fatal and almost always seriously debilitating. It is caused by a protozoan parasite of the genus Plasmodium, which is transmitted to humans by Anopheles mosquitoes. Transmission occurs during the bite of an infected female mosquito, or, more rarely, through the direct inoculation of infected red blood cells. The illness is variable but is generally characterized by episodes of fever, chills, severe anemia, and enlargement of the spleen. Malaria transmission occurs in over one hundred countries throughout Africa, Asia, and Latin America and on certain Caribbean and Pacific islands.

The estimated annual global incidence of the disease is 300-500 million communicable cases. In sub-Saharan Africa alone, it causes an estimated one million deaths each year. Since German soldiers in World War II were being deployed to areas where exposure to malaria infection was possible, the Nazis attached great importance to finding effective immunizations and treatments for the disease.

Experiments to this end were conducted at the Dachau concentration camp, with more than 1,200 inmates as test subjects.[26] Dr. Claus Schilling [also Klaus Schilling] supervised the experiments, with the assistance of Dr. Wolfram Sievers and others. The evidence shows that healthy persons were infected by mosquitoes or by injections made from the glands of mosquitoes. After the victims had been infected, they were variously treated with Quinine, Neosalvarsan, Pyramidon, Antipyrin, and several combinations of these drugs. Many deaths occurred from excessive doses of Neosalvarsan and Pyramidon.

26 Opening Statement of the Prosecution by Brig. General Telford Taylor, 9 Dec. 1946, in *Trials NMT,* vol. 1, pp. 43–44.

The purpose of these experiments was apparently two-fold, first to test various substitutes for quinine, the supply of which was limited, and second to find a method of immunization against malaria.

In the four years during which the experiments were conducted (1941–45), prisoners were deliberately and involuntarily infected with malaria.[27] The disease was produced either by the bite of infected insects or by direct inoculation of blood from infected patients. Prisoners thus infected were permitted to develop typical clinical malaria and were treated with Neosalvarsan, Atabrine and certain Atabrine-like drugs. By repeated inoculation, many prisoners were kept infected for periods of two to three years. In an attempt to immunize against malaria, a state of chronic infection was induced and Pyramidar [Pyramidon] was used to suppress the clinical manifestations of the disease. Certain groups of prisoners served merely as hosts to perpetuate malaria strains for the experiments.

In subjects already exposed to the starvation and disease rampant at Dachau, the debilitating effect of repeated attacks of malaria was tantamount to signing their death warrant. These prisoners were defenseless against opportunistic secondary infections such as pneumonia, tuberculosis and typhus. Moreover, the drugs themselves caused fatal reactions in perhaps one hundred cases: specifically granulocytosis produced by Pyramidon and hemorrhagic conditions caused by Neosalvarsan. The suffering of those who survived is immeasurable but manifest in the words of the victims who testified at Dr. Schilling's trial.

The former prisoner-physician Fritz Blaha testified before the International Nuremberg Tribunal on 13–14 January 1946, there reiterating in essence the statements he made in an earlier affidavit taken at Dachau.

Translation of Document No-3249-PS[28]

Dachau, Germany
24 November 1945
Excerpt from Affidavit of Franz Blaha
I, Franz Blaha, being duly sworn, depose and state as follows:

27 *Report of the Atrocities Committed at the Dachau Concentration Camp,* Vol. 1, YVA, JM/10046, pp. 16–17.

28 Testimony of Dr. Franz Blaha before the International Military Tribunal, Nuremberg, [beginning] 11 January 1946, Document No-3249-PS, in *Trial IMT,* vol. 5, pp. 167–174. On the web, see The Avalon Project at Yale Law School at www.yale.edu/lawweb/avalon/imt/proc/v20.

I studied medicine in Prague, Vienna, Strasbourg and Paris and received my diploma in 1920. From 1920 to 1926 I was a clinical assistant. In 1926 I became chief physician of the Iglau Hospital in Moravia, Czechoslovakia. I held this position until 1939 when the Germans entered Czechoslovakia and I was seized as a hostage and held a prisoner for cooperating with the Czech government. I was sent as a prisoner to the Dachau Concentration Camp in April 1941 and remained there until the liberation of the camp in April 1945. While there I performed approximately 7,000 autopsies. Altogether 12,000 autopsies were performed under my direction.

...During my time at Dachau I was familiar with the many kinds of medical experiments carried out there on human victims. These persons were never volunteers but were forced to submit to such acts. Malaria experiments on about 1,200 people were conducted by Dr. Klaus Schilling between 1941 and 1945. Schilling was personally asked by Himmler to conduct these experiments. The victims were either bitten by mosquitoes or given injections of malaria sporozoites taken from mosquitoes. Different kinds of treatment were applied including Quinine, Pyrifer, Neosalvarsan, Antipyrin, Pyramidon and a drug called 2516 Bohring. I autopsied bodies of people who died from these malaria experiments. 30 to 40 died from the malaria itself, 300 to 400 died later from diseases which were fatal because of the physical condition resulting from the malaria attacks. In addition there were deaths resulting from poisoning due to overdoses of Neosalvarsan and Pyramidon. Dr. Schilling was present at the time of my autopsies on the bodies of his patients.

Translation of Document No-2428-PS
Office of U.S. Chief Counsel

Excerpt from the Testimony of Witness Marion Dabrowski[29]

Q. Your name is Marion Dabrowski?
A. Yes.

Q. You are a Roman Catholic priest?
A. Yes.

Q. When were you brought to the Dachau prison camp?
A. 5 July 1942.

29 Testimony of Marion Dabrowski, Document No-2428-PS, Office of U.S. Chief Counsel, in RG-30.001M.

Q. Where were you arrested originally?
A. In Warsaw.

Q. By whom?
A. Gestapo.

Q. What crime or offense did you commit to warrant the Gestapo taking you in custody and arresting you?
A. I was accused of having been in charge of a printing press which was allegedly used to print anti-Nazi propaganda. That was a fabricated reason. In reality I was arrested simply as a member of the Polish intelligentsia. I could even prove that it was impossible for me to have been connected with a printing press for illegal propaganda in Warsaw, as I had been living in Dublin, yet I was arrested on that account.

Q. Were there other Catholic priests confined in prison at Dachau at the time you arrived?
A. Very many.

Q. Approximately how many Catholic priests have been confined at Dachau?
A. Altogether about 1,700.

Q. Are those 1,700 priests alive today?
A. Approximately 900 died.

Q. What was the cause of their death?
A. I would say most of them died from hunger and over work, also from disease contracted while working in the very cold weather without sufficient protection and many died from phlegmone. A few were also executed or tortured to death.

Q. Were you forced to submit to the malaria experiment while you were a prisoner at Dachau?
A. Yes, three times by mosquitoes and once by an injection of blood from a malaria patient.

Q. Did you volunteer or offer yourself for the experiment?
A. Never.

Q. How did it happen that these experiments were performed upon you?
A. It happened through the camp secretaries' office. At that station, prisoners who were communists were told to present the names of 100 pris-

oners for the malaria injections. These communists said that the priests are the most useless among the prisoners, so we priests were told that 100 of us had to go forward to get the malaria injections. The hundred names were finally chosen from among the priests by alphabet.

Q. Were the 100 Catholic priests forced to submit to the malaria experiments?
A. Yes.

Q. What result did this malaria injection have upon you and the other priests who were subjected to malaria infections?
A. At first we got a fever for about three hours. After three hours, we felt extremely cold and started shaking with cold. Then the fever started again, and the whole process continued sometimes for as many as nine days. My own brother, who is also a priest, had, for nine days, daily higher fever, as high as 41 or 42 centigrade. Generally they were in a very bad state of health and there were several cases of death.

Q. Over what period of time were you subjected to these four experiments?
A. They began the experiment on me in December 1942 and the last was in June of 1943.

Q. Who performed these experiments upon you and the other priests?
A. That was SS Obergruppenführer, Professor Schilling.

Q. Did Dr. Schilling ever tell you by whose order he was making these experiments?
A. No, he never said anything to us. He treated us like dogs. When I protested to Dr. Schilling in person, I tried, at first, to talk French to him, because he knew that language; and it is easier for me than to talk German. He told me, in fact, he stopped me at once, and said, "In this camp we speak German!" When, after that, I protested in German language against further experiments on my body, he said, "You have no right to protest, you are a prisoner here, and I shall report you to the Commander of this camp for your protest, and you will see how hard the consequences will be for you." Nevertheless, I kept on protesting. I had an order from the Camp Commander later on that, every time Dr. Schilling wanted me at the hospital, I had to appear without fail at his disposal. I have witnesses that the facts I just related are exact.

Q. Upon how many prisoners did Dr. Schilling perform these experiments?
A. I understand, 1,100.

Q. What would you say if I were to tell you that Dr. Schilling admitted that he had inoculated some 2,000 prisoners?
A. Yes, that figure may be exact, because his experimenting had started before I arrived to this camp.

The witness was then cross-examined by Capt. Clyde L. Walker.

Q. Father, is there anything else that you would like to tell us?
A. I would like to give statistical proof for my testimony. There were exactly 846 Catholic Polish Priests who died in this camp. 794 Roman Catholic Polish Priests lived the day when the Americans entered this camp. 260 Polish priests were sent out on invalid transports and never returned. Those transports contained altogether, 5,000 prisoners approximately. They started on 6 May 1942, and the last ones left in October 1942. Nobody ever returned from those transports. As to the number of non-Polish Catholic Priests there were approximately 450 since 1940. Of that number, approximately 100 died. 41 German priests were still in the camp when the Americans arrived, but that figure includes 11 Austrians and 4 Germans from Czechoslovakia, who were brought among the German priests into this camp. As to the malaria experiments, 200 Polish priests received injections, and were subjected to this experiment, and 21 died from experiments. 40 Polish priests were subjected to the phlegmone experiments, 11 of them died.

The above deposition was signed by Investigator-Examiner, Col. DAVID CHAVEZ, Jr., JAGD., and Assistant Investigator-Examiner, Capt. of Information, CLYDE L. WALKER.

■

The next two documents elaborate on Father Dabrowski's assertion that participation in the experiments was compulsory, that protest was useless. They also provide graphic evidence of the suffering inflicted on experimental subjects.

Translation of National Archives Document RG 238, M887[30]

Excerpt from the Testimony of Father Leo Miechalowski [Michalowski], also a Former Prisoner in Dachau

Q. Now, father will you tell the Tribunal what happened to you after your arrest?
A. When I was arrested I was first kept in prison for two months. From there we were sent into a cloister. There other priests were assembled until about ninety priests had been assembled altogether, and from there were sent to Strutthof near Danzig into the concentration camp. From there on the fifth or ninth of February we were transferred to Sachsenhausen-Oranienburg which is located near Berlin. On the 13th of December 1940, we were transferred to Dachau. I was confined in Dachau until the arrival of the Americans – until we were liberated – that was on the 29th of April 1945.

Q. Now, father, were you a political prisoner in Dachau?
A. Yes. I wore a red insignia. All those who had been arrested for political reasons had to wear this insignia.

Q. Now, father, were you experimented on in the concentration camp at Dachau?
A. Yes. I was involved in malaria experiments and also on one occasion in high altitude experiments.

Q. Now, father, will you tell the Tribunal just what happened when you were experimented on with malaria? That is, when did it happen and how you happened to be selected?
A. I was so weak from hunger that I fell down on the road. I wanted to be transferred to another assignment where we would get some bread between meals so my health could improve by additional food. One man arrived and selected about thirty people for some easy labor. I also wanted to be selected for this assignment. Those of us who had been selected were led away. We went in the direction where the work was located and at the very last moment instead of going to that place of work we were led to the camp hospital. We did not know what was going to happen to us there. I thought that perhaps this was going to be some detail for easier work in the hospital. We were told to undress and our numbers were

30 Testimony of Father Leo Miechalowski [Michalowski], in RG-238, M887 (also on The United States Holocaust Memorial Museum Web Site), pp. 874–877.

taken down. We were not told what they were going to do with us. Then the doctor came and told us that we were to be x-rayed and then go to our block. After two days, I was again called to the hospital and there I was given malaria. There were little cages with infected mosquitoes and I had to put my hand into one of them. A mosquito stung me and afterwards I was ill in the hospital for five weeks. Somewhat later, I don't exactly recall, two or three weeks later, I had my first malaria attack. Such attacks recurred frequently and several medicines were given to us. I was given Neosalvarsan, two injections of Quinine, on one occasion Atabrine and the worst was that one time when I had an attack, I was given so-called Perifer. It was by injections, one every hour. All of a sudden my heart felt like it was going to be torn out. I became insane. I completely lost my ability to speak. This lasted until the evening. In the evening a nurse arrived and wanted to give me more injections. I resisted. The nurse had already prepared the injection and said that he would report this to Dr. Schilling. After approximately ten minutes another nurse arrived and said that he would have to give me the injection after all. I kept resisting but finally they gave me the injection anyway.

Q. Father, do I understand you to say that you were injected with malaria in the middle of 1942?
A. It was approximately in the middle of 1942 when I was infected with malaria.

Q. And you were asked to consent to the malaria experiment?
A. No. I was not asked for my consent.

Q. And you did not volunteer for this experiment?
A. No. I was taken in the manner which I have just described.

Q. Did you make any protest?
A. In 1942, it was very difficult in the camp to lodge any protest. When I protested, I clearly realized that protesting could have the most serious consequences for me.

Q. Now how many people were experimented on in the malaria experiments?
A. In the hospital when I had my attacks, there were approximately fifty to sixty people; the numbers changed.

Q. And do you know the approximate total number of inmates experimented on with malaria in Dachau?

A. Towards the end I heard that approximately one thousand two hundred prisoners were subjected to these experiments.

Q. How many recurrences of malaria fever did you have, Father?
A. I cannot give you the exact number any more. However, those attacks recurred frequently, I think about five times, and then I still had treatment in bed for some time, and then there were several more. Altogether I had about ten attacks.

Q. Do you still suffer any effects from the malaria?
A. I still have some after-effects, but I do not know if this is only due to malaria because I was also subjected to another experiment.

Father Miechalowski [Michalowski] had already given a deposition at Dachau, on 13 May 1945.[31]

Q. How much did you weigh in civilian life?
A. Approximately 90 kilos.

Q. How much did you weigh at the time that you were undergoing the experiment?
A. Approximately 47 kilos.

Q. And how much do you weigh today?
A. I should say about 60 kilos.

The above deposition, part of the evidence introduced to the General Military Court at Dachau, in the case of United States vs. Weiss, Ruppert, et al., was signed by Investigator-Examiner, Col. DAVID CHAVEZ, Jr., Jagd., and Assistant Investigator-Examiner, Capt. of Information, CLYDE L. WALKER.

■

Whereas Father Michalowsky was forced to allow malarial mosquitoes to bite him, witness August H. Vieweg received direct injections of malaria-infected blood. The testimony follows.

31 Deposition of Father Miechalowski [Michalowski], 13 May 1945, to American Investigators at Dachau, Translation of Document No-2428-PS, Office of U.S. Chief of Counsel, in RG-30.001M.

Excerpt from Testimony by Prosecution Witness August H. Vieweg[32]

Mr. Hardy: While you were an inmate at the concentration camp, did you ever undergo any medical experiments?
Witness Vieweg: I was used for malaria experiments by Professor Dachfinney at the Dachau concentration camp.

Q. How many times were you subjected to the malaria experiments by Dr. Schilling?
A. On five occasions I received injections of 5 cubic centimeters of highly infectious malaria blood.

Q. Would you kindly tell the Tribunal what effect these experiments had on you; that is, did you have high fever, serious illness, and so forth?
A. Quite often I ran a very high temperature. I got into a very exhausted condition, and after the injection I received large doses of medical drugs, Quinine, Ephedrine, and many others. I was in bed for weeks, and after one treatment there were 20 to 26 occasions in the course of the years 1943, 1944, and 1946, when I had malaria attacks, so that for a long time I was unable to work.

Q. At the present time, do you have recurrences of this malaria fever?
A. This last year I was in the hospital from August 1st to 15th, again with malaria attack.

Q. How many recurrences of malaria have you endured since you were experimented on by Dr. Schilling?
A. After my treatments in the experimental station had been concluded I stayed with Dr. Schilling, and there were about 20 occasions when I was treated for recurrences.

Q. Are you completely cured now, Witness?
A. No.

32 Testimony of Prosecution Witness August H. Vieweg, 13, 16 December 1946, in *Trials NMT,* vol. 1, p. 303.

Extracts from the Review of the Proceedings of the General Military Court in the Case of the United States vs. Weiss, Ruppert, et al., held at Dachau, Germany[33]

A series of experiments concerning the treatment of malaria were conducted under the supervision of Dr. Schilling. Three hundred to four hundred persons died as a result.

An inmate, a priest named Father Koch, related his experience. He was first X-rayed and then sent to the malaria station. He was put into a little room where he received a box with mosquitoes, in which he had to put in his hands for about half an hour. That went on every day for one week. Every afternoon another box of mosquitoes was put in between his legs while he was in bed. Each morning a blood smear was taken from his ear and his temperature was measured each day and night. He was given Quinine. In about 17 days he left the hospital. After being released from the hospital he had to report back every Saturday. Eight months later he had an attack of malaria, which recurred precisely every 3 weeks for 6 months (R 359, 363, 364, 365). The symptoms he felt were high fever, chills, and pains in the joints (R 359). Koch did not volunteer for the experiments nor did the other prisoners who were mostly Poles and Russians, who underwent the treatment with him.

The prisoners were infected with malaria by the injections of the mosquitoes themselves or the injections of extracts of the mucous glands of the mosquitoes. After having contracted malaria the prisoners were treated in different ways. Some, as Father Koch, were given Quinine. Others were given Neosalvarsan, Pyramidon, Antipyrin, a drug numbered 92516, and several combinations of these. Some people died as a result of these experiments.

At the trial, an affidavit by Schilling, executed in his own handwriting on 30 October 1945 before 2nd Lieutenant Werner Conn, was admitted into evidence.

My name is Professor Dr. Claus Schilling. I have already worked on tropical diseases for 45 years. I came to the experimental station in Dachau in February 1942. I judge that I inoculated between 900 and 1,000 prisoners. Those were mostly inoculations for protection. These

33 Extracts from the Review of the Proceedings of the General Military Court in the Case of the "United States vs. Weiss, Ruppert, et al.", held at Dachau, Germany, in *Trials NMT,* Vol. 1, pp. 289–308. Documents from the Dachau trials were admitted as evidence in the Nuremberg Doctors' Trial.

> people, however, were not volunteers. The inmates whom I gave protective inoculations were not examined by me but by the current camp doctor.[34]

The accused Doctor Schilling elected to testify further, thus providing a more detailed record of his personal history. He stated that he was seventy-four years old, married, had one son, and was a physician; that he had specialized in tropical diseases, particularly malaria; that he had studied under Professor Koch of Berlin, and had received his medical doctor's degree in Munich in 1894. He did research work in Africa on malaria, sleeping sickness, and tsetse fly disease, then worked for the Rockefeller Foundation in Berlin, receiving a grant in 1911 for the study of various tropical diseases. In December 1941, in Italy, Dr. Schilling met Leonardo Conti, Reichgesundheitsführer and Reichärzteführer, who invited him to see Himmler. Himmler asked Schilling, who had retired, to undertake research for effective drugs against malaria and sent him to Dachau for that purpose.

In assessing the evidence that had been used at Dachau to convict Schilling, the Nuremberg Military Tribunal prosecutor argued that Schilling was "the most reprehensible [of the persons who had been tried and condemned at Dachau]. He voluntarily came to Dachau fully cognizant of the nature of the work he intended to perform. Being the educated and learned person that he was, Schilling undoubtedly must have realized the manner in which his work suited the needs of the Nazis. Although his personal motives may have stemmed from his desire to aid humanity, he permitted himself to utilize their methods in contrast to other eminent German artists and scientists who either fled or refused to make themselves a part of the Nazi system. It is believed that the sentence of the Court, which was aware of Schilling's position in the scientific world, should be approved."[35]

Dr. Schilling's records of his experiments on August Vieweg reveal a physician methodically subjecting a "patient" to procedures that could kill.

34 Extract from the Review of Proceedings of the General Military Court in the Case of the "United States vs. Weiss, Ruppert, et al.", held at Dachau, Germany, Document No-856, Prosecution Exhibit No-125, in *Trials NMT,* vol. 1, pp. 289 ff.; here pp. 291–292. This document from Nuremberg summarizes and cites extracts from Dr. Schilling's testimony in "United States [vs.] Weiss, Ruppert, et al.", one of the Dachau trials. The entire text of the document can be viewed on the Internet at www.mazal.org/archives/nmt/01/NMT289 ff.

35 Ibid.

Document No-983[36]

Sample of Dr. Schilling's Treatment Record[37]

Vieweg, August H No. 20196 Block 24/1

2.IV.42 [2 April 1942] 5 ccm Venenblut von Pecker (Stamm Rose) subkutan

12.IV–37.4; 12.IV. Chinin 2, Ogr. Per os; 14.IV.[Chinin] 2, Ogr. [Per os] kein Fieber bis 21.IV. 5ccm Blut Stamm Rose s.c.v. Zahn.

2.V. [2 May] Chinin. 1.0 gr. Im [i.m.] Urin Chinin #; 3.V. [3 May] Chinin 1.0 gr. Im [i.m.] Urin: Chinin plus, #; 4.V. [4 May] Urin: Chinin plus I; 5.V. [5 May] Urin: Chinin 0.

13.V. [13 May] 5 ccm Blut von Ableiter (St. Rose) s.c.Par. O; 21.v. [21 May] Par. 0.

24.V. [24 May] 1.0 gr. Chinin 1.m. [i.m.]; 25.V. [25 May] 1.0 gr. Chinin i.m.; 26.V. [26 May] 1.0 gr. i.m.; 3.VI. [3 June] 5.0 ccm Blut v. Altmann (St. Rose) s.c.; 4.VI. [4 June] Hgl b. 73%; 8.VI. [8 June] Par.0.

13.VI. [13 June] Par. 0; 1.0 gr, Chinin i.m.; 14.VI. [14 June] 1.0 gr. Chinin i.m; 18.VI. [18 June] 5Jnj. 5.0 ccm Blut v. Martin (Stamm Rose) s.c; 30.VI. [30 June] Par.0.

Cont._____

Vieweg August H. No. 20196, Block 24/1, Gi: 25

2 April 42 5 ccm venous blood from Becker (Rose's culture subcutaneous.

12 April–37.4.

13.April–Quinine 2.0 gr. by mouth.

14 April–2.0 gr. [by mouth], no fever till 21 April, 5 ccm Blood, Rose's culture subcut, by Za.

2 May–*Quinine 1.0g* i.m. Urine Quinine 11; 3.V. [3 May]–Quinine 1.0 gr. i.m. Urine: Quinine 1.11; 4 May Urine: Quinine 1; 5 May–Urine Quinine 0.

13 May–5 ccm Blood by Ableiter (Rose's culture) p.c.Par.0; 21 May–Par 0.

24 May–1.0 gr. Quinine i.m; 25 May–*1.0 gr. Quinine i.m;* 26 May–*1.0* gr. Quinine i.m.

36 Inpatient Records, Dachau Hospital, Dachau, Germany, Document No-983, in RG-30.001M, Malaria.

37 Quantities have been converted to the decimal format used in the United States, i.e., 0.x, or x.xx; the German "ccm" has been converted to "cc". Dates have been left European style, i.e., "day.month.year".

3 June–5.0 ccm Blood by Altmann (Rose's culture) p.c; 4 June–Hgl b 73%, 8 June–Par. 0.

9/10 June–37.4; 13 June–Par. 0, *1. 0 gr. Quinine i.m;* 14 June–1.0 gr. Quinine i.m.

18 June 5 Inj. 5.0 ccm Blood by Martin (Rose's culture) s.c. 30 June Par. O. 37.0.

Cont.____

Vieweg August–*MALARIA*

1 July I, 37.8; 2 July Par.–plus gam 0; 3 July Par.–plus 40.0.

4 July Par. + gam I.

6 July Par. + Gam + 0.6 gr. Neosalvarsan I.v. 18 Par.

7 July Par. Gam 0 temp 0, 20 gr. *Quinine by mouth;* 8 July Par 0, *0,3 gr. Atebrine i.m.*

9 July Par. 0 Temp 0.

10 July in observation R; 11 Aug P Q = –37.4; 12 Aug 0.6: Neosalv. I.v.–37.8

13 August 0.45 Neosalv. I.v; 14 Aug 0.3 Neosalv. I.v. PO; 15 Aug *2x 1g 2x 1g Quin by mouth;* 16 Aug; *2g Quin by mouth;* 18 Aug; PO.

29 Aug New infection?

19 Dec 39.3 Par +/*–0.45 Neosalv. I.v;* 30 Dec. with 1 Jan. 43 Iva Qin by mouth.

20 Dec. 38.4 *0.8 Quinine i.m.*

21 Dec. 37.4 *1.0 g. Quinine i.m.*

22 Dec 37.1 *1.0 g. Quinine by mouth.*

23 Dec Tempo *1,0 g. Quinine by mouth;* 13 Jan Temp. 0. *0.3 Atebrine i.m.*

24 Dec with *28 Dec Atebrine.*

9 Jan. [1943] 38.2.

11 Jan 40.4.

12 Jan Par +/– 0.45 Neosalv. Iv. 40.8.

14 Jan with 18 Jan 1.0 g Quinine by mouth.

HIGH ALTITUDE EXPERIMENTS

The possibility of using concentration camp prisoners for high altitude tests needed by the Luftwaffe (the German Air Force), with all the dangers they entailed, was first broached in a letter of 15 May 1941 to the Reichsführer SS, Heinrich Himmler, by Dr. Sigmund Rascher, who was an officer in both the SS and the Air Force Medical Corps. In the letter, Rascher argues the importance of the experiments for the war effort and also for the necessity of using human subjects.

Translation of Document No-1602-PS[38]
Prosecution Exhibit No-44

Letter from Rascher to Himmler, 15 May 1941, Concerning High-Altitude Experiments on Human Beings

Sigmund Rascher, M.D. (stamp)

Personal Staff Reich Leader SS
Archives File No. Secret/58
München
Trägerstrasse, 56 15 May 1941

Highly esteemed Reich Leader,
...For the time being, have been assigned to the Luftgau Kommando VII, München, for a medical selection course. During this course, where research on high-altitude flying plays a prominent part, determined by the somewhat higher ceiling of the English fighter planes, considerable regret was expressed that no experiments on human beings have so far been possible for us because such experiments are very dangerous and nobody is volunteering. I therefore put the serious question: is there any possibility that two or three professional criminals can be made available for these experiments. The experiments are being performed at the Ground Station for High-Altitude Experiments of the Luftwaffe (Bodenständige Prüfstelle für Höhenforschung der Luftwaffe) at München. The experiments, in which the experimental subject of course may die, would take place with my collaboration. They are absolutely essential for the research on high-altitude flying and cannot, as it has been tried until now, be carried out on monkeys, because monkeys offer entirely different test conditions. I had an absolutely confidential talk with the representative of the Luftwaffe physician who is conducting these experiments. He also is of the opin-

38 "Letter from Rascher to Himmler, 15 May 1941, Concerning High-Altitude Experiments on Human Beings", Translation of Document No-1602-PS, Prosecution Exhibit No-44, in RG-30.001M. See also *Trial IMT,* vols. 1, 5, 20.

ion that the problems in question can only be solved by experiments on human beings. (Feeble-minded individuals also could be used as experimental material.)

The report from Himmler's office represents the first instance in which Himmler agreed to experiments on human subjects.

Translation of Document No-1582-PS Prosecution Exhibit 45[39]

Letter from Rudolf Brandt to Rascher, undated

AK/104a/LO Bra/V

(Stamp illegible May 2 (?) 1941)

SS Untersturmführer Sigmund Rascher M.D.
München
Trägerstr, 56

Dear Dr. Rascher:
Shortly before flying to Oslo, the Reich Leader SS gave me your letter of 15 May 1941, for partial reply.

I can inform you that prisoners will, of course, be gladly made available for the high-flight researches. I have informed the Chief of the Security Police of this agreement of the Reich Leader SS, and requested that the competent official be instructed to get in touch with you.

I want to use this opportunity to extend my cordial wishes to you on the birth of your son.

I shall refer as soon as possible to the second part of your letter.

By order

Heil Hitler!
(initials) R Br (Rudolph Brandt)
SS Sturmbannführer

The next document is a letter of authorization for Rascher, including Himmler's consent for both high-altitude and hypothermia experiments.

39 Letter from Rudolf Brandt to Rascher, undated, Office of the U.S. Chief of Counsel for War Crimes, Evidence Division, Document No-1582-PS, Prosecution Exhibit 45, in *PTT*.

Translation of Document No-1612-PS
Office of U.S. Chief of Counsel[40]

Der Reichsführer SS
Field Command Post
Rubber Stamp: Personal Staff of Reich[s]führer SS
Documentation Section
File No. Confidential.
Field Command Post 13 December 1941
Der Reichsführer SS
Personal Staff
Journal No. 19/10/43 g
Bra/Secret

1. Hauptsturmführer Dr. med Rascher
   (illegible) SS
2. (illegible) Berlin
3. Medical officer in SS Führungshauptamt (Leadership Central Office) Berlin
   SS Obergruppenführer POHL Berlin
4. Ahnenerbe (ancestry heritage) Berlin-Dahlen [Dahlem]

Enclosed I am sending you a letter of the Reichsführer SS (copy of same) with an order for SS Hauptsturmführer Dr. Rascher.

You are requested to duly note and accord needed assistance to Hauptsturmführer Dr. Rascher in the carrying through of his experiments.

By order(s) B
SS Obersturmbannführer

Translation of Document 1612-PS (contd.)
Office of U.S. Chief of Counsel

Prinz-Albrechtstrasse
(rubber stamp) Personal Staff of
Reich[s]führer SS
Documentation Section
Journal No. Confidential

40 Memo on Rascher from Himmler, undated, Translation of Document No-1612-PS, in RG-30.001M. Office of U.S. Chief of Counsel, RG-30.001M; first used as evidence at the Dachau trial before the U.S. Military Government Court, Dachau, Germany, 2 November 1945.

SS Hauptsturmführer Dr. Rascher is being assigned to me to carry through the following experiments:

1. Low pressure chamber experiments – to be carried out under conditions corresponding to those actually prevailing under normal operating conditions – for rescue from high and extremely high altitudes. Determination of change in chemical equilibrium, as well as gas equilibrium of human body. Experiments are to be repeated until a scientifically incontestable basis for findings is established. Testing of pressure-proof protection garments for the highest altitudes to be carried out with the assistance of manufacturers of such protective suits.

2. Testing for reimparting warmth after total chilling of the human body – recording all changes of chemical and gas characteristics are to be further continued until complete clarification of doubtful questions. I attach particular value to conditions for experiments as close to actual conditions as possible, quite particularly as regards reimpartation of warmth. SAUNA equipment available in Dachau should be used in connection with experiments on reimpartation of warmth.

3. Experiments on removal of effects due to freezing of parts of human system, especially the extremities, to be carried through in suitable form (e.g. applications with Gastoir water).

4. Experiments concerned with adaptation to freezing cold in snow huts (igloos) to be carried out under varying diets in order to establish whether adaptation to cold and resistance increase against freezing is possible. These experiments are to be carried out on the site of SS Berghaus (SS Mountain-retreat) Sudelfeld.

5. The procurement of the apparatus needed for all the experiments should be discussed in detail with the offices of the Reicharzt SS, of SS Wirtsschafts-Verwaltungshauptamt (SS Main Office for Economics and Administration) and with Ahnenerbe c.V. (ancestry heritage, registered society). The necessary chemical products, medical supplies and glass wire will be available by SS-Sanitätsamt (SS Medical Office) Berlin.

6. Publication of results obtained in such tests subject to my approval only.

(s) H. Himmler

In the following letter to State Secretary of the Air Force, Field Marshal Milch, Himmler explains that he assumed responsibility for the selection and use of experimental subjects from among the Dachau concentration camp prisoner population. He also expresses his intense dislike of the "Christian medical circle", and their views.

Translation of Document No-1617-PS[41]
Office of U.S. Chief of Counsel

The Reichsführer SS
Berlin, SW 11, D.
Prinz-Albrechtstrasse I
November 1941
Field Command Test

SECRET

Dear Comrade Milch:

You will recall that through General Wolff I particularly recommended to you for your consideration the work of a certain Dr. Rascher, who is a physician of the Air Force on leave (Arzt des Beurlaubtenstandes der Luftwaffe).

These researches which deal with the behavior of the human organism at great heights, as well as with manifestations caused by prolonged cooling of the human body in cold water, and similar problems which are of vital importance to the air force in particular, can be performed by us with particular efficiency because I personally assume the responsibility for supplying asocial individuals and criminals who serve only to die (todeswürdig) from concentration camps for these experiments.

Unfortunately, you had no time recently when Dr. Rascher wanted to report on the experiments at the Ministry for Aviation. I had put great hopes in that report, because I believed that in this way the difficulties, based mainly on religious objections, which oppose Dr. Rascher's experiments for which I assumed responsibility – could be eliminated.

The difficulties are still the same now as before. In these "Christian medical circles" the standpoint is being taken that it goes without saying that a young German aviator should be allowed to risk his life but that the life of a criminal – who is not drafted into military service – is too sacred for this purpose and one should not stain oneself with this guilt; at the same time it is interesting to note that creed is taken for the results of the experiments while excluding the scientist who performed them.

41 Office of U.S. Chief of Counsel, Translation of Document No-1617-PS, "Letter from Himmler to Milch", in RG-30.001M.

I personally have inspected the experiments, and have, I can say this without exaggeration, participated in every phase of this scientific work in a helpful and inspiring manner.

We too should not get angry about these difficulties. It will take at least another ten years until we can get such narrow-mindedness out of our people. But this should not affect the research work which is necessary for our young and splendid soldiers and aviators.

I ask you to release Dr. Rascher, Stabsarzt in reserve, from the Air Force and to transfer him to me to the Waffen SS. I would then resume the sole responsibility for having those experiments made, in this field, and would put the results, of which we in the SS need only a part for the frost injuries in the test, entirely at the disposal of the Air Force.

However, in this connection I suggest that with the liaison between you and Wolff, a "non-Christian" physician should be charged, who should be at the same time honorable as a scientist and not prone to intellectual theft and who could be informed of the results. This physician should also have good contacts with the administrative authorities, so that the results would really obtain a hearing.

I believe that this solution – to transfer Dr. Rascher to the SS, so that he could carry out the experiments under responsibility and under my orders – is the best way. The experiments should not be stopped; we owe that to our men. If Dr. Rascher remained with the Air Force, there would certainly be much annoyance; because then I would have to bring a series of unpleasant details to you, because of the arrogance and assumption which Professor Dr. Holzloehner has displayed in the post of Dachau – who is under my command – about me in utterances delivered to SS Colonel Sievers. In order to save both of us this trouble, I suggest again that Dr. Rascher should be transferred to the Waffen SS as quickly as possible.

I would be grateful to you if you would give the order to put the low pressure chamber at our disposal again, together with step-up pumps (Stufenaggregatpumpen), because the experiments should be extended to include even greater altitudes.

Cordial greetings and Heil Hitler!

Rascher wrote to Himmler's personal assistant, Rudolf Herman Brandt, requesting that the experiments be carried out at Dachau concentration camp, on the outskirts of Munich.

Translation of Document No-217[42]
Office of U.S. Chief of Counsel

My dear Doctor BRANDT,

...May I also ask that you grant soon the perhaps possible permission for carrying out the experiments (high altitude-pressure) (reported to Hauptsturmführer FAELSCHLIEN) within the camp of Dachau itself. I forgot to mention to Haupsturmführer FAELSCHLEIN, that a movable pressure chamber has been provided for this purpose out of the Research Fund of the RLM.

Heil Hitler!

Yours thankfully,
Devoted

Sig/S. RASCHER

By May 1942 Rascher was ready to provide his first report on the experiment to Himmler.

Translation of Document No-220a[43]
Office of U.S. Chief of Counsel

SIGMUND RASCHER, M.D.
München
Trägerstr 56
11 May 1942

Highly esteemed Reichsführer:

Enclosed I am forwarding a short summary on the principal experiments conducted up to date. A detailed report on the practical as well as the theoretical results will take some more time. I shall hurry.

Heil Hitler
Yours gratefully
/s/ S. Rascher

42 Document No-217, in RG-30.001M.
43 Document No-220a, in RG-30.001M.

Translation of Document No-220b[44]
Office of U.S. Chief of Counsel

München, 11 May 1942

Secret Report

Based on results of experiments which up to now various scientists had conducted on animals only, the experiments in Dachau were to prove whether these results would maintain their validity on human beings.

1. The first experiments were to show whether the human being can gradually adapt himself to higher altitudes. Some ten tests showed that a slower ascent without oxygen taking from six to eight hours keep the functions of the senses of the various VPs (Versuchspersonen – human experimental subjects) fully normal up to a height of 8,000 meters. Within 8 hours several VPs had reached a height of 9.5 kilometers without oxygen when bends (Hohenkrankheit) occurred suddenly (schlagartig).
2. Normally it is impossible to stay without oxygen at altitudes higher than six kilometers. Experiments showed however that after ascent to 8000 meters without oxygen, bends combined with unconsciousness lasted only about 25 minutes. After this period the VPs had mostly become accustomed to that altitude: Consciousness returned, they could make knee bends, showed a normal electrocardiograph and were able to work (60 to 70% of the cases examined).
3. Descending tests on parachutes (suspended) without oxygen.

These experiments proved that from 14 kilometers on down severest bends occurred which remained until the ground was reached. The detrimental effects caused by these experiments manifested themselves at the beginning as unconsciousness and subsequently as spastic and limb paralysis, catetomy, stereortypy, and as retrograde amnesia lasting several hours. About one hour after the end of the experiment the VPs for the most part were still disoriented as to time and locality. The blood picture often showed a shift to the left; albumen and red and white blood corpuscles were regularly found in the urine after the experiment; cylinders were sometimes found. After several hours or days the blood and urine returned to normal. The changes of the electrocardiograph were reversible.

44 Office of U.S. Chief of Counsel, Translation of Document No-220b, in RG-30.001M.

Contrary to descending tests on parachutes without oxygen, descending tests with oxygen were carried out from heights up to 18 kilometers. It was proven that on the average the VPs regained the normal function of their senses at 12 to 13 kilometers. No disturbances of general conditions occurred during any of these experiments. Brief unconsciousness at the beginning of the experiment caused no lasting disturbances. Urine and blood showed only a slight change.

4. As the long time of descent on parachutes, under actual conditions, would cause severe freezing even if no detrimental effects were caused by lack of oxygen, VPs were brought by sudden decreases in pressure (Druchsturz) with a cutting torch (Sauerstoffgeblase) from 8 to 20 kilometers, simulating the damage to the pressure machine of the high altitude airplane. After a waiting period of 10 seconds, corresponding to stepping out of the machine, the VPs were made to fall from this height with oxygen to a height where breathing is possible. The VPs awoke between 10 and 12 kilometers and at about 8 kilometers pulled the parachute lever.

5. In experiments of falling from the same height without oxygen the VP's regained normal function of their senses only between two and five kilometers.

6. Experiments testing the effect of Pervitin on the organism during parachute jumps, provide the severe after effects, as mentioned under No. 3, were considerably milder. The "Hohenfestigkeit" (ability to withstand the conditions at high altitudes) was only slightly improved, while the bends (Hohenkrankheit) since they were not noticed occurred suddenly (schlagartig) (restraint-loosening effects of Pervitin–Lemmungslosende Wirkung des Pervitin).

7. Dr. Kilches, Karls-University in Prague, reports in the publication of the Reich Research Council (Reichsforschungsrat): "By prolonged breathing of oxygen, human beings should theoretically be kept fully fit up to 13 kilometers. Practically the limit is around 11 kilometers."

Experiments which I carried out in this connection proved that with pure oxygen no lowering of the measurable raw energy (ergometer) was noticeable up to 13.3 kilometers. The VPs merely became unwilling since pains of the body cavities grew too severe, due to the lowering of pressure between body and thin air. When pure oxygen was inhaled bends occurred in all 25 cases only at heights above 14.2 kilometers.

As practical result of the more than 200 experiments conducted at Dachau the following can be assumed:

Flying in altitudes higher than 12 kilometers without pressure-cabin or pressure-suit is impossible even while breathing pure oxygen. If the airplane pressure machine is damaged at altitudes of 13 kilometers and higher the crew will not be able to bail out of the damaged plane themselves since at that height the bends appear rather suddenly (Schlagartig). It must be requested that the crew should be removed automatically from the plane, for instance, by catapulting the seats by means of compressed air. Descending with opened parachute without oxygen would cause severe injuries due to the lack of oxygen besides causing severe freezing; consciousness would not be regained until the ground was reached. Therefore the following need be requested: 1. A parachute with barometrically controlled opening. 2. A portable oxygen apparatus for the jump.

For the following experiments Jewish professional criminals who had committed "Rassenschande" (race pollution) were used: The question of the formation of embolism was investigated in 10 cases. Some of the VPs died during a continued high altitude experiment; for instance, after one-half hour at a height of 12 kilometers. After the skull had been opened under water an ample amount of air embolism was found in the brain vessels and, in part, free air in the brain ventricles.

To find out whether the severe psychological and physical effects, as mentioned under No. 3, are due to the formation of embolism, the following was done: After relative recuperation from such a parachute descending test had taken place, however before regaining of consciousness, some VPs were kept under water until they died. When the skull and the cavities of the chest and of the abdomen had been opened under water an enormous amount of air embolism was found in the vessels of the brain, the coronary vessels, and the vessels of the liver and the intestines.

That proves that air embolism, so far considered as absolutely fatal, is not fatal at all, but that it is reversible as shown by the return to normal conditions of all the other VPs.

It was also proved by experiments that air embolism occurs in practically all vessels even while pure oxygen is being inhaled. One VP was made to breathe pure oxygen for two and one-half hours before the experiment started. After six minute at a height of 20 kilometers he died and at dissection also showed ample air embolism as was the case in all other experiments.

At sudden decreases in pressure (Drucksturze) and subsequent immediate falls to heights where breathing is possible no deep reaching damages due to air embolism could be noted. The formation of air embolism always needs a certain amount of time.

(Signed) Dr. Rascher

In August 1942, Rascher sent Himmler his second progress report.[45]

[margin note
very interesting 8-4-42
Apparently by Himmler]

Sigmund Rascher, M.D.

Highly esteemed Reichsführer:
Enclosed is an interim report on the low pressure experiments so far conducted in the concentration camp of Dachau. May I ask you respectfully to treat the report as secret.

A few days ago Reich Physician SS (Reichsarzt SS) Professor Dr. Grawitz made a brief inspection of the experimentation plant. Since his time was very limited no experiment could be demonstrated to him. SS-Obersturmbannführer Sievers took a whole day off to watch some of the interesting standard experiments and may have given you a brief report. I believe highly esteemed Reichsführer, that you would be extraordinarily interested in those experiments. Is it not possible that on the occasion of a trip to Southern Germany you have some of the experiments demonstrated to you? If the results so obtained by the experiments are confirmed by further experimentation, entirely new data will be secured for science; simultaneously entirely new aspects will be opened to the Luftwaffe.

I hope that thanks to the intended efforts of SS Obersturmbannführer Sievers, the Luftwaffe will make no difficulties from now on. I am very much indebted to Obersturmbannführer Sievers as he has shown a very active interest in my work in every respect.

I thank you specifically highly esteemed Reichsführer for the generous realization of my proposition to conduct such experiments in the concentration camp.

With my best wishes for your personal well-being,

Gratefully yours,
(Signed) S. Rascher

45 Document No-1971-a-PS, RG-30.001M.

Translation of Document 1971-a-PS[46]
Office of U.S. Chief of Counsel

First Interim Report on the Low Pressure Chamber Experiments in the Concentration Camp of Dachau

1. The object is to solve the problem of whether the theoretically established norms pertaining to the length of life of human beings breathing air with only a small proportion of oxygen and subjected to low pressure correspond with the results obtained by practical experiments. It has been asserted that a parachutist, who jumps from a height of 12 km would suffer very severe injuries – probably even die – on account of the lack of oxygen. Practical experiments on this subject have always been discontinued after a maximum of 53 seconds, since very severe bends (Hohenkrankheit) occurred.

2. Experiments testing the length of life of a human being, above the normal breathing limits (4, 5, 6 km) have not been conducted at all, since it has been a foregone conclusion that the human experimental subject (Versuchsperson – VP) would suffer death.

The experiments conducted by myself and Dr. Romberg proved the following:

Experiments on parachute jumps proved that the lack of oxygen and the low atmospheric pressure at 12 or 13 km altitude did not cause death. Altogether 15 extreme experiments of this type were carried out in which none of the VP died. Very severe bends together with unconsciousness occurred, but completely normal functions of the senses returned when a height of 7 km was reached on descent. Electrocardiograms registering during the experiments did show certain irregularities, but by the time the experiments were over the curve had returned to normal and they did not indicate any abnormal changes during the following days. The extent to which deterioration of the organism may occur due to continuously repeated experiments can only be established at the end of the series of experiments. The extreme, fatal experiments will be carried out on especially selected VPs otherwise it would not be possible to exercise the rigid control so extraordinarily important for practical purposes.

The VPs were brought to a height of 8 km under oxygen and to make 5 knee bends with and without oxygen. After a certain lapse of time, moderate to severe bends occurred and the VPs became unconscious.

46 Ibid.

However, after a certain period of accustoming themselves to the height of 8 km, all the VPs recuperated and regained their consciousness and the normal functions of their senses.

Only continuous experiments at altitudes higher than 10.5 km resulted in death. These experiments showed that breathing stopped after about 30 minutes, while in 2 cases the electrocardiographically charted action of the heart continued for another 20 minutes.

The third experiment of this type took such an extraordinary course that I called an SS physician of the camp as witness, since I had worked on these experiments all by myself. It was a continuous experiment without oxygen at a height of 12 km conducted on a 37 year old Jew in good general condition. Breathing continued up to 30 minutes. After 4 minutes the VP began to perspire and wiggle his head, after 5 minutes cramps occurred, between 6 and 10 minutes breathing increased in speed and the VP became unconscious; from 11 to 30 minutes breathing slowed down to three breaths per minute, finally stopping altogether.

Severest cyanosis developed in between and foam appeared at the mouth.

At five minute intervals electrocardiograms from 3 leads were taken. After breathing had stopped EKG (electrocardiogram) was continuously taken until the action of the heart had come to a complete standstill. About 1/2 hour after the breathing had stopped, autopsy was started.

Autopsy Report

When the cavity of the chest was opened the pericardium was filled tightly (heart tamponade). Upon opening of the pericardium 80 ccm of clear yellowish liquid gushed forth. The moment the tamponade had stopped, the right auricle began to beat heavily, at first at the rate of 60 actions per minute, then progressively slower. 20 minutes after the pericardium had been opened, the right auricle was opened by puncturing it. For about 15 minutes a thin stream of blood spurted forth. Thereafter clogging of the puncture wound in the auricle by coagulation of the blood and renewed acceleration of the action of the right auricle occurred.

One hour after breathing had stopped, the spinal cord was completely severed and the brain removed. Thereupon the action of the auricle stopped for 40 seconds. It then renewed its action coming to a complete standstill 8 minutes later. A heavy subarchnoid edema was found in the brain. In the veins and arteries of the brain a considerable quantity of air was discovered. Furthermore, the blood vessels in the heart and liver were enormously obstructed by embolism.

The anatomical preparations will be preserved so I'll be able to evaluate them later.

The last mentioned case is to my knowledge the first one of this type observed on men. The above described heart actions will gain particular scientific interest since they were written down with EKG to the very end.

The experiments will be continued and extended. Another interim report will follow after new results have been obtained.

(Signed) Dr. Rascher

In view of this report, Himmler ordered the condemned prisoners who survived the experiments to have their sentences commuted to life imprisonment in a concentration camp. Rascher sought clarification of this directive. See below Rascher's letter and the most interesting answer.

Translation of Document 1971-d-PS[47]
Office of U.S. Chief of Counsel

Reich Main Security Office
Communication
20 October 1942, 5:25 PM

URGENT

Communication No. 1194
RFSS Munich–Teletype

To: SS Obersturmbannführer Dr. BRANDT
Field Command Post (Feldkommandostelle) Hegewald

Highly esteemed Obersturmbannführer

Will you please clarify the following case with the Reichsführer SS as soon as possible.

In communication RFSS of B-4-42 and r S3 it is ordered that if prisoners in Dachau condemned to death live through experiments which have endangered their lives, they should be pardoned. As up to now only Poles and Russians were available, some of who had been condemned to death, it is not quite clear to me yet as to whether the

47 Document 1971-d-PS, in RG-30.001M.

above mentioned paragraph also applies to them, and whether they may be pardoned to concentration camp for life after having lived through several very severe experiments.

Please answer to teletype via Adjutants Office RFSS Munich.

Obedient Greetings, Heil Hitler, yours,

(Signed) S. Rascher

Translation of Document No-1971-e-PS[48]
Office of U.S. Chief of Counsel

Teletype
To SS Obersturmführer SCHNITZLER
München

Please inform SS Untersturmführer Dr. Rascher with regard to his teletype inquiry that the instruction given some time ago by the Reichsführer SS concerning amnesty of test persons does not apply to Poles and Russians.

(Signed) Brandt
SS Obersturmbannführer

Dr. Hans Wolfgang Romberg and Dr. Siegfried Ruff, who also participated in the high altitude experiments in Dachau, sent separate reports to Himmler.

Partial Translation of Document No-402, Prosecution Exhibit 66[49]

Letter (29 September 1942) and Report (28 July 1942) from Romberg and Ruff to Himmler concerning Experiments on Rescue from High Altitudes

German Aviation Research Institute
Berlin-Adlershof, Rudower Ch. 16-23

(Stamp) Secret

48 Document 1971-e-PS, RG-30.001M.

49 Letter, 29 September 1942 and Report, 28 July 1942, from Romberg and Ruff to Himmler concerning "Experiments on Rescue from High Altitudes", Document No-402, Prosecution Exhibit 66, in *PTT.*

To the Reich Leader SS
Berlin SW 11
Prinz-Albrechtstr. 8
Your Ref.
Your communication of DVL-Ref. Day
R/Ru/Ko 2098/42, 22 September 1942
Military Secret

RE: Report "Experiments on Rescue from High Altitudes"

(handwritten) to files
B (initial)

Enclosed we submit copies Nos. 2, 3, and 4 of the report "Experiments on Rescue from High Altitudes" for your files.

German Aviation Research Institute
Per procura

(Signed) Dr. Romberg
L. Ruff

(handwritten)
Report 3–received 2 November
(Signed) Sievers, SS Oberführer

SUMMARY

Experiments were instituted upon the possibility of rescue from altitudes up to 21 km (68,900 ft).

Without parachute oxygen equipment, rescue in descending experiments is still possible from 13 km (42,700 ft), with equipment, from 18 km (59,100 ft). The danger arising from cold must be considered.

In falling experiments, rescue from 21 km (68,900 ft) altitude with and without oxygen was proved possible. Automatic parachute opening is necessary. Ebullition of the blood does not yet occur at 21 km (68,900 ft) altitude.

Oxygen must be breathed before explosive decompression. Abandonment must be by means of ejection seat. The dive to safe altitude offers good possibilities of rescue if abandonment of the plane isn't necessary after loss of the cabin pressure.

The following excerpt from the deposition of Rudolf Herman Brandt gives further evidence that the Dachau experiments were conducted with the full knowledge and approval of Himmler. It also discusses the commutation of death sentences for survivors of the experiments. Eventually, only one prisoner's sentence was commuted.

Translation of Document No-191 Office of Chief of Counsel for War Crimes[50]

Deposition of Rudolf Hermann Brandt

I, Rudolf Hermann Brandt, swear, depose and state

1. I was born on 2 June 1909 at Frankfurt, Germany and studied law at the universities of Berlin and Jena. In 1932 I became a member of the National Socialist German Labor Party. In October 1933, I became a member of the SS. In 1936 or 1937, I became personal consultant (Referent) to Heinrich HIMMLER, Reichsfuehrer of the SS. This position was of an administrative nature as a personal assistant to HIMMLER.

2. By reason of my above mentioned position and experiences, I also obtained insight in the medical experiments on human beings and I am in the position to give the following testimony on this subject.

In May 1941, I heard for the first time of the plan to conduct experiments on human beings. The idea came from Dr. Sigmund RASCHER, Stabsarzt of the Lufwaffe and later Hauptsturmfuehrer of the SS. At that time, RASCHER participated in a course of aviation medicine at the Luftgaukommando VII (Air Force District Command) in Munich. He wrote to HIMMLER and suggested that concentration camp inmates be placed at his disposal in order to establish the altitude reaction on the human body. Volunteers could not very well be expected since the experiments could be fatal. RASCHER further declared, that the Test Station for High Altitude Research of the Air Force... whose director was Dr. G. K. WELTZ, was ready to conduct such experiments.

HIMMLER had me answer this letter. RASCHER was informed in this answer that prisoners would be made available for the purpose of experiments. Later on, in July 1941, HIMMLER authorized Dr. WELTZ, Dr. RASCHER, and Dr. KOTTENHOFF to conduct the tests of low pressure experiments in the concentration camp Dachau.

50 Deposition of Rudolf Hermann Brandt, Office of U.S. Chief of Counsel, Translation of Document No-191, in RG-30.001M.

On 2 April 1942 RASCHER sent a report draft on the progress of the experiments to HIMMLER. This report stated, that the experiments were conducted with the aim to ascertain how long human beings could live if subjected to the variations occurring in high altitudes (lack of oxygen, low pressure). Many experiments ended with the death of the experimental subject. RASCHER declared in an accompanying letter that SIEVERS had been at some of the experiments.

After HIMMLER had read the report, he ordered RASCHER to continue the experiments on persons who were sentenced to death. If the experimental subjects survived the experiments their sentence should be commuted to life imprisonment. He also requested him to invite Dr. FAHNENKAMP to his experiments. In the meantime, SIEVERS had reported to HIMMLER on his visitation to Dachau and his knowledge of the participation in the low pressure experiments. For subjects who volunteered the prison sentences were to be reduced.

RASCHER inquired later on, whether Poles and Russians who survived the experiments were to have their death sentences commuted. I answered Obersturmführer SCHNITABER, by order of the Reichsführer SS that the death sentence of the Russians were not to be commuted.

There is no doubt that numerous mishaps occurred in the course of these experiments. I remember that Mrs. RASCHER wrote to me asking for permission to take color photos of newly disposed bodies; this permission was granted.

(Signature) R. BRANDT

Dr. Siegfried Ruff, who was Head of the Medical Department of the Aviation Research Institute (DVL), testified concerning the set-up of the experiments.

Translation of Document No-437[51]
Office of U.S. Chief of Counsel

Deposition of Siegfried Ruff

I, Siegfried Ruff, being duly sworn, depose and state: I studied medicine at Bonn and Berlin Universities and was a doctor in the University Hospital at Bonn until January 1932, when I joined the staff of the German Experimental Institute for Aviation (hereinafter called the DVL).

51 Deposition of Siegfried Ruff, Office of U.S. Chief of Counsel, Translation of Document No-437, in RG-30.001M.

Late in 1941, I believe December, Dr. G. W. Weltz of the Institute for Aviation Medicine at Munich told me that Dr. Sigmund Rascher was to make certain low-pressure experiments at the Dachau Concentration Camp.

Early in 1942, about January or February, a conference was held in Dachau in which Dr. Weltz, Dr. Rascher, Dr. Romberg, two officers who were apparently of the concentration camp staff, and I took part. We discussed the arrangements for conducting the experiments.

In due course, a movable low-pressure chamber was taken from the DVL in Berlin to Munich. It was taken to Munich instead of directly to Dachau so that the driver would not learn of its final destination.

The experiments were actually conducted in Dachau during the spring or summer of 1942. They lasted from 2 to 3 months.

Dr. Weltz was informed about these experiments as were a number of doctors in the medical service of the Luftwaffe. A motion picture of the experiments was shown in the Reich Ministry of Aviation (RMA). Dr. Weltz certainly never told me that he considered the experiments immoral or criminal or that his superiors thought so.

Dr. Romberg, another participant in the experiments, gave the following affidavit.

Translation of Document No-476[52]
Office of U.S. Chief of Counsel

Affidavit of Hans Wolfgang Romberg

I, Hans Wolfgang Romberg, being duly sworn, depose and state: On January 1, 1938 I became an associate scientist in the Department for Aviation Medicine at the German Experimental Institute for Aviation (Deutsche Versuchsanstalt für Luftfahrt, hereinafter called the DVL).

From about the first part of March 1942 to about the end of May 1942 experiments were conducted at the Dachau Concentration Camp to determine the effects of extreme high altitudes on the human body. These experiments were conducted for the benefit of the Luftwaffe.

A low pressure chamber was sent from the DVL in Berlin first to Weltz's Institute in Munich and from there to Dachau. This chamber could duplicate atmospheric conditions and pressures prevailing at high

52 Affidavit of Hans Wolfgang Romberg, Office of U.S. Chief of Counsel, Translation of Document No-476, in RG-30.001M

altitudes. It consisted of two parts, one of which was used for low ascensions and descensions and could accommodate as many as twelve people at a time, while the other was used for explosive decompression and could accommodate only one or two people. This low pressure chamber was set up in one of the blocks at the Concentration Camp. The experiments actually started around the first part of March and the initial experiments were conducted on twelve prisoners. When prisoners were requested, we asked that they be in a physical condition which compared with members of the Luftwaffe. The experimental subjects were tested in either the large or small part of the chamber, usually one at a time, and their reactions to high altitudes were checked with an electrocardiograph. Four series of experiments were conducted:

a) Slow descent without oxygen,
b) Slow descent with oxygen,
c) Falling without oxygen,
d) Falling with oxygen.

The latter two tests were designed to simulate a free fall from an airplane before the parachute opens. Several tests were from time to time conducted on the same experimental subject.

I witnessed the death of three of Dr. Rascher's human experimental subjects during the experiments. The first death occurred in the latter part of April. On this particular occasion I was studying the electrocardiograph of the human experimental subject then being tested. After the death of this human experimental subject I rushed to Rascher and also informed Ruff concerning the matter.

Thereafter two other deaths occurred on different days in May. I also reported these to Dr. Ruff. I know that other experimental subjects were killed while I was not present and I would estimate that they totaled between five and ten.

After a human experimental subject died as a result of the low pressure experiments, an autopsy was performed. The purpose of this was to determine the exact cause of death. Once, to my knowledge, the autopsy was performed under water in order to observe the air bubbles which might have formed in various parts of the human experimental subject's body.

No one in the Luftwaffe ever made any objection concerning these experiments.

I have read the foregoing deposition consisting of four pages, in the German language, and declare that it is the full truth to the best of my knowledge and belief. I have had the opportunity to make changes and corrections in the above statement. I made this declaration voluntarily without any promise of reward, and I was not subjected to an duress or threat whatsoever.

Nürnberg, 1 November 1946

(Signature) Dr. Romberg

The following excerpts about the altitude tests have been extracted from the *Report of the Atrocities Committed at the Dachau Concentration Camp*, and are part of the collection of the Yad Vashem Archives.[53]

Military Government Court, Dachau, Germany, 2 November 1946

Direct Examination of Franz Blaha
(Pathologist, Former Prisoner at Dachau)

Q. You mentioned, Doctor, that Doctor Rascher was in charge of the experiments for the Luftwaffe; what was the nature of these experiments?
A. There were two groups of experiments; one with air pressure, and one with cold water.

Q. Now, this first experiment, the air pressure experiment; how was that conducted?
A. A bell-like thing was brought in.

Q. How was that bell-like thing used?
A. Twenty or twenty-five prisoners were locked up in one of them, then by means of machines the air pressure was raised and lowered suddenly.

Q. And what was the effect on the persons in the chamber?
A. Many were dead, and some of them died shortly after that. Some of them had hemorrhages, or several other injuries, for instance, from the ear or from the nose.

Q. You saw they had hemorrhages from the ears and nose – is that right?
A. Yes.

Q. Did you ever perform the autopsies on any of the person[s] who died from these experiments?
A. All of these dead ones were autopsied.

Q. Will you state to the court the causes that produced those deaths?
A. Most of them died of brain hemorrhages or of embolism; of infarctions of the heart and lungs. This is due to the sudden difference of from high to low blood pressure. That's the sudden change in air pressure.

53 *Report of the Atrocities Committed at the Dachau Concentration Camp*, Vol. I., YVA, JM/1004,7, pp. 4–6.

> Q. Do you have any judgment as to the number of persons that died as a result of these experiments?
> A. I think above a hundred.

Dr. Blaha also testified at the Trial of the Major War Criminals by the International Military Tribunal.[54]

> BLAHA: Dr. Rascher made exclusively so-called Air Force experiments in the camp. According to scientific standards, insofar as I can judge, this was all to no purpose. Like all the other experiments, it was simply useless murder; and it is amazing that learned university professors and physicians, particularly, were capable of carrying out these experiments according to plan. These experiments were much worse than all the liquidations and executions, because all the victims of these experiments simply had their suffering prolonged, as various medicines such as vitamins, hormones, tonics, and injections, which were not available for the ordinary patients, were provided for these patients so that the experiments might last longer and give those people more time to observe their victims.

The following excerpt has been taken from the summary of the testimony given by Wolfram Sievers at his interrogation by the Office of the U.S. Chief Counsel for War Crimes.[55]

> RESTRICTED CLASSIFICATION
> Removed per
> Executive Order 10501

Evidence Division, Interrogation Branch
Interrogation Summary No-374
Office of the U.S. Chief Counsel for War Crimes APO 124 A

> Interrogation of: Wolfram SIEVERS
> Interrogated by: Capt. Koch, 28 October 1946, Nuremberg
> Section & Att'y: High Command – Mr. King and Mr. Hayman

54 Testimony of Dr. Franz Blaha before the International Military Tribunal, Nuremberg, 11 January 1946, in *Trial IMT,* vol. 5, p. 184. On the web, see the "Avalon Project at Yale Law School".

55 Office of the U.S. Chief Counsel for War Crimes, APO 124 A, Evidence Division, Interrogations Branch, Interrogation Summary No-374, YVA, JM/6027.

Excerpt From Summary

High Altitude tests were made in a mobile pressure chamber, which had been supplied by the Air Crops. RASCHER's final report went to the DVL, where it was published. Sources saw this report later in the Reich Research Council. The DVL also had the distribution list. The use of KZ inmates was made necessary, since experiments were at a stage where fatal results were to be expected. GRAWITZ personally witnessed high altitude experiments. HIMMLER was also repeatedly in Dachau. It is clear that RASCHER conducted experiments far beyond the bounds of his authority. Several deaths occurred during the high altitude experiments. Photographs of autopsies on fatal cases were made by the camp photographer. The film on Altitude tests was shown at he Air Ministry upon MILCH's invitation, however, MILCH was unable to attend at the last minute having to go to a meeting with GOERING.

Analysis of the Experiments at the Nuremberg Trial
(Excerpts)
by Expert Witness Ivy[56]

"I do not believe that it was necessary to do this experiment in order to determine the equipment to supply aviators who have to bail out of an airplane at high altitude."

Ivy maintained that the information obtained by these experiments on concentration camp inmates could have been gained from animal experiments, as indicated by the results of Lutz's and Wendt's animal work. The differences in the reactions of human subjects and animals, as reported by Lutz and Wendt, were not sufficient to warrant these hazardous experiments on human beings.

Former prisoner Pacholegg, a witness for the prosecution, gave the following, most dramatic description of the experiment.[57]

Testimony of Former Prisoner Pacholegg

I have personally seen, through the observation window of the chamber, when a prisoner inside would stand a vacuum until his lungs ruptured. Some experiments gave men such pressure in their heads that they

56 Expert Witness at the Nuremberg Trial.
57 Testimony of Former Prisoner Pacholegg, in *Trial IMT*, vol. 20, pp. 535–537.

> would go mad and pull out their hair in an effort to relieve the pressure. They would tear their heads and faces with their fingers and nails in an attempt to maim themselves in their madness. They would beat the walls with their hands and head and scream in an effort to relieve pressure on their eardrums. These cases of extremes of vacuums generally ended in the death of the subject. An extreme experiment was so certain to result in death that in many instances the chamber was used for routine execution purposes rather than as an experiment. I have known Rascher's experiments to subject a prisoner to vacuum conditions or extreme pressure conditions, or combinations of both, for as long as 30 minutes. The experiments were generally classified into two groups, one known as the living experiments, and the other simply as the "X" experiment, which was a way of saying execution experiment.

In *Doctors of Infamy: The Story of the Nazi Medical Crimes,* Alexander Mitscherlich and Fred Mielke note, "Insofar as the documentary evidence permits an opinion, the Dachau experiments suggested and conducted by Dr. Rascher, appear to be the earliest human experiments of a new category, with the 'terminal experiments...,' as Dr. Rascher put it – in other words, the death of the test person – part and parcel of the experimental plan."[58]

HYPOTHERMIA EXPERIMENTS

In their attempt to conceal the atrocities of the concentration camp experiments from the Allied forces, the Nazis destroyed most of the documentation of the procedures before the camps were liberated. Himmler's files, which contained secret reports and other records of the camp experiments, survived, however; they had been buried in a cave in Germany and were found after hostilities ended. The American military transferred these documents to the Nuremberg courts for use in the war crimes trials.

Immediately after the war, U.S. Army Medical Corps Major Leo Alexander reviewed the records of the Dachau hypothermia experiments and prepared a

58 Mitscherlich and Mielke, eds., *Doctors of Infamy,* which cites the translation of Document No-1602-PS, Prosecution Exhibit 44. Rascher's letter to Himmler (15 May 1941) is the first in which he indicates that the experiments may be fatal: "The experiments, in which the experimental subject may die, would take place with my collaboration."

228-page report, which is the principal primary source available to historians.[59] The Alexander report includes sixty-eight pages of personal commentary about the background and substance of the study and a reproduction of a fifty-six-page comprehensive report on the Dachau proceedings, dated 21 October 1942, signed by Drs. Ernst Holzlöhner, Sigmund Rascher and Erich Finke, and forwarded to Himmler.[60] A separate communication notes that the 1942 report, hereafter named the "Dachau Comprehensive Report", had been prepared by Rascher for presentation at a medical conference for military personnel on hypothermia.

Hypothermia was a threat faced by German soldiers in all branches of the military. Experiments with both guinea pigs and adult domestic pigs had shown that the effects of exposure to intense cold could be reversed by immersing the animals in warm (40 °C) water. It was assumed, however, that heat regulation mechanisms in guinea pigs differ from those in humans, so the value of the findings for human beings was questioned. Rascher therefore requested Himmler's permission to conduct experiments on humans. The Alexander report contains an interesting detail about a July 1942 meeting with Himmler during which Rascher first broached the subject of such experiments. With him was Dr. Hans Wolfgang Romberg of the Deutsche Versuchsanstalt für Luftfahrt (German Research Institute for Aviation, or DVL). Rascher and Romberg had just finished a series of experiments on the effects of high altitude and oxygen deprivation on human beings, and they were presenting their results:

> We had to report to the SS headquarters and here Rascher introduced me to Himmler. Himmler was very friendly to Rascher, who had given me instructions as to how to behave beforehand. When Rascher had delivered his report, Himmler told him to present himself to Goering and inform him of the results of the Dachau experiments.
>
> He also gave orders to effect preparations for cold experiments and talked about popular methods of warming up near-drowned and frozen people. In particular, the story of a fisherwoman who warmed her half-frozen husband up in bed seemed to please him. I entered into the conversation and said that it was not so much the method by which a person was warmed up as the speed in which this was done.

59 Major Leo Alexander, "The Treatment of Shock from Prolonged Exposure to Cold, Especially in Water", Combined Intelligence Objectives Subcommittee, Target No. 24, Report No. 250 (Washington, D.C.: Office of Publications Board, Dept of Commerce, 1946).

60 Robert L. Berger, "Nazi Science: The Dachau Hypothermia Experiments", *New England Journal of Medicine* 322: 20 (17 May 1990), pp. 1438–1439.

> A painful silence ensued and I realized that this was not the moment to speak to Himmler. Afterwards Rascher asked me whether I did not have a screw loose, talking like that to Himmler, his "Reichs-Heini!" Himmler also took this opportunity to explain that in an all-out war, concentration camp prisoners had to be used for medical experiments. He added that those who did not understand this failed to understand the whole war; for it meant life or death for Germany.[61]

Himmler readily consented to the hypothermia experiments and appointed Rascher the principal researcher for the experiments. Rascher, however, lacked the proper training for this work, and therefore the prominent scientists Holzlöhner and Finke were ordered to join him for the project.

This trio, along with assistants, conducted two sets of experiments, one in which they studied how humans react to being immersed into freezing water and the other in which they evaluated the human response to various rewarming methods. Later Rascher, working alone, carried out some "cold air" experiments. According to the Alexander report, 130 experiments were performed. Rascher's assistant, Walter Neff estimated that 300 inmates served as experimental subjects, of whom 80 to 90 died. The actual number of deaths will never be known for sure.

The details of Rascher's professional and personal life, which are summarized in an article by Robert L. Berger, also provide insight into the ethics and value of Nazi science.[62] Sigmund Rascher was born in 1909. He started his medical studies in 1930 and joined both the Nazi party and the Storm Troopers (the SA) three years later. After a volunteer internship, Rascher served for three years as an unpaid surgical assistant. He was barred temporarily from the University of Munich for suspected Communist sympathies. In 1939, the young doctor denounced his physician father, joined the SS, and was inducted into the Luftwaffe. A liaison with and eventual marriage to Nini Diehl, a widow fifteen years his senior who was a one-time cabaret singer but also the former secretary and possibly the mistress of the Reichsführer, gained for Rascher direct access to Himmler; a strange partnership evolved between the junior medical officer and one of the highest officials of the Third Reich. One week after his first meeting with Himmler, Rascher presented a "Report on the Development and Solution to Some of the Reichsführer's Assigned Tasks during a Discussion held on 24 April 1939". The title of this paper foretold the character of the relationship between the two men. Rascher's servile and ingratiating approach to

61 Cited in Hoedeman, *Hitler or Hippocrates.*
62 Berger, "Nazi Science".

Himmler brought the junior medical officer power much greater than his position would have warranted.

The frequent references to Rascher in top-level documents indicate that he did indeed attract extraordinary attention from Germany's highest officials. His work was reported even to Hitler, who was pleased with the accounts. Rascher was not well-regarded in professional circles, however, and his superiors repeatedly expressed reservations about his performance. In one encounter, Professor Karl Gebhardt, a general in the SS and Himmler's personal physician, told Rascher, in connection with his experiments on hypothermia through exposure to cold air, that "the report was unscientific; if a student of the second term dared submit a treatise of the kind he [Gebhardt] would throw him out".[63] Despite Himmler's strong support, Rascher was rejected for faculty positions at several universities and his name and results are ignored in the standard scientific work on the wartime accomplishments of German aviation medicine.

Although Rascher's private ventures rivaled his scientific exploits in grotesqueness, the story that emerges as the most fateful deception of his life involves his claim to have had three children; they were in fact not his own. In an attempt to please Himmler by proving that the growth of the Aryan population could be accelerated by extending a woman's childbearing years, Rascher made it known that his wife had given birth to three children in quick succession after turning forty-eight. During her fourth "pregnancy", Mrs. Rascher was, it seems, arrested for attempting to kidnap an infant. The ensuing investigation disclosed that the other three Rascher children were not hers but had been bought or abducted. Himmler felt betrayed, and in April 1944 had his protégé arrested. Besides complicity in the kidnapping, Dr. Rascher was accused of financial irregularities, the murder of a German assistant, and scientific fraud. Dr. and Mrs. Rascher were subsequently executed, presumably on Himmler's orders.

■

Himmler requested regular reports on the progress of the hypothermia experiments. One of these "intermediate" reports follows, along with Himmler's reply.

63 Ibid.

Translation of Document No-1618-PS Prosecution Exhibit 84[64]

Intermediate Report, 10 September 1942, on Intense Chilling Experiments in Dachau Concentration Camp
S. Rascher
Intermediate report on intense chilling experiments in the Dachau Camp, started on 15 August 1942

Experimental procedure

The experimental subjects (VP) were placed in the water, dressed in complete flying uniform, winter or summer combination, and with an aviator's helmet. A life jacket made of rubber or kapok was to prevent submerging. The experiments were carried out at water temperatures varying from 2.5° to 12°. In one experimental series, the occiput (brain stem) protruded above the water, while in another series of experiments the occiput (brain stem) and back of the head were submerged in water.

Electrical measurements gave low temperature readings of 26.4° in the stomach and 26.5° in the rectum. Fatalities occurred only when the brain stem and the back of the head were also chilled. Autopsies of such fatal cases always revealed large amounts of free blood, up to one-half liter, in the cranial cavity. The heart invariably showed extreme dilation of the right chamber. As soon as the temperature in these experiments reached 28°, the experimental subjects died invariably, despite all attempts at resuscitation. The above discussed autopsy finding conclusively proved the importance of a warming protective device for head and occiput when designing the planned protective clothing of the foam type.

Other important findings, common in all experiments, should be mentioned, marked increase of the viscosity of the blood, marked increase of hemoglobin, an approximate five-fold increase of the leukocytes, invariable rise of blood sugar to twice its normal value. Auricular fibrillation made its appearance regularly at 30°.

During attempts to save severely chilled persons [Unterkuehlte], it was shown that rapid rewarming was in all cases preferable to slow rewarming, because after removal from the cold water, the body temperature continued to sink rapidly. I think that for this reason we can dispense with the attempt to save intensely chilled subjects by means of animal heat.

Rewarming by animal warmth – animal bodies or women's bodies – would be too slow. As auxiliary measures for the prevention of intense

64 Translation of Document No-1618-PS, Prosecution Exhibit 84, in RG-30.001M. Temperatures are centigrade, unless specifically indicated.

chilling, improvements in the clothing of aviators come alone into consideration. The foam suit with suitable neck protector which is being prepared by the German Institute for Textile Research, Munich-Gladbach, deserves first priority in this connection. The experiments have shown that pharmaceutical measures are probably unnecessary if the flier is still alive at the time of rescue.

(Signed) Dr. S. RASCHER
Munich–Dachau, 10 September 1942

Translation of Document No-1611-PS, Prosecution Exhibit 85[65]

SECRET

Reich Leader SS
Rf/Dr. AR/19/30/42
Personal Headquarters
Reich Leader SS
22 September 1942

1. Dr. Rascher
Munich–Dachau

I have received the intermediate report on the chilling experiments in Camp Dachau.

Despite everything, I would so arrange the experiments that all possibilities, prompt warming, medicine, body warming, will be executed in positive experiment orders.

(Signed) H. Himmler

2. SS–Lt. Col. Sievers
Berlin
A carbon copy with the request for acknowledgement.

SS Lt. Col.
25 Sep 42

65 Letter from Himmler to Rascher and Sievers, 22 September 1942, Translation of Document No-1611-PS, Prosecution Exhibit 85, in Ibid.

Of course, Rascher eagerly followed through on any request that Himmler made.

Partial Translation of Document No-285
Prosecution Exhibit 86[66]

Letter from Rascher to Rudolf Brandt, 3 October 1942

Dr med. Sigmund Rascher
Munich
Trägerstr. 56
3 October 42

Most honored Obersturmbannführer!

...Today I received your letter of 22 September 1942 in which the Reich Leader orders that the experiments on warming through body heat must absolutely be conducted. Because of incomplete address it was delayed. Today I asked Obersturmbannführer Sievers to send a telegram to the camp commander immediately to the effect that four gypsy women be procured at once from another camp.

With best wishes,

Heil Hitler!
Yours most sincerely,
(Signed) S. Rascher

Rascher sent the following memorandum to his immediate superior, in order to provide further evidence of his devotion to the ideology of "racial purity".[67]

Sigmund Rascher, M.D.
Munich, Trägerstr. 56
5 November 1942

Subject: Requested report about concentration camp prostitutes

From the Women's Concentration Camp Ravensbrück, 4 women were assigned to me for the prescribed re-warming experiments with animal heat after a sub-normal cooling had taken place.

66 Letter from Sigmund Rascher to Rudolf Brandt, 3 October 1942, Partial Translation of Document No-285, Prosecution Exhibit 86, in RG-30.001M, p. 257

67 Memo from Rascher, "Requested Report on Concentration Camp Prostitutes", Document No-323, in RG-30.001M.

One of the women assigned to me shows indisputably Nordic racial characteristics: blond hair, blue eyes, corresponding shape of the head and frame of the body, 21-3/4 years old. I asked this girl the question why she had volunteered for the brothel. I received the answer: "To get out of the concentration camp because it was promised that all those who signed up for half a year in the brothel would in exchange for this be released from the concentration camp." Upon my remark that it was a terrific shame to volunteer as a brothel-girl, I was informed, "Rather half a year of brothel than 6 months of concentration camp." Then followed an account of a series of strange conditions from the Camp R. The described conditions were for the major part confirmed by the 3 other brothel-girls and by the female supervisor, who had come along from Ravensbrück. It offends my racial feelings to deliver this girl, who, as to her looks, is pure Nordic and could perhaps be led on the right way through a corresponding labor assignment, as a prostitute to racially inferior concentration camp elements.

For this reason I reject the utilization of this girl for my experiments and make a corresponding report to the camp commander and the adjutant to the Reichsführer SS.

(S) Dr. S. RASCHER

Rascher did not hesitate to denounce his colleagues, thus endangering their careers. In the following letter, Holzloehner is singled out for criticism. Rascher's servility is evident in this denunciation as it also is in his apologetic excuses for delays in the re-warming-by-body-heat experiments.

Partial Translation of Document No-1610-PS[68]

Dr. med. Sigmund Rascher
Munich, Trägerstr. 46
9 October 1942

Most honorable Reichsführer,

As in the interest of his scientific renown, Prof. HOLZLOEHNER declined to carry out the scientific utilization of the experiments (experiments made on human beings): for shame. I shall take over the

68 Letter from Rascher to Himmler, 9 October 1942, Office of the U.S. Chief Counsel, Partial Translation of Document No-1610-PS, in RG-30.001M.

exploitation of them through the University Institute of SS Obersturmführer Prof. Dr. Pfannenstiel, Hamburg.

...The final report concerning the freezing experiments with all the charts will be ready in about 6 days and will be sent at once to Berlin.

The experiments of rewarming by body heat, which were ordered, will be carried out as soon as the women necessary for this experiment arrive, in about 2 days. I shall report the results of this experiment separately.

With best wishes,
Heil Hitler!

(Handwritten) I remain your most obedient
(Signature) S. RASCHER

Rascher did not have to wait long for a predictable response from Himmler.

Translation of Document No-1609-PS[69]
Office of U.S. Chief of Counsel

Reichsführer-SS
Field Command Post
NR 1397/42
24 Oct 1942

Dr. SIGMUND RASCHER
Munich
Träger St. 56

TOP SECRET
3 copies
2nd copy

Dear Rascher!

I... regard those people as high and national traitors who, still today, reject these experiments on humans and would instead let sturdy German soldiers die as a result of these cooling methods. I shall not hesitate to report these men to the Offices concerned. I empower you to make my opinion on this known to the concerned offices.

69 Office of U.S. Chief of Counsel, Translation of Document No-1609-PS, in RG-30.001M.

...I am very curious as to the experiments with body warmth. I personally take it that these experiments will probably bring the best and lasting results. Naturally, I could be mistaken.

Keep me informed on the findings. Of course we will see each other in November.

Heil Hitler!
Your
(Signed) H. Himmler

The following is the description of the practical details of the experiments, followed by the summary of the findings and conclusions.

Partial Translation of Document No-428[70]
Prosecution Exhibit 91

Report of 10 October 1942, on Cooling Experiments on Human Beings

Stabsarzt [Captain in the Medical Corps] Prof. Dr. E. Holzloehner
Stabsarzt Dr. S. Rascher
Stabsarzt Dr. E. Finke

The effect of water temperatures of 2°, 3°, to 12° C [34°, 37°, to 54° F] were investigated. A tank 2 × 2 × 2 m [6-2/3 × 6-2/3 × 6-2/3 ft.] served as an experimental basin. The water temperature was attained by addition of ice, and remained constant during the experiment. The experimental subjects were generally dressed in equipment such as the flier wears, consisting of underclothing, uniform, a one-piece summer or winter protective suit, helmet, and aviators fur-lined boots. In addition they wore a life preserver of rubber or kapok. The effect of additional protective clothing against water-cold was tested in a special series of experiments, and in another series the cooling of the unclothed person was studied.

The bodily warmth was measured thermoelectrically. Following preliminary experiments in which gastric temperatures were measured by a thermic sound, we adopted the procedure of continuously registering

70 Partial Translation of Document No-428, Prosecution Exhibit 91, *The Trial of Major German War Criminals: Proceedings of the International Military Tribunal Sitting at Nuremberg, Germany,* Part 8, 27 February 1946–11 March 1946, Official Transcription (London: His Majesty's Stationery Officer, 1947), p. 7.

rectally the body temperature [Kerntemperatur]. Parallel with this, the recording of the skin temperature was undertaken. The point of measurement was the skin of the back at the level of the fifth thoracic vertebral process. The thermoelectrical measurements were controlled before, during, and after the experiments by thermometric tests of the cheek and rectal temperature.

In severe cooling, checking of the pulse is difficult. The pulse becomes weaker, the musculature become stiff, and shivering sets in. Auscultation during the experiment by means of a tube stethoscope fastened over the tip of the heart proved effective. The tubes were led out of the uniform and made possible the continuous listening to the heart during the stay in the water.

Electrocardiographic controls were not possible in the water. After removal from the water they were possible only in those cases in which a too severe muscle shivering did not disturb the electrocardiograph records.

The following chemical studies were carried out: following up of the blood sugar picture (continuous); the sodium, chloride picture in the serum; the nonprotein nitrogen (Rest-N) the alkali reserve; the alkali reserve of the venous and arterial blood and sedimentation rate (before and after the experiment). Besides this the general blood condition and viscosity were followed during the experiment, and before and after the experiment the resistance of the red blood cells and the protein content of the blood plasma (this refractometrically) were measured.

The following urinalyses were made regularly: sediment, albumen, sugar, sodium chloride, acetone, acetic acid, as well as a qualitative albumen determination.

In part of the experiment lumbar and suboccipital punctures were made as well as corresponding spinal fluid studies.

Among physical and therapeutic measures the following were tested:

a) Rapid warming by means of a hot bath.
b) Warming by means of a light cradle.
c) Warming in a heated sleeping bag.
d) Vigorous massage of the whole body.
e) Wrapping in covers.
f) Diathermy of the heart.

In addition the following drugs were given: Strophanthin i.v. Cardiaz 1 i.v. and i.c.; Lobelin and Coramin i.v. and i.c. In other experiments alcohol or grape sugar was given.

A part of the experiment was begun under narcosis (8 cc Evipan i.v.).

X Summary

1. The curve of rectal temperature of human beings chilled in water of 2 °C [35.6 °F] to 12 °C [53.6 °] shows a gradual drop to about 35 °C [95 °F], after which the drop becomes rapid. Death may occur at rectal temperatures below 30 °C [86 °F].

2. Death results from heart failure. The direct damage to the heart becomes evident from the total irregularity observed in all cases, setting in at approximately 30 °C [86 °F]. This cardiac damage is due to overloading of the heart, caused by the marked and regular increase in the viscosity of the blood, as well as by the marked throttling of large peripheral vascular areas; besides, a direct injury to the heart by the cold is also probable.

3. If the neck is also chilled, the lowering of the temperature is more rapid. This is due to interference with the temperature-regulating and vascular centers; cerebral oedema also makes its appearance.

4. The blood sugar rises as the temperature falls, and the blood sugar does not drop again as long as the body temperature continues to fall. This fact suggests an intermediary disturbance of metabolism.

5. Respiration of the chilled subject is rendered difficult due to the rigor of the respiratory musculature.

6. After removal from the cold water, the body temperature may continue to fall for 15 minutes or longer. This may be an explanation of deaths which occur after successful rescue from the sea.

7. Intensive rewarming never injures the severely chilled person.

8. Strophanthin treatment was not observed to have been successful. The question of the use of strophanthin remains open, however. Remedies which influence the peripheral circulation are definitely not advisable.

9. The most effective therapeutic measure is rapid and intensive heat treatment, best applied by immersion in a hot bath.

10. By means of special protective clothing, the survival time after immersion in tepid water could be extended to double-the survival time of subjects who were immersed without protective clothing.

11. Certain proposals for improvement of life jackets are being made.

Concluded on 10 October 1942.

(Signed) Prof. Dr. Holzlöhner
Dr. Rascher
Dr. Finke

Prof. Holzlöhner presented the final report on the freezing experiment at a conference in Nuremberg, 26–27 October 1942. Ninety-five prominent physicians participated in the meeting. None objected or made any critical remarks or raised any questions about the ethics of the presented experiments.

Translation of Document No-401[71]
Office of Chief of Counsel for War Crimes

(Luftwaffen Eagle)

RESTRICTED

Report from the Field of Aviation Medicine
Published by the Inspector of Medical Service of the Luftwaffe

---

Minutes of Meeting 7/43
REPORT
on a scientific conference
on 26 and 27 October 1942 in Nuremberg
on
Medical Problems Arising from Distress at Sea
And Winter Hardships
Sponsored by the Inspector of Medical Service of the Luftwaffe
Chairman of the Conference: Stabsarzt Professor Dr. A. J. Anthony

In January 1943, Rascher, working alone, began the last phase of the freezing experiments, the so-called "dry freezing" experiment: naked inmates bound to a stretcher and left outside in the cold throughout the night.

Rascher suggested two modifications to Himmler: to move this experiment to a new locale, Auschwitz, where the nights were colder than in southern Germany; and to relocate them to an area far from other settlements, so that the screams of the subjects would not be heard. For some unknown reason, these recommendations were never implemented.

■

71 Translation of Document No-401, Office of Chief of Counsel for War Crimes, in RG-30.001M.

Walter Neff, Rascher's aide, provided a description of the "experimental" procedures:[72]

> A prisoner was placed naked on a stretcher outside the barracks. This was in the evening. He was covered with a sheet, and every hour a bucket of cold water was poured over him. The test subject lay out in the open like this until the morning. The temperature of these test subjects was taken with a thermometer. Later, Dr Rascher said it was a mistake to cover the subject with a sheet and to drench him with water. This caused the wrong effect since the air could not reach the test subject.

Rascher's letter to Himmler, requesting the move to Auschwitz, was quoted by the Russian prosecutor, Colonel Smirnov, at Nuremberg.[73]

> If it is agreeable to you, Reichsfurhrer [sic], to have these experiments so important for our land forces, quickly carried out at Auschwitz (in Lublin or any other Eastern camp), I would respectfully beg you to give the necessary orders for my transfer in the near future, so that we could still profit by the cold winter weather.
>
> With most respectful greeting, I am, in sincere gratitude, with Heil Hitler, your always devoted ever-obedient servant, S. Rascher

Here is Himmler's response to the proposal to move the "dry-cold" experiments to Auschwitz. As mentioned before the move never took place.

Translation of Document No-1580-PS Prosecution Exhibit 107[74]

> *Letter from Himmler to Rascher, 26 February 1943, on Freezing Experiments in the Concentration Camps Auschwitz and Lublin*
>
> The Reich Leader SS
> 1516/43
> 26 February 1943
> *Secret*

72 *The Trial of Major German War Criminals: Proceedings of the International Military Tribunal Sitting at Nuremberg Germany,* Part 8, 27 February 1946–11 March 1946, Official Transcription (London: His Majesty's Stationery Officer, 1947), p. 7.

73 Ibid.

74 Letter from Himmler to Rascher, 26 February 1943, on "Freezing Experiments in the Concentration Camps Auschwitz and Lublin", Office of the Chief of Counsel for War Crimes, Document No-1580-PS, Prosecution Exhibit 107, in *Trials NMT,* vol. 1.

Dear Rascher:

Best thanks for your letter of 17 February with report on warming-up experiments. I agree to experiments being made at Auschwitz or Lublin, although I believe that the time for the cooling-off and warming-up tests under natural conditions of cold weather has nearly passed for this winter.

I am sending this letter at the same time to SS Obergruppenführer Pohl, whom I request to order the execution of your experiments at Lublin or Auschwitz.

Kind greetings and

Heil Hitler!
Yours
(Signed) H. Himmler

2. SS Obergruppenführer Pohl
Transmitted with request to take note and to take the necessary steps.
By order,

(Signature illegible)
SS Obersturmbannführer

The following is the last available report on experiments that Rascher sent to Himmler. It discusses the rewarming of hypothermic subjects by body heat, one of Himmler's favorite ideas.

Translation of Document No-1616-PS Prosecution Exhibit 105[75]

Dr. S. Rascher
SS Hauptsturmführer
Munich
17 February 1943

To the Reich Leader SS and Chief of the German Police Heinrich Himmler
Berlin SW 11, Prinz-Albrechtst. 8

75 Letter from Rascher to Himmler, 17 February 1943, Translation of Document 1616-PS, Prosecution Exhibit 105, in RG-30.001M.

Dear Reich Leader,

Enclosed I present to you in condensed form a summary of the results of the experiments made in warming up people who have been cooled off by using animal heat.

Right now I am attempting to prove through experiments on human beings that it is possible to warm up people cooled off by dry cold just as fast as people who were cooled off by remaining in cold water. The Reich Physician SS, SS Gruppenführer Dr. Grawitz, doubted very much that that would be possible, and said that I would have to prove it first by 100 experiments. Up to now I have cooled off about 30 people stripped in the open air during 9–14 hours at 27°–29°...

With most obedient greetings and sincere gratitude and

Heil Hitler!
Yours very devotedly
RASCHER

The above letter contained an enclosure to Himmler, marked "SECRET". This enclosure describes the experiments on rewarming intensely chilled human beings by animal warmth.

Summary of Experiments for Rewarming of Chilled Human Beings by Animal Warmth, 12 February 1943[76]

A) Purpose of the Experiments

To ascertain whether the rewarming of intensely chilled human beings by animal warmth, i.e., the warmth of animals or human beings, is as good or better than rewarming by physical or medical means.

B) Method of the Experiments

The experimental subjects were cooled in the usual way – clad or unclad – in cold water of temperatures varying between 4 °C and 9 °C. The rectal temperature of every experimental subject was recorded thermoelectrically. The reduction of temperature occurred within the usual span of time varying in accordance with the general condition of the body of the experimental subject and the temperature of the water. The experimental subjects were removed from the water when their rectal

76 "Summary of Experiments for Rewarming of Chilled Human Beings by Animal Warmth", 12 February 1943, in RG-30.001M.

temperature reached 30 °C. At this time the experimental subjects had all lost consciousness. In eight cases the experimental subjects were then placed between two naked women in a spacious bed. The women were supposed to nestle as closely as possible to the chilled person. Then all three persons were covered with blankets. A speeding up of rewarming by light cradles or by medicines was not attempted.

C) Results

1. When the temperature of the experimental subjects was recorded, it was striking that an after-drop of temperature up to 3 °C occurred, which is greater after-drop than seen with any other method of rewarming. It was observed, however that consciousness returned at an earlier point, that is, that is, at a lower body methods of rewarming. Once the subjects regained consciousness, they did not lose it again, but very quickly snuggled up to the naked female bodies. The rise of body temperature then occurred at about the same speed as had been rewarmed by packing in blankets. Exceptions were four experimental subjects who, at body temperatures between 30 °C and 32 °C, performed the act of sexual intercourse. In these experimental subjects the temperature rose very rapidly after sexual intercourse, which could be compared with the speedy rise in temperature in a hot bath.

2. Another set of experiments concerns the rewarming of intensely chilled persons by one woman. In all these cases, rewarming was significantly quicker than could be accomplished by two women. The cause of this seems to me that in warming by one woman only, personal inhibitions are removed, and the woman nestles up to the chilled individual much more intimately. Also in these cases, the return of complete consciousness was strikingly rapid. Only one experimental subject did not return to consciousness and the warming effect was only slight. This person died with symptoms suggesting cerebral hemorrhage, as was confirmed by subsequent autopsy.

D) Summary

Rewarming experiments of intensely chilled experimental subjects demonstrated that rewarming with animal warmth was very slow. Only such experimental subjects whose physical condition permitted sexual intercourse rewarmed themselves remarkably quickly and showed an equally striking rapid return to complete physical well-being. Since excessively long exposure of the body to low temperatures implies danger of internal damage, that method must be chosen for rewarming which guarantees the quickest relief from dangerously low temperatures. This method, according to our experiences, is a massive and rapid supply of warmth by means of a hot bath.

Rewarming of intensely chilled human beings by human or animal warmth can therefore be recommended only in such cases in which other possibilities for rewarming are not available, or in the cases of specially tender individuals who possibly may not be able to stand a massive and rapid supply of warmth. As for example, I am thinking of intensely chilled small children, who are best rewarmed by the body of their mothers, with the aid of hot water bottles.

Dachau, 12 February 1943.

(Signature) Dr. S. RASCHER
SS Hauptsturmführer

Rascher also proposed trying different diets on hypothermic subjects to determine which diets optimize survival chances. It is not known for sure whether the following study was ever conducted.

Translation of Document No-1579-PS[77]
Office of U.S. Chief of Counsel

Dr. med. Sigmund Rascher

Personal Staff
Reichsführer SS
Document Administration
Secret

MEMORANDUM

Subject: Joint research work of Dr. Rascher and Medical Research Station for Mountain Medical Troops.

Oberstabsarzt Dr. Craemer asked whether there were a possibility of collaborating with me.

The most urgent problem to be solved is the adaptability of the troops to winter cold and the diet best suited for it. Since the solution of this problem is also of great importance to the SS troops, I have reached the following conclusions after careful consideration:

Since there are concentration camp inmates in the region of the SS mountain house near Bayrischzell, it should be possible to carry out the adaptability tests in that region, which can be isolated to a certain degree.

77 Memo from Rascher, 6 November 1942, Office of U.S. Chief of Counsel, Translation of Document No-1579-PS, in RG-30.001M.

The most realistic adaptation would have to be carried out in igloos in ordinary troop clothing.

To be tried are: a) diet rich in fat,
b) vitamin-rich, meatless diet,
c) meat-fat diet of the inhabitants of the Arctic regions.

After the adaptability tests it would be important to investigate whether injuries to the extremities due to freezing have a better prognosis in persons accustomed to cold than in persons unaccustomed to cold.

The reason for this idea of adaptability are: 1. that by tests in Dachau I could prove that individuals accustomed to cold live from 3–4 times longer under the same conditions of intense cooling as persons unaccustomed to cold; 2. that in the central sector (abschnitt Mitte), mountain troops who have been, from the beginning, fighting at –40 °C in ordinary clothing without suffering from frost injuries, whereas as many as 50% of the unhabituated reserve troops drawn from Western France succumbed to the cold while on their way to the front.

The proposals for carrying out the above-mentioned series of tests seem therefore justified.

I request that this matter be looked into and that I receive proper instructions.

Munich, 6 November 1942

(Signature) Dr. Rascher

Walter Neff worked with Rascher on all his experiments and testified at the Nuremberg Trial about his experiences.

Extracts from the Testimony of Tribunal Witness Walter Neff[78]

Examination by Prosecution

Mr. McHaney (Q): When did the freezing experiments start?
Neff (A): The first freezing experiments started during August or at the end of July. They were conducted by Prof. Holzloehner, Dr. Finke and Dr. Rascher. The freezing experiments can be divided into two separate classes, the Holzloehner-Finke series, which were later dropped, and a series where Dr. Rascher conducted these experiments himself.

78 Testimony of Tribunal Witness Walter Neff, Mimeographed Trancript, 17–18 December 1946, in *Trials NMT*, vol. 1, pp. 595–695.

Q. All right. Suppose you describe the experimental basin.
A. The experimental basin was built of wood. It was 2 meters long and 2 meters high. It was raised about 50 centimeters above the floor and it was in Block No. 5. In the experimental chamber and basin there were many lighting instruments and other apparatus which were used in order to carry out measurements.

Q. Now, you have stated that you can divide the freezing experiment into two groups, one where Holzloehner and Finke were working with Rascher and then the period after Holzloehner and Finke had left.
A. Yes.

Q. Now, will you tell the Tribunal approximately how many persons were used over the whole period? That is, including both groups that you have mentioned?
A. Two hundred and eighty to three hundred experimental subjects were used for these freezing experiments. There were really 360 to 400 experiments that were conducted, since many experimental subjects were used for more than one such experiment – sometimes even for three.

Q. Now, out of the total of 280 or 300 prisoners used, approximately how many died?
A. Approximately 80 to 90 subjects died as a result of these freezing experiments.

Q. Now, how many experimental subjects do you remember that they used in the Holzloehner-Finke-Rascher experiments?
A. During that period of time approximately 50 to 60 subjects were used for experimental purposes.

Q. Did any of these experimental subjects die?
A. Yes. During that period of time there were about 15, maybe even 18 cases of death.

Q. When was that experimental series concluded?
A. It was concluded in the month of October. I think it was at the end of October. At that time Holzloehner and Finke discontinued these experiments, giving the reason that they had accomplished their purpose and that it was useless to carry out further experiments of that kind.

Q. And then Rascher continued experiments on his own?
A. Yes. Rascher conducted these experiments saying that he had to build a scientific basis for them and he prepared a lecture for Marburg University on the subject.

Q. How long did Rascher continue to experiment with freezing by cold water?
A. Until May 1943.

Q. Suppose you describe to the Tribunal exactly how these freezing experiments were carried out.
A. The basins were filled with water and ice was added until the water measured 3° and the experimental subjects were either dressed in a flying suit or were placed in the ice water naked. During the period where Holzloehner and Finke were active, most experiments were conducted under narcotics, because they maintained that you could not find the exact condition of the blood, and that you would exclude the will power of the experimental subject if he was under an anaesthetic. [NOTE: When Rascher worked alone, no anesthetic was given.] Now, whenever the experimental subjects were conscious, it took some time until so-called freezing narcosis set in. The temperature was measured rectally and through the stomach through the Galvanometer apparatus. The lowering of the temperature to 3° was terrible for the experimental subject. At 32° the experimental subjects lost consciousness. These persons were frozen down to 25° body temperature and now in order to enable you to understand the problem, I should like to tell you something about the Holzloehner and Finke period. During the period when Holzloehner and Finke were active, no experimental subject was actually killed in the water. Deaths occurred all the more readily because during revival the temperature dropped even further and so heart failure resulted. This was also caused by wrongly applied therapy.

Q. Witness, how long did it normally take to kill a person in these freezing experiments?
A. The length of the experiment varied, according to the individual case. Whether the subject was clothed or unclothed also made a difference. If he was slight in build and if in addition to that he was naked, death often occurred after only 80 minutes. There were a number of cases where the experimental subject lived up to 3 hours, and remained in the water until finally death occurred.

Q. Will you describe to the Tribunal the method used for rewarming the victims of the freezing experiments?
A. During the period where Rascher, Holzloehner and Finke were there, rewarming was in the beginning carried out by massage and partly by means of injection of drugs affecting the heart, and also by means of rewarming by electrical heaters and sometimes by means of a warm bath. At the end of the Holzloehner period, the hot water rewarming method was introduced, and that was carried out until the end of the rewarming experiments with the exception of a few special experiments with animal

heat. About 10 women from the concentration camp at Ravensbrueck were ordered to report to Dachau to supply the heat and were forced to press themselves against the body of the frozen person in order to rewarm him in that manner. These are the methods which were employed to rewarm the frozen body.

A survivor of the freezing experiments, Leo Miechalowski, a Roman Catholic priest, gave the following testimony.

Translation of Document No-2428-PS[79]
Office of U.S. Chief of Counsel

Mr. Leo Mi[e]chalowski appeared before the Investigator-Examiner and testified as follows:

Q. Your name is Leo Mi[e]chalowski?
A. Yes.

Q. You are a Roman Catholic Priest?
A. Yes.

Q. Father were you subjected to an experiment while you were held as a prisoner at Dachau?
A. Yes. To several.

Q. What were they?
A. At first malaria and then the water bath experiment.

Q. Do you mean the freezing water experiment?
A. Yes.

Q. When were you were subject to the freezing water experiment?
A. On October 7, 1942, in the afternoon.

Q. Can you briefly describe the freezing water experiment?
A. I was taken to room No. 4 on Block 5 where there was a basin about 2 meters by 2 meters in dimension. I was undressed and two medical apparatuses were tied to my body. The wires were introduced into my rectum and affixed to my body with scotch tape. I was then dressed in a flyer's uniform, flyer's boots, and a safety life-saving belt. I was then dropped in the water in which ice blocks were floating. I was conscious for one hour

79 Testimony of Leo Mi[e]chalowski, taken at Dachau, Germany, 0800 hrs 13 May 1945, Document No-2428-PS, Office of the U.S. Chief Counsel, in RG-30.001M. This witness's name appears in the records with the spellings "Michalowski" and "Miechalowski".

> during which I was at first given a cigarette and some rum. I still remember when the doctor put some drops of yellow fluid into my mouth. Shortly afterwards, I lost consciousness. But I remember that, at that time, my legs and arms were absolutely like frozen iron, and that cold sweat came down from my forehead.
>
> Q. Do you know exactly how long you were in this frozen water after you become unconscious?
> A. I know only that, at 8 o'clock in the evening, I regained consciousness and was, at that time, outside of the water basin.
>
> Q. Did you later find out how long you were in the basin of ice-cold water?
> A. I think approximately two hours.

Dr. Franz Blaha, an inmate from Czechoslovakia, worked as a pathologist at Dachau. He gave the following affidavit.

Affidavit of Dr. Franz Blaha[80]

> Rascher conducted experiments on the effects of cold water on human beings. This was done to find a way for reviving airmen who had fallen into the ocean. The subject was placed in ice cold water and kept there until he was unconscious. Blood was taken from his neck and tested each time his body temperature dropped one degree. This drop was determined by a rectal thermometer. Urine was also periodically tested. Some men stood it as long as 24 to 36 hours. The lowest body temperature reached was 19 degrees centigrade, but most men died at 25 or 26 degrees. When the men were removed from the ice water, attempts were made to revive them by artificial sunshine, with hot water, by electrotherapy, or by animal warmth. For this last experiment, prostitutes were used and the body of the unconscious man was placed between the bodies of two women.
>
> Himmler was present at one such experiment. I could see him from one of the windows in the street between the blocks. I have personally been present at some of these cold water experiments when Rascher was absent, and I have seen notes and diagrams on them in Rascher's laboratory. About 300 persons were used in these experiments. The majority died. Of those who survived, many became mentally deranged. Those

80 Affidavit of Dr. Franz Blaha (witness), 11 January 1946, Document No-3249-PS, Exhibit No. USA-663, in *Trial IMT,* vol. 5, pp. 167–174, here p. 170.

> who did not die were sent to invalid blocks and were killed just as were the victims of the air pressure experiments. I know only two who survived, a Yugoslav and a Pole, both of whom are mental cases.

Dr. Robert L. Berger has reviewed and analyzed the hypothermia experiments conducted at Dachau. He reports that his review of the Dachau hypothermia experiments

> ...reveals critical shortcoming[s] in scientific content and credibility. The project was conducted without an orderly experimental protocol, with inadequate methods and an erratic execution. The report is riddled with inconsistencies. There is also evidence of data falsification and suggestions of fabrication. Many conclusions are not supported by the facts presented. The flawed science is compounded by evidence that the director of the project showed a consistent pattern of dishonesty and deception in his professional as well as his personal life, thereby stripping the study of the last vestige of credibility. On analysis, the Dachau hypothermia study has all the ingredients of a scientific fraud, and rejection of the data on purely scientific grounds is inevitable. They cannot advance science or save human lives.[81]

SEAWATER EXPERIMENTS

On 16 February 1946, an officer at the Vienna State Police completed a report that stated the following: "The State police has received information from the wife of the Vienna University Professor Wilhelm Beiglböck in 1944, which states that the experiments her husband conducts at the concentration camp in Dachau are a threat to his life and well being since the prisoners often become insane and frantic." The letter also stated that a few other famous university professors, including Professor Hans Eppinger, were involved in the experiments.[82] What were these experiments?

The German Navy and Air Force (Luftwaffe) were interested in discovering a method for making seawater potable, so that shipwrecked sailors, or pilots who had been shot down into the sea, might have improved chances of surviving. At the time, two methods for converting seawater into drinking water were

81 Berger, "Nazi Science", pp. 1439–1440.
82 Klee, *Auschwitz*, pp. 243–255.

known. One method, devised by the Air Force engineer Dr. Edward Berka, consisted of adding "Berkatit" to seawater, changing its taste but not its composition. The other, developed by the Viennese doctor and chemist D. Konrad Schäfer, used the substance "Wofatit", which, when added to seawater, actually removed the salt. The latter was undoubtedly the better method but also by far the more expensive. Its manufacture required a great deal of silver, and, more important, the construction of enormous factories. Thus its use was limited. Berkatit, meanwhile, was known to cause serious side effects rather quickly: after just six days painful cramps and hallucinations occurred, and after just twelve days use, it could even cause death. A less dangerous method was clearly needed.

On 7 June 1944, Oskar Schröder, Medical Inspector of the Air Force, approached Himmler with a request for an experimental laboratory at Dachau. There the search for an effective and safe additive to seawater would be conducted.

Translation of Document No-185[83]
Office of U.S. Chief of Counsel

(handwritten) *Top Secret (Military)*

CHIEF MEDICAL SERVICE OF THE LUFTWAFFE
File: 55 Nr.510/44 top secret (military) (2F)
Über Zossen/Lend
7 June 1944

2 copies *SAALOW*
1st copy Über Zossen/Lend
13 (handwritten)
44

To the Reich Minister of the Interior and Reichsführer SS
through Reichsarzt SS and Police

Berlin W
Knesebeckstr. 51

83 Request of Schroeder, Medical Inspector of the Air Force, to SS Chief, Heinrich Himmler, 7 June 1944, Document No-185, in RG-30.001M.

The Reichsführer SS
Reichsarzt SS and Police-Adjutant
12 June 1944

Arzt	Adjutant	Illegible
Initialed	*initialed*	*initialed*

Highly Respected Reich Minister:

Earlier already you made it possible for the Luftwaffe to settle urgent medical matters through experiments on human beings. Today I again stand before a decision, which, after numerous experiments on animals and also on voluntary human subjects, demands final resolution: the Luftwaffe has simultaneously developed two methods for making seawater potable. The one method, developed by a Medical Officer, removes the salt from the seawater and transforms it into real drinking water; the second method, suggested by an engineer, leaves the salt content unchanged, and only removes the unpleasant taste from the seawater. The later method, in contrast to the first, requires no critical raw material (Engpassrohstoffe). From the medical point of view this method must be viewed critically, as the administration of concentrated salt solutions can produce severe symptoms of poisoning.

As the experiments on human beings could thus far only be carried out for a period of four days, and as practical demands require a remedy for those who are in distress at sea up to 12 days, appropriate experiments are necessary.

Required are 40 healthy test subjects, who must be available for 4 whole weeks. As it is known from previous experiments, that necessary laboratories exist in the concentration camp Dachau, this camp would be very suitable.

Direction of the experiments shall be taken over by Stabsarzt, lecturer (Dozent) Dr. BEIGLBOECK, civilian profession: Chief Physician of the Medical University Clinic in Vienna (Prof. Dr. EPPINGER). After receipt of the basic approval, I shall list by name the two other physicians who are to participate in the experiments.

Due to the enormous importance which a solution of this problem has for soldiers of the Luftwaffe and Navy who have become shipwrecked, I would be greatly obliged to you, my dear Reich Minister, if you would decide to comply with my request.

Heil Hitler!
(Signature) Schroeder

Although earlier experiments by Dr. Sirany in Vienna had already demonstrated that Berkatit was injurious to health, it remained attractive because it was cheap and simple to manufacture, especially in comparison with Wofatit. The Dachau experiments aimed at finding a safe way to use Berkatit.[84]

Office of U.S. Chief of Counsel for War Crimes APO 124a Evidence Division, Interrogation Branch Interrogation Summary No-576[85]

Interrogation of:	Dr. Konrad SCHAEFER, 2nd Lt.M.C. (Unterarzt) Air Force–Index No. 341
Interrogation by:	Mr.v.Halle, 22 November 1946, Nuremberg
Section & Att'y:	I.G. Farben – Mr. Heath, Mr. Kove
Compiled by:	HEW

Excerpt from Summary

SCHAEFFER was sent to Vienna in order to examine the experiments which Dr. SIRANY conducted there. SCHAEFFER, after having concluded his examination submitted a report stating that the SIRANY experiments had been carried out and that they proved the Berka Method to be inadequate. The sea-water which was treated according to the Berka Method had proven injurious to health. This report was submitted to BECKER-FREYSENG and as a result the Chief of the Medical Corps disapproved of the Berka Method. The informant states that nevertheless the Technical Department tried forcibly to adapt the Berka Method.

BECKER-FREYSENG suggested that further experiments be conducted on human beings in the Dachau concentration camp. It was decided to appoint a commission of experts. The Berka Method was to be applied for such a period of time as would permit the first symptoms to be noticed, then the Wolfatit method was to be applied, generally for a period of twelve days.

In September SCHAEFER concluded from a report by Beigelboeck that the experiments had been executed. This report stated, among other things, that persons on whom the Berka Method had been tried showed the following symptoms: on the 6th or 7th day: dry skin, drying out of the

84 Hoedeman, *Hitler or Hippocrates*, pp. 174–182.

85 Interrogation of Nuremberg Defendant Konrad Schaefer, Office of U.S. Chief Counsel for War Crimes, Evidence Division, Interrogation Branch, Interrogation Summary No-576, YVA, JM/6021

> muscular system, swelling of the liver, general mental irritation, hallucinations. Also the persons on whom the experiments had been conducted started to quarrel with each other and suffered pain.

Thus despite knowledge that the ingestion of seawater with the Berkatit additive for periods of six days would cause permanent injury leading to death within twelve days, plans were made to conduct further experiments that would last from six to twelve days. Himmler responded positively to the Luftwaffe's request and ordered a conference of high-ranking SS officers to determine which prisoners would be used.

Translation of Document No-179[86]
Office of Chief of Counsel for War Crimes

The Reichsführer SS
Berlin W. 15, 28 June 1944
Reich Physician of the SS and Police
Knesebeckstr. 50/51
Telefon: 924249.924351 924373.924406
Journal Number 13/44 Top Secret
(handwritten) FS

Concerning: Experiments in the concentration camp instigated by the Chief of the Medical Service of the Luftwaffe
Refer: Order RF-SS of 15 May 44
Enclosure: 1

2 copies
1. copy

To the
Reichsführer SS H. HIMMLER
Field Command Post.
————————————————
Top Secret (Military)

86 Letter to Himmler from Grawitz, Head of the SS Medical Service, Document No-179, in RG-30.001M.

Reichsführer!

The Chief of the Medical Service of the Luftwaffe requests in the top secret (military) letter, enclosed herewith, that experiments be performed on prisoners in order to test two simple methods which seem to promise success for seawater potable.

In accordance with your order of 15 May 1944, Reichsführer, I have requested the opinion of SS Gruppenführer Prof. Dr. GEBHARDT, SS Gruppenführer GLUECKS and SS Gruppenführer NEBE. They read as follows:

1. SS Gruppenführer Prof. Dr. GEBHARDT:

"I deem it absolutely right to support the Luftwaffe in every way and to place a general physician of the Waffen SS at disposal to supervise the experiments."

2. SS Gruppenführer GLUECKS:

"Referring to the above letter, we report that we have no objections whatsoever to the experiments requested by the Chief of the Medical Service of the Luftwaffe to be conducted at the experimental station RASCHER in the concentration camp Dachau. If possible, Jews or prisoners held in quarantine are to be used."

3. SS Gruppenführer NEBE:

"I agree with the proposal to conduct experiments on prisoners of concentration camps in order to evolve a method for making seawater potable. I propose taking for this purpose the asocial Gypsy half breeds (asozialen Zigeunermischlinge). There are people among them, who, although healthy, are out of the question as regards labor commitment. Regarding these Gypsies, I shall shortly make a special proposal to the Reichsführer, but I think it right to select from among these people the necessary number of test subjects."

Should the Reichsführer agree to this, I shall list by name the persons to be used. To the proposal of the SS Gruppenführer NEBE to use Gypsies for the experiment, I beg to raise an objection to wit that the Gypsies being of somewhat different racial composition might possibly provide experimental results, which might not apply entirely to our men. It would therefore be desirable, if such prisoners could be used for these experiments, as are racially comparable to European peoples.

I request most humbly being granted your approval in order to start with the experiments.

Zz–yes (handwritten) Heil Hitler!
Grawitz (Signature)

(handwritten)
Gipsies and for control 3 others
HH (Signature)

30 June 1944 (stamp)
1962/44 (handwritten)
RF (")

Himmler agreed with SS Gruppenführer Nebe's suggestion to use gypsies for the experiments.

Translation of Document No-183[87]
Office of U.S. Chief of Counsel

(stamp) Top Secret (Military)
Teletype: VI.M 21 608
Acc. Bg 27/7
(handwritten remark) to previous correspondence.

To the Reichsarzt SS and Police
SS Obergruppenführer Dr. GRAWITZ,

Berlin
Subject: Experiments by the Chief of the Medical Service of the Luftwaffe.
Reference: Your letter of June 28th 1944 – Journal Number 13/44
Military secret.
Obergruppenführer!

87 Teletype from Brandt to Grawitz, Document No-183, in RG-30.001M.

The Reichsführer SS decided, that according to suggestion of SS Gruppenführer NEBE gipsies should be used for the experiments. In addition three other prisoners shall be made available.

Heil Hitler!
(Signed) BRANDT
SS Standartenführer
(Dispatched by F.S.)

Hm (handwritten initials)

S. [8.] 7.1944
Bg./Hm
(8. 7. 18:05)

(Rubber stamp: Day. Month. Time)

The experiments began in August 1944 and continued until the middle of September. The following are details of the procedures according to the chart kept by Professor Beiglboeck:[88]

Subjects 1–6: ...deprived of all food and water from 5 1/2 – 7 1/2 days.

Subjects 7–10: ...were given 1000 cc of water treated by the Schaefer method for 12, 13, 12, days respectively, and hungered for 7, 8, and 9 days, respectively. (Subject #9 was not used for health reasons.)

Subjects 11–18: ...were given 500 cc of seawater plus sea rations for a total of 2400 calories. These experiments lasted from 5–10 days. They hungered for 6 1/2 days.

Subjects 19–25: ...were given 500 cc of Berka-treated water plus the emergency sea ration. These experiments lasted 5–9 1/2 days with periods of hunger of up to 6 1/2 days.

Subjects 26–30: ...were given 1000 cc of Berka-treated water plus the emergency sea ration for 5–9 1/2 days with periods of hunger up to 6 1/2 days.

Subjects 31 and 32: ...were given 1000 cc of seawater for 8 and 6 days respectively.

Subject 33: ...was given 500 cc of Berka water for 6 days.

Subject 34: ...was given 1000 cc of Schaefer water for 12 days.

Subjects 35, 36, 37, 39, 41, 42: ...were given 500 cc of seawater for periods of 4–6 days.

Subjects 38, 40, 43: ...were given 1000 cc of seawater for 6, 5, 6 days respectively.

Subject 44: ...was given Schaefer water for 12 days.

88 Details of the experiments according to the charts kept by Prof. Beiglboek, in *Trials NMT,* pp. 423–424.

Excerpts from the Testimony of Prosecution Witness, Former Prisoner Karl Hoellenrainer[89]

Q. Did you at any time volunteer for these experiments?
A. No.

Q. Were any of the other inmates asked if they would like to volunteer?
A. No.

Q. Did the professor or any of the other Luftwaffe physicians talk to the inmates and advise them as to the hazards of the experiment prior to the commencement of the actual experiments?
A. No.

Q. Now, will you, in detail, tell the Tribunal just what food the experimental subjects received prior to the experiments, during the course of the experiments, and after the experiments.
A. Yes. At first we got potatoes, milk, and then we got these cookies and dextrose and rusks. That lasted about 1 week. Then we got nothing at all. Then the doctor from the Luftwaffe said, "Now you have to drink seawater on an empty stomach." That lasted about 1 or 2 weeks. This Rudi Taubmann, as I already said, got excited and didn't want to participate; and the doctor from the Luftwaffe said, "If you get excited and mutiny, I will shoot you", and then we were all quiet. Then we began to drink seawater. I drank the worst kind, that was yellowish. We drank two or three times a day, and then in the evening we drank the yellow kind. There were three kinds of water, white water, and yellow water; and I drank the yellow kind. After a few days the people became raving mad; they foamed at the mouth. The doctor from the Luftwaffe came with a cynical laugh and said, "Now it is time to make the liver punctures [liver biopsies]."

I remember one very well... He went crazy and barked like a dog. He foamed at the mouth. The doctor from the Luftwaffe took him down on a stretcher with a white sheet over him, and then he stuck a needle about this long [indicating] into his right side and there was a hypodermic needle on it, and it bled, and it was very painful. We were all quiet and excited. When that was over, the other inmates took their turn. The people were crazy from thirst and hunger; we were so hungry – but the doctor had no pity on us. He was as cold as ice. He didn't take any interest in us. Then, one gypsy – I don't know his name any more – ate a little piece of bread once, or drank some water; I don't remember just what he did. The

89 Testimony of Karl Hoellenrainer, in *Trials of War Criminals*, Green Series, vol. 1, pp. 457–463, on the Mazal Library website.

doctor from the Luftwaffe got very angry and mad. He took the gypsy and tied him to a bedpost and sealed his mouth.

Q. Witness, do you mean that he put adhesive tape over this Gypsy's mouth?
A. Yes... Then a gypsy, he was lying on the right, a big, strong, husky fellow, he refused to drink the water. He asked the doctor from the Luftwaffe to let him go. He said he couldn't stand the water. He was sick. The doctor from the Luftwaffe had no pity and he said, "No, you have to drink it." The doctor from the Luftwaffe told one of his assistants to go and get a sun. Naturally, we didn't know what a sun was. Then one of his assistants came with a red tube about this long... And then the doctor from the Luftwaffe took this red tube and put it in the gypsy's mouth and into his stomach. And then he pumped water down the tube. The gypsy kneeled in front of him and beseeched him for mercy but the doctor had none.

Q. Were any of the experimental subjects ever taken out of the station room to the yard outside the experimental barracks?
A. Yes, at the end when the experiments were finished; and three people were carried out with white sheets over them on a stretcher... We thought they were dead.

Excerpts from the Testimony of Prosecution Witness, Former Prisoner Joseph Laubinger[90]

Q. Then you were to drink sea water. Do you know whether or not the water you were drinking was specially treated?
A. Yes, this was the second sort that had been mixed with something.

Q. Can you relate how much you received of this water during one day?
A. In the morning, noon and night, we received a glassful but how much was in each glass I can't tell you. It was about the size of a beer glass.

Q. What effect did the drinking of this water have on you?
A. It tasted very salty. After drinking it one became thirsty and tired.

90 Testimony of Joseph Laubinger, in *Trials of War Criminals before the Nuremberg Military Tribunals,* Simon Weisenthal Archives, pp. 10197–10209.

Q. Did you feel very sick?
A. We got so weak that we could hardly stand up.

Q. Did you have a fever at all?
A. Yes.

Q. Did you ever become so weak that you were unable to stand up?
A. Well, I could stand up, but I had to hold onto something. Otherwise I would have fallen down.

Q. How long were you subjected to drinking this particular water?
A. For eleven or twelve days we drank this water.

Q. Well, now, did you ever at any time receive a liver puncture [biopsy]?
A. Yes.

Q. Do you remember when you received this?
A. After the experiment, that is, when the experiments were over.

Q. Did you also receive a lumbar puncture?
A. I don't know what that word means.

Q. Well, that would be a puncture in your back?
A. Yes.

Q. And you received that also at the completion of the experiments, you think?
A. Yes.

Q. ...Well, now after the experiments were completed, that is, the entire experimental program had been completed, did you then go to the hospital for rest?
A. No. Here is the way it was. Beiglboeck said that whoever felt weak would have a chance to convalesce in the hospital. A friend of mind told me that those who went to the hospital for convalescence would never come out again. I asked, how come. He said they would get injections and would die. Of course, hearing this, I declined to enter the hospital. I said I was quite strong enough to work.

Translation of Document No-910[91]
Office of U.S. Chief of Counsel

Testimony of an Eyewitness

Ignaz Bauer
Vahringerstrasse 162
Born on 8 June 1908
Interned I Dachau Concentration Camp from June 1944 to June 1945
Prisoner #73059

REPORT

Experiments of the Luftwaffe performed under the
Direction of the academic lecturer, Dr. BEIGLBOECK
in the Dachau Prisoners' Hospital barracks in Summer 1944

In the summer 1944, shortly after my transfer to Dachau from a French prison, I worked in the infirmary of the Light station where I did physical therapy and male electrocardiogram.

I think that about the end of July a sick-room for experimental purposes was made available to the Luftwaffe. Several series of experiments were carried out forcibly...

...I had, apart from some electrocardiograms, to test the electric excitability of muscles and nerves of the patients and therefore had the opportunity to watch part of what was happening and to draw my own conclusions.

...Visible deterioration of the patients, nervousness, agitation, which, in some cases, mounted to the point of madness. (The raving people were tied to their beds.) Some of the patients showed signs of apathy and unconsciousness. In many instances, weakness of the hearing could be observed.

Subjectively, the patients suffered from gnawing hunger and above all, from terrible thirst, which, through the drinking of saltwater, became even more painful. The thirst was so terrible that some patients did not hesitate to drink dirty water used for washing the floor. I saw one of these poor devils falling on his knees, begging in vain for water. Doctor Beiglboeck was pitiless. One youth, who had succeeded in getting some water to drink, was bound to his bed for punishment.

91 Testimony of Ignaz Bauer, in Ibid., pp. 10197–10209, and RG-30.001M.

The Fate of the Perpetrators of the Seawater Experiments[92]

Beiglböck was sentenced to fifteen years imprisonment at the Nuremberg Medical Trial in 1947, but he was set free in 1951. In 1952 he began working as the lead physician at a clinic in Buxtehude. He died in 1963 at the age of fifty-eight.

Erich Hippke disappeared underground and Hubertus Strughold was traced to Texas by the American secret police. It is assumed that following Strughold's lead, at least thirty-four physicians of the Luftwaffe fled to Texas.

The other participants in the experiments were sentenced on 20 August 1947 as follows: Siegfried Handloser and Oskar Schröder to life and Hermann Becker-Freyseng to twenty years. Luftwaffe experts Siegfried Ruff, Hans Wolfgang Romberg, Konrad Schäfer and Georg August Weltz were acquitted. Schäfer and Becker-Freyseng left for the U.S.A after the hearing. It is interesting that Hubertus Strughold was repeatedly honored for his work, not only with the title "Father of Space Medicine", but also with papal audiences in Paris and Rome, and with honorary membership in the German Air and Space Society of Munich!

POLYGAL EXPERIMENTS

Robert Feix was known in Germany as an expert on blood coagulation.[93] He was caught up in a sinister deal, tried for corruption and acquitted, but as he was leaving the courtroom, he was rearrested, this time on Bormann's orders, with Himmler's permission: his research skills were needed by the SS. He was interned consequently in Dachau, where he was ordered to do research under the direction of Sigmund Rascher.

Feix immediately set to work. In May 1943 Rascher returned from a vacation to find that, in his absence, Feix had perfected a coagulating tablet that effectively stopped hemorrhage and had begun producing it under the name "Homtag".

Rascher was enthusiastic and immediately notified Reichsführer Himmler of the promising findings. He knew that Himmler was always interested in new remedies that might help the soldiers on the front. Himmler was indeed

92 Klee, *Auschwitz*, pp. 243–255.
93 Aziz, *Doctors of Death*, vol. 3, pp. 78–81.

delighted with the news and encouraged Rascher to use the tablets on patients undergoing surgery. The pills were dispatched immediately to the Dachau dental service and to operating rooms. But that was not enough for the ambitious director of the Dachau laboratory, who decided also to test the substance in another form called "Polygal". His report of 7 February 1944, to Dr. Graue, Director of War Economy of the Research Council, describes the composition and qualities of this alternative form of the remedy.

Letter from "R" [Sigmund Rascher] to Dr. Graue, 7 February 1944 Document No-613[94]

> 1. The basic components are slices of beet, pectin extracted from apples, and dextrose.
> 2. The use of [sic] haemostatic *polygal* in tablet form is especially useful in the prevention of hemorrhages. It can be particularly useful for flight crews, in shock troop actions, etc... and in case of long delays between the infliction of a wound and the dressing of it.
> 3. No other haemostatic preparations offer the following advantages: The use of it in tablet form is very simple. You merely allow it to melt in the mouth, and then swallow it slowly. Effects last from one to six hours. The remedy is not affected by temperature changes.
> 4. The remedy is in no way toxic, and can consequently be taken frequently without risk. (Absolutely no danger of thrombosis or embolism.)
> 5. The cost of this mass produced drug is lower than that of any other haemostatic presently available; it is almost negligible.

Another SS physician, Dr. Kurt Blome, assisted Rascher with the Polygal research.

Extract from the Closing Brief Against Defendant Blome[95]

> In order to test the effectiveness of the blood coagulant "Polygal", Rascher carried out experiments in which inmates of the Dachau concentration camp were shot to induce bleeding. Rascher's uncle, in an affi-

94 Letter from "R" [Rascher] to Graue, 7 Feb 1944, Document No-613, in RG-30.001M.

95 Extract from the Closing Brief against Defendant Blome: Selection from the Argumentation of the Prosecution, in *Trials NMT,* vol 1, no. 10, pp. 669–670, referring in part to Document No-1424, Prosecution Exhibit 462.

davit, describes the murderous experiments which were carried out by his nephew. In August 1943, he visited Rascher in Dachau and, while Rascher was away from his office, he saw a report which he described as follows:

It referred to the shooting (execution) of four people for the purpose of experimenting with the haemostatic preparation "Polygal 10". As far as I remember they were a Russian commissar and a cretin, I do not remember who the other two were. The Russian was shot in the right shoulder from above by an SS man who stood on a chair. The bullet emerged near the spleen. It was described how the Russian twitched convulsively, then sat down on a chair and died after about 20 minutes. In the autopsy report the rupture of the pulmonary vessels and the aorta was described. It was further described that the ruptures were tamponed by hard blood clots. That could have been the only explanation for the comparatively long span of life after the shot.

This evidence is corroborated by the testimony of witness Stoehr and the affidavit of Pohl (No-065, Prosecution Exhibit 221). Even the defendant Gebhardt admitted, during his testimony, that he knew that Rascher had carried out blood coagulation experiments on concentration camp inmates who had been shot for the purpose.

Several documents on clinical experiments with Polygal follow.

Translation of Document No-656[96] Office of the Chief Counsel for War Crimes

Concentration Camp Dachau
The camp physician
Dachau, 10 December 1943

Subject: Administering "Polygal" upon amputation of the thigh of a 40 years [sic] old male patient

To Stabsarzt Dr. RASCHER
Dachau

96 Memo from Dr. Kahr to Rascher, 10 December 1943, Document No-656, Office of the Chief Counsel for War Crimes, in RG-30.001M.

On 10 December 1943 the effectiveness of "Polygal" in the case of the amputation of a thigh was tested. The drug was administered 45 minutes before the operation was placed in the patient's mouth to be dissolved. A blood transfusion of 500 ccm had been made the previous day in preparation for the operation. Blood pressure on the day of the operation was 130/80.

As regards to the effectiveness of "Polygal" one can say that it was absolutely evident how little the tissues bled. After the first rush of blood from the vessels which had been cut when completely emptied of blood, no more bleeding occurred after their first issuing of accumulated blood, so that it was not necessary to apply any ligatures to the surface of the muscles and the fatty tissues, or the subcutaneous tissues, as had always been the case with other amputations. The effectiveness of "Polygal" must in this case be described as complete.

The First Camp Physician Concentration Camp Dachau
On order (Signed) Dr. KAHR
SS Obersturmführer

Translation of Document No-586[97]
Office of Chief Counsel for War Crimes

Concentration Camp Dachau
The Camp Physician
Dachau 13 December 1943

To SS Hauptsturmführer Dr. RASCHER
Dachau

"Polygal 10" was used for herniotomies. The patients were men of 35 and 42 years of age respectively. In both cases the tablets were administered to the patients 40 minutes before the operation. Both patients tolerated "Polygal 10" without complaint, nor were there any unpleasant accompanying symptoms in the stomach.

It is to be said that the loss of blood was conspicuously slight in the both cases...

The favorable effect of "Polygal 10" in surgical operations consists not only in it preventing great loss of blood, but also in that it makes

97 Memo from Dr. Kahr to Rascher, 13 December 1943, Document No-586, in Ibid.

possible considerably faster operations. Because the application of clips and later ligatures always takes up a certain time, which can be saved by the use of "Polygal 10".

(Signed) Dr. KAHR
SS Obersturmführer

To publicize his successes with Polygal, Rascher had the following report printed in the *Münchner Medizinischen Wochenschrift* (Munich Medical Weekly), 28 January 1944.

Translation of Document No-438[98]
Office of Chief of Counsel for War Crimes

(handwritten) Mue.Med.Wo.Schri.
delivered 20 Dec. 1943.

From the Institute for Military Scientific Research. (Department Dr. Rascher)
"Polygal 10", hemostat to be administered orally
Dr.med. S. Rascher, Munich, and Dr.med.Haferkamp, Walters in Usen (Thuringia).

Excerpt:

A good *hemostat* has to have the following qualifications:

1. Must be harmless.
2. Must be administered easily (orally).
3. Must not have a bad taste.
4. Must have a deep and long lasting effect on the bleeding and clotting time.
5. After the effect wears off it must be possible to administer another dose without any danger.

The currently commercially available hemostats only partially meet these requirements. Especially no unobjectionable hemostat is known which is in form of tablets is durable, unimpaired by cold temperature and therefore easily transportable. But it would be worthwhile to produce a preparation which would have the following important advantages:

98 Notice from Drs. Rascher and Haferkamp, printed in the *Münchner Medizinischen Wochenschrift,* Document No-438, in Ibid.

1. It would be given prophylactically to the combat troops before an attack and to air crews before action. Great blood loss could be avoided when tending to wounds is delayed; similarly it could be avoided that the wounded become incapacitated by a delay of loss of blood.

2. Before operations in which great area bleeding is to be expected, it could be used to keep the operative area clear of interfering bleeding.

3. Persons having a high blood clotting time could benefit inestimatably from such a remedy in cases of teeth extractions, etc.

4. In severe cases of lung or stomach hemorrhage which cannot be treated surgically at once, such a remedy could be life saving.

We believe to have such a remedy in "Polygal 10", a preparation composed and tested in our institute, which does fulfill the above requirements. "Polygal 10" is a drug composed of a "Pectin" base; its new method, differentiating it from other hemostats of a Pectin basis is to be found in the activation of Pectin before composing it into the hemostat.

Before we tried the clinical use of the drug, it was tested on *human beings* by thorough experiments as to its influence on clotting and bleeding. The period of clotting was occasionally established in short intervals by 10 parallel definitions of free flowing venous blood according to the method of Burcker. The period of bleeding was measured by a stopwatch after a wound at the ear had been inflicted by a "Frankeschen Schnepper".

Summary

A report is submitted on a new hemostat based on Pectin and to be administered orally, which after a short time causes an extremely strong and long-lasting regular reduction of the bleeding and blood clotting time. The practical tests of this medicine "Polygal 10" showed under the most varied circumstances no failures up to now. No contraindications on the part of the heart or the circulation could be found, as was expected considering the composition of the drug.

Rascher's ambitious action evoked a negative response from his superiors, who were concerned lest the facts about the experiments in the camps be made public.

Translation of Document No-614[99]
Office of Chief of Counsel for War Crimes

The Reichsführer-SS
The Reich Physician SS and Police
Berlin W 15, 17 February 1944
File–No: 189/XVI/44

RE: Your article in No. 3/4 of the Munich Medical Weekly
(*Münchner Mediz. Wochenschrift* of 28 January 1944)

To SS Hauptsturmführer Dr. RASCHER
Dachau/Obb.

In the *Munich Medical Weekly,* 10.3/4 of 28 January 1944, there is an article on "Polygal 10", a haemostatic to be taken "per os" by Dr. RASCHER and Dr. HAFENKAMP. "Dachau 3 K" is indicated as the address and human experimental subjects are mentioned in the article.

The publication of scientific treatises is subject to the granting of the authorization to print by the senior professional authority (for SS physicians, the Reich Physician SS and Police) as well as the High Command of the Wehrmacht.

This subjection to censorship is also known to the editorial office of professional periodicals.

You are requested to let us know why you did not apply for the necessary consent for publication.

Heil Hitler!

(Signed) GRAWITZ

99 Memo from Grawitz to Rascher, Document No-614, in Ibid.

Translation of Document No-615[100]
Office of Chief of Counsel for War Crimes

The Chief of the Economic and Administrative Main Office
Berlin-Lichterfelde West, Unter den Eichen
Ch.Pa (illegible)

To:
Stabsarzt Dr. Sigmund RASCHER

Date illegible (stamp)
001533 16 Feb 1944
E/R/8 (crossed out)
File No. G/P/19
Illegible margin notation

Dear Rascher:

In the *Munich Medical Weekly Journal* (Münchner Medizinischen Wochenschrift) of 26 January 1944 you published an article about "Poligal 10".

I deem it necessary that in future publications you avoid carefully everything which could induce people who are familiar with the subject (and one must always consider that such people exist) to the conclusion that experiments on prisoners are involved.

This is possible from various passages in the above mentioned article. It is paramount that you do not use "Dachau 3 K" as the authors address.

Heil Hitler!

(handwritten) Yours,
P (initial for POHL)

Copy to:
SS Obersturmbannführer
Dr. BRANDT, Personal
Staff Reichsführer SS
SS Standartenführer SIEVERS
Ahnenerbe-Berlin

SS Obergrupprenführer
And General of the Waffen SS.

100 Memo from Pohl to Rascher, 16 February 1944, Document No-615, in Ibid.

Translation of Document No-616[101]
Office of Chief of Counsel for War Crimes

THE "AHNENERBE"
The Reich Business Manager

Waischenfeld/Ofr., 10 Feb 1944
No. 135 Tel No 2 PLZ: 13?
(handwritten) G/R/8 S/St.

Note:

Subject: Publication RASCHER–HAFERKAMP in the Munich Medical Weekly

On the occasion of my presence in Munich at the beginning of January, SS Hauptsturmführer Dr. RASCHER and Dr. HAFERKAMP informed me about the publication of an article which they wrote together and which they planned for the Munich Medical Weekly. Dr. RASCHER received the necessary authorization from me, as he had left the Luftwaffe and had not yet been taken over by the Waffen SS and thus had to obtain the authorization from the competent office, namely the "Ahnenerbe". The article planned was also known to deputy Reichsarzteführer, SA-Gruppenführer Professor Dr. BLOME and had met with his approval. Dr. HAFERKAMP, declared that he did not need an authorization as he was leaving the Waffen SS. On 12 Jan. 1944, a discussion took place between SS Standartenführer, Dr. BEWING, SS Hauptsturmführer Dr. RASCHER and myself, in the course of which Dr. HAFERKAMP was mentioned. On that occasion it was revealed that Dr. HAFERKAMP had not yet left and certainly had to have the authorization of the Reichsarzt SS for the publication. Following this discussion, I immediately sent this teletype to the Munich Medical Weekly (Lehmann Publications Munich): "Publication RASCHER/HAFERKAMP must by no means take place as HAFENKAMP was without prescribed authorization."

On 4 Feb. 1944, I was informed by SS Hauptsturmführer Dr. RASCHER that the publication had already taken place when my teletype was received.

(Signature) SIEVERS
SS Standartenführer

Distribution:
1. Files
2. Dr. Rascher for his information

101 Memo from Sievers, 10 February 1944, Document No-616, in Ibid.

Apparently, subsequent experience with Polygal significantly decreased the optimism and excitement about its effectiveness. This must have been the stimulus for the following letter.

Translation of Document No-612[102]
Office of Chief of Counsel for War Crimes

The Reichsführer SS	Field Command Post, 29 November 1943
Personal Staff	
Diary No.	Stamp 001339–3 December 1943
Bra/H.	Reference No. 9L/8-S/P/AG
	Handwritten (initials illegible)

To: SS Standartenführer SIEVERS
Waischenfeld/Oberfranken
No. 132

Dear Comrade Sievers:

The matter of Polygal No. 10 did not develop as quickly as you and SS Hauptsturmführer Dr. RASCHER expected. The Reichsführer SS has talked to SS Gruppenführer Professor Dr. GEBHARDT. He allowed himself to be convinced that for various reasons it is still necessary to make thorough tests at Hohenlychen which are previously to be discussed by SS Hauptsturmführer Dr. RASCHER with the competent physician at Hohenlychen and/or SS Gruppenführer Professor Dr. GEBHARDT personally. I shall also write a few lines to that effect to SS Hauptsturmführer Dr. RASCHER and I shall ask him now to remain really objective and not to get excited because things cannot be done as quickly as he originally thought. SS Hauptsturmführer Dr. RASCHER will furthermore be given the opportunity to get in touch with a competent specialist in Berlin, as far as I know, Professor SEITZ, in order to discuss the whole problem and possibly further experiments.

Heil, Hitler!

(Signature) R. BRANDT
SS Obersturmbannführer

102 Letter from Rudolf Brandt to Sievers, 3 December 1943, Document No-612, in Ibid.

THE SEARCH FOR THE TREATMENT OF PHLEGMONE AND SEPSIS

The report entitled *Atrocities Committed at the Dachau Concentration Camp,* in the Yad Vashem Archives, notes that the Nazis authorized a series of experiments to study ways of treating a particularly serious infection called phlegmone.

> The so-called "phlegmone" experiments were apparently also one of the attempts on the part of the Nazis to find an antibiotic similar to our penicillin and form some of the most inhuman and horrible pages of Dachau history. The experiments involved the intravenous and intramuscular injection of pus followed by attempts at chemotherapeutic treatment of the resulting infections.
>
> Some 800 prisoners were subjected to these experiments in the years 1942–43. Following the injection, patients developed overwhelming septicemia or massive multiple abscesses of the extremities which required repeated incisions and drainage and in many cases amputation. Ninety percent of the subjects of these experiments died and the remaining ten percent were crippled or permanently disabled. The majority were sent out on the inevitably fatal "invalid" transports.[109]

These experiments, performed in Dachau with various traditional, natural, hence "*bio*chemical" remedies, complemented the sulfanilamide experiments conducted by Karl Gebhardt in Ravensbrück.[104] That the two sets of experiments were related is shown by the fact that in September 1942, while the sulfanilamide experiments were still in progress, Gebhardt received a copy of a report on the Dachau biochemical experiments from Reichsarzt-SS Ernst-Robert von Grawitz, who was charged with overseeing all SS medical experiments.[105] The report presented the results of experiments with treatments for various types of infection, such as sepsis, phlegmone, furuncle, and abscess, which had been carried out on forty Dachau inmates. All the infections, including the eight cases of sepsis, had been artificially inflicted on unwilling subjects,

103 "Report of the Atrocities Committed at the Dachau Concentration Camp," vol. 1, YVA JM/10046, p. 17.

104 The terms "sulfanilamide" and "sulfonamide" appear here and later in this chapter, in the section devoted directly to testing sulfa preparations. The term "sulfonamide" is the formal generic name for all sulfa-containing drugs. A "sulfanilamide" is a topical sulfa preparation.

105 This report became Document No-409, Prosecution Exhibit 249, at the Nuremberg Doctors' Trial.

and ten of the subjects had died. The report also covered three fatal sepsis cases in Auschwitz. It concluded with the bland statement that the experiments were being continued.

Further evidence that the connection between the Dachau and Ravensbrück experiments was more than a casual one was found in Himmler's papers; specifically, a 7 September 1942 letter from Grawitz to Himmler, with a marginal notation written and signed by Gebhardt! Copies of both Gebhardt's preliminary report on his Ravensbrück sulfanilamide experiments and the report on the Dachau sepsis experiments accompanied this letter. Gebhardt's handwritten note reads as follows: "16 September 1942. Settled, after conversation with Reich Leader SS. Obersturmführer F. Fischer has been given new instructions for Ravensbrück and Dachau. Gebhardt."[106]

Gebhardt's testimony at Nuremberg, which was of course self-serving, intends to demonstrate that the doctors involved in the experiments were simply following higher orders. The testimony is particularly notable in its attempt to present Himmler as open to medical opinions from different schools of thought. Gebhardt mentioned the fact that Himmler was known to prefer homeopathic medicine and "natural" remedies to the methods and drugs of the medical establishment. Himmler's position in this matter was consistent with the tendency among Nazis to prefer organic, "folk" healing to modern, "mechanized" "academic" medicine. In approving the Dachau experiments with sepsis and phlegmone, two potentially fatal forms of infection, he was following the advice of a biochemist, not a physician.

Extract from the Testimony of Defendant Gebhardt, Direct Examination[107]

> I request permission of the Tribunal to permit me here to describe what Himmler thought with regard to such experiments, and to show, therefore, how impossible it was in certain cases, in spite of obtaining knowledge, to effect any change. For a person who has studied school medicine it is impossible to believe that through the homeopathic administration of sulphur and phosphorus, surgical case histories, as well as internal case histories, and metabolic diseases can be influenced. However, in medicine one can, of course, take a completely different point of view,

106 Mitscherlich and Mielke, eds., *The Death Doctors,* pp. 205–212.

107 Testimony of Defendant Gebhardt, in *Trials NMT,* vol. 1. The Kieselwetter mentioned here is likely the Dr. Kiesewetter/Kiesswetter noted in the appendix to the present work.

and that is the basic conception of biochemistry up to homeopathy, to which Himmler completely adhered. And here in two sentences we have described how all the elements which appear in nature also have traces in the human body. Now, if one small trace of an element is lacking, then the human being is susceptible to and suffering from some disease or other.

The therapy and method of treatment by the biochemist is the exact contrast of medicine as practiced by a person who has studied it at school. They make test experiments on human beings and discover what element is lacking in that human being, and no matter from what disease he is suffering, the patient is treated with minimum doses of the element which he lacks. Never in the world has it been possible for a typical school practitioner and a biochemist to agree, because they want to treat the human being completely in contrast to each other. From this example you can see now that when I went to Himmler and said that it was madness for not only an experiment to be performed on out-patients, but that also simultaneously ten or twelve different cases should be treated with the same medicine – when I told Himmler this, he said that he had one of the most experienced biochemists, and a layman, Herr Laue with him, and that he was absolutely convinced that this method of treatment was correct. Himmler always attempted to discover old-fashioned popular remedies.

In spite of my objection and in spite of my proof that my own surgical patients would suffer from it, these experiments were performed until I succeeded in bringing this [problem] to Dr. Laue and Dr. Kieselwetter [sic] from Marburg (who enjoyed Himmler's complete confidence on this question) to Hohenlychen. There we performed a similar experiment together on my patients in order to show that this method of treatment was impossible. But even in this way I was not able to achieve my purpose with Himmler, because afterwards it was said we had not applied the drugs properly, and so on. Therefore, one can conclude from this that it was not the case that Himmler adhered to one certain medical concept, and if one accidentally heard of an experiment, one could convince him. Himmler maintained a hostile attitude toward school medicine, and from nature cures to biochemistry he was accessible to every thought, and when Laue convinced him of the fact that this drug was of decisive importance, then the experiment was performed.

On 12 September 1942 SS Standartenführer Dr. Theodor Laue, one of those responsible for the parallel experiments in therapy by allopathic and traditional biochemical methods, wrote to Rudolf Brandt, Himmler's personal consultant.

Letter to Rudolf Brandt from Dr. Theodor Laue[108]

> I was particularly gratified to find that as a direct consequence of certain failures recently experienced at Dachau Gruppenführer Dr. Grawitz now intends to concentrate on the purely scientific side, so as to drive a wedge once and for all into the tradition of mineral salt therapy. I believe that his plans can only meet with general satisfaction, as no better field for their realization can be found than at Dachau. Since the key to the lock has now been discovered, in other words the collaboration of a physician experienced in that direction – This was Dr. Kiesewetter, a biochemist – I am sure that success will not be long delayed.

Gebhardt, who knew of the experiments, stated in his evidence that he had protested against them to Himmler. But he added that the latter, as an opponent of academic medicine eager "to dig up old popular remedies out of the rubbish heap", had been convinced of the propriety and urgency of the tests in question.

Excerpts from Direct Examination of Dr. Franz Blaha[109]

> Q. What was the nature of these phlegmone experiments?
> A. For that purpose, entirely healthy people were selected. They received in the operation room injections from the pus of phlegmone diseased people into the rectum muscles and sometimes into the rectum itself.
>
> Q. What prisoners, if they were prisoners, were used in these experiments?
> A. Firstly, the priests.
>
> Q. Is this phlegmone calculated to produce pain?
> A. Yes.
>
> Q. What is the nature of the pain?
> A. Large pains, great pains.

108 Mitscherlich and Mielke, eds., *The Death Doctors,* citing Document No-409, Prosecution Exhibit 626, from the Nuremberg Doctors' Trial.

109 Direct Examination of Dr. Franz Blaha, Military Government Court, Dachau, Germany, 2 November 1945, YVA JM/10047, pp. 13–15.

Q. How is the phlegmone usually treated in order to effect a cure?
A. First, by surgical methods and then through injections.

Q. Injections of what, Doctor?
A. Either sulfanilamide or penicillin.

Q. After these prisoners had been given this disease of phlegmone how were they treated?
A. At first, for about three or four days, they were not treated at all. Only after the infection had formed and there was pus they were either given sulfanilamide injections or surgical methods or the biochemicals. They were pills containing calcium phosphate, barium phosphate.

Q. Can you tell us, Doctor, whether or not any people died as a result of these experiments?
A. Many people died, and the others were mostly turned into invalids.

Q. Doctor, what position did you hold here in Camp Dachau beginning with July 1942?
A. I was taken into the hospital by the chief physician.

Q. What were your duties in the hospital?
A. As a surgeon, first.

Q. And then what did you do?
A. Because I didn't want to do the operation that I was ordered to do I was, as punishment, sent into the death chamber.

Q. What do you mean, the death chamber?
A. That was the room where the corpses were kept and the autopsies were performed.

The following quote is from another of Dr. Blaha's testimonies.[110]

Document No-3249-PS, Exhibit No. USA-663

Phlegmone experiments were conducted by Dr. Schutz, Dr. Babor, Dr. Kieselwetter and Professor Laue. Forty healthy men were used at a time, of which twenty were given intramuscular and twenty intravenous injections of pus from diseased persons. All treatment was forbidden for 3 days, by which time serious inflammation and in many cases general

110 Affidavit of Dr. Franz Blaha, Document No-3249-PS, Exhibit No. USA-663, in *PTT [Trial IMT]*, p. 171.

blood poisoning had occurred. Then each group was divided again into groups of 10. Half were given chemical treatment with liquid and special pills every 10 minutes for 24 hours. The remainder were treated with sulfonamide and surgery.

In some cases all the limbs were amputated. My autopsy also showed that the chemical treatment had been harmful and had even caused perforations of the stomach wall. For these experiments Polish, Czech, and Dutch priests were ordinarily used. Pain was intense in such experiments. Most of the 600 to 800 persons who were used finally died. Most of the others became permanent invalids and were later killed.

INFECTIOUS HEPATITIS

Infectious hepatitis was a significant problem for the German military, particularly on the Russian front. Even though the fatality from the disease was relatively low, it caused high rates of disability among stricken soldiers, which in turn affected the strength of the fighting forces. Combating the disease was a matter of great urgency; research designed to identify the etiology and mode of transmission of the disease, also to discover an effective preventive vaccine, was thus authorized.

Reich Health Commissioner of the Führer, SS Brigadenführer Professor Karl Brandt sponsored the experiments. He asked Dr. Ernst Robert Grawitz to obtain the approval and assistance of Himmler. On 1 June 1943 Grawitz wrote to Himmler.

Translation of Document No-01[111]

The Reichsführer SS
Reichs Physician SS and Police

Berlin W 15, 1 June 1943
Knesebeck Str. 50/51
Phone: 924249-924351
924373-924466

File Note: 42o/IV/3
(Handwritten)
Journal No. 6/42 Top Secret (Mil.)

111 *Nazi Conspiracy and Aggression,* Supp. A, Document No-01, pp. 1270–1271.

Subject: Experiments to determine the cause of Infectious Jaundice (Hepatitis Epidemics)
Top Secret (Mil.)
(stamped) Top Secret (Mil.)
(Initialed) H. H.

Reichsführer:

The General Commissioner of the Führer, SS Brigadeführer Prof. Dr. Brandt, has approached me with a request to help him in the research on the causes of infectious jaundice (Hepatitis epidemics), which has been to a large extent, promoted by him, by placing prisoners at his disposal. To date, research has been conducted by a Stabsarzt Dr. Dohman within the Research Laboratory of the Army Medical Inspectorate (Forschungsstätte der Heeres-Sanitäts-Inspektion) and with the cooperation of the Robert Koch Institute. In conformity with results obtained by other German scientists, this research led to the discovery that infectious jaundice is not caused by bacteria but by a virus. In order to extend our knowledge, which to date is based only on inoculation of animals with germs taken from human beings, the reverse is now necessary, namely the inoculation of human beings with virus cultures.

Cases of death (Todesfälle) must be anticipated.

Therapeutic and prophylactic conclusions, in particular, will to a great extent depend on this final experimental step.

Eight Prisoners condemned to death, young if possible, are needed in the prison hospital of the concentration camp Sachsenhausen.

I respectfully request your decision, Reichsführer,

1. As to whether I may have the experiments started in the manner described.
2. As to whether the experiments may be conducted in the prison hospital of the concentration camp Sachsenhausen by Stabsarzt Dr. Dohman himself.

Although Mr. Dohman is not a member of the SS (he is an AS Führer and a Party Member), I would recommend an exception in this case in the interest of continuity of the Experiments and thus the exactness of the results.

The practical importance of the matter in questions for our troops, especially in Southern Russia, results from the fact that this disease has spread so extensively during the past years, both among us in the Waffen SS and Police and in the army, that up to 605 casualties for a period of up to six weeks suffered in some companies. On the other hand, however, this disease generally has had a relatively favorable prognosis when treated quickly and properly. The possibilities of a prophylactic inoculation would be of great tactical importance.

(Signature) Grawitz

Of particular interest is the fact that Grawitz felt compelled to assure Himmler that Dohman is reliable, even though he is not a member of the SS. Grawitz had written earlier to SS Obergruppenführer Pohl.

Letter from Grawitz to Pohl, 19 May 1944[112]

The Führer's Commissioner-General, SS Brigadeführer Professor D [?] Brandt, called me with the request that I should assist him by placing prisoners at his disposal for research work into the cause of contagious jaundice (Hepatitis epidemica) which he was furthering considerably.

The work has been carried out up to now by a medical captain, Dr. Dohman, within the framework of the research place of the army medical inspectorate, with the participation of the Robert Koch Institute. It has up to now led to the result, in agreement with the result of other German research workers, that contagious jaundice is not carried by bacteria, but by a virus. In order to increase our knowledge, which is based up to now only on vaccination experiments from men to animals, the reverse way is now necessary, namely the vaccination of the cultivated virus germ into humans. One must reckon on cases of death.

Himmler's answer, is dated 16 June 1943.

Document re: No-11[113]
Office of U.S. Chief of Counsel

(Page 1 of original)
XIa -/- 43

112 Ibid. See also "Documented Report of the Sachsenhausen Trial" (Berlin: SWA Verlag, 1948).

113 Mitscherlich and Mielke, eds., *The Death Doctors,* pp. 165–169.

The Reichsführer SS
Day Book No. 1652/43
RF/BN

Field H.Q., 16 June 1943

Subject: Investigation of the cause of the infectious jaundice (Hepatitis epidemica).
Reference: Yours of 1 June 1953 [1943] – Az.: 420/IV/43 – Day Book No. 6/43 g.Kdos.

Top Secret

Reich Doctor SS and Police

4 Copies
3rd Copy

Berlin

I acknowledge the receipt of your letter of 1 June 1943.

1. I approve that 8 criminals condemned in Auschwitz (8 Jews of the Polish resistance movement condemned to death) should be used for experiments.
2. I agree that Dr. DOHMAN should make these experiments in Sachsenhausen.
3. I agree with your opinion that a real fight against the infectious jaundice would be of unheard value.

(S) H. HIMMLER

SS Obergruppenführer POHL, Berlin
Carbon copy forwarded with request that you duly note.
Signature
SS Obergruppenführer

Sachsenhausen and Natzweiler were the two concentration camps designated for the infectious hepatitis experiments. The men involved in the experiments, in addition to Grawitz, were Professor Kurt Gutzeit, consultant to the Army Medical Service Academy, Dr. Arnold Dohman, a bacteriologist, also a member of the Academy, an officer of the Army Medical Inspectorate, and Professor Dr. Eugen Haagen of the Air Force Medical Service. The Army Medical Service Academy was subordinated to Professor Handloser as Army Medical Inspector. Dr. Dohman previously had worked in Professor Gildemeister's laboratory in the Robert Koch Institute and had discovered a virus, not the expected bacterium is the causative agent of infectious hepatitis.

Haagen was anxious to start the experiments, as the following letter to the Office of the Chief of Luftwaffe Medical Service demonstrates.

Document re: No-126[114]
Office of U.S. Chief of Counsel

Oberstabsarzt Prof. Dr. Haagen
Consulting Hygienist
To the Physician for Air Fleet Reich
Strasbourg, 27/ 6/44

(To) Oberstabsarzt Prof. Dr. Kalk
With the Chief of the Luftwaffe Medical Service
Saalow

Dear Herr Kalk,

In the enclosure I send you a copy of a letter from Gutzeit and my reply. We must proceed as soon as possible with the experiments on human beings. These experiments of course should be carried out in Strasbourg or in its vicinity.* Could you in your official position take the necessary steps to obtain the required experimental subjects? I don't know what sort of subjects Gutzeit has at his disposal, whether they are soldiers or other people.**

I shall appreciate a prompt reply.

With cordial greetings,

Heil Hitler!
Yours
(Signed) Oberstabsarzt Prof. Dr. E. Haagen
Consulting Hygienist with Reich Luftflottenarzt
(Reich Air Force Physician)

* "Vicinity of Strasbourg" meant the Natzweiler camps.
** "Other people" meant concentration camp inmates

At the same time that Grawitz wrote to Himmler, Dohman, who previously had transferred tissue taken by liver biopsy of hepatitis patients into mice and chicken embryos, expressed a desire to inject substances taken from mice into human subjects.

After receiving Himmler's approval, Dohman traveled to Auschwitz and selected not eight but eleven prisoners between the ages of nine and nineteen whom he took back to Sachsenhausen.

114 Ibid.

Dr. Kurt Gutzeit, Professor of Internal Medicine in Breslau, who previously had worked on a vaccine for hepatitis in Crete, assisted Dohman. Gutzeit seems to have felt that the research was urgent, for he noted in a letter to Professor Wilhelm Fändrich, that he had attempted to persuade Dohman to "wake up from his lethargy" and speed up the experiments.[115]

Bruno Krieger, head of the block where Jewish children were isolated for research, reported that Dohman brought ampules onto the block, the contents of which he pumped through a narrow rubber tube into the gastrointestinal tracts of his young subjects.

Prof. Dr. Siegfried Handloser was connected with yet another series of jaundice experiments. These were carried out with his knowledge and approval in Buchenwald, by his subordinates. On 29 January 1945 Dr. Joachim Mrugowsky wrote to Grawitz as follows.

Document No-1303, Prosecution Exhibit 467[116]

> Haupsturmführer Professor Dr. Dressel, Director of the Hygienic Institute of the University of Leipzig, has cultivated a virus from persons suffering from hepatitis and succeeded in transplanting it to animals.
>
> It is necessary to make experiments on human beings in order to determine the fact that this virus is indeed the effective virus hepatitis epidemica. The plenipotentiary for research on epidemics in the Reich Research Council therefore addressed himself to me with the request to carry out the above experiments.
>
> I am asking you to obtain authorization from the Reich Leader SS to carry out the necessary experiments on 20 suitable prisoners who have hitherto never suffered from hepatitis epidemica, at the typhus experimental station of the concentration camp in Buchenwald.

The plenipotentiary for research on epidemics in the Reich Research Council who requested these experiments on concentration camp inmates was Generalarzt Schreiber, at the same time commander of Lehrgruppe C of the Military Medical Academy under Handloser *(Tr. P. 5402).* Handloser had given Schreiber the responsibility of coordinating jaundice research.

At Nuremberg, Dr. Rudolf Emil Brandt gave details of the organization of these experiments.

115 Klee, *Auschwitz*, pp. 259–268.

116 Letter from Mrugowsky to Grawitz, 29 January 1945, Document No-1303, Prosecution Exhibit 467, in *Trials NMT,* vol. 1, pp. 494–495.

Translation of Document No-371[117] Office of U.S. Chief of Counsel

I, Rudolf Emil Herman Brandt, being duly sworn, depose and state:

1. I am the same Rudolf Brandt who has heretofore sworn to an affidavit on the 30th day of August 1946 concerning low pressure experiments performed on involuntary human beings in the Dachau Concentration Camps and to certain other affidavits concerning medical experiments on involuntary human subjects.

2. For the same reasons set forth in paragraphs 1, 2 and 3 of my affidavit of 30 August 1946, I am able to make this statement concerning experiments performed on human beings.

Experiments to determine the cause of epidemic Jaundice (Hepatitis Epidemica)

3. About the middle of 1943, Dr. Grawitz, Reichsarzt SS, wrote Himmler that Dr. Karl Brandt wished to obtain prisoners for experimentation on the causes of a jaundice epidemic. He had been doing research on this problem with the assistance of Dr. Dohman, a medical officer attached to the Army Medical Inspectorate and the Robert Koch Institute. Experiments had thus far disclosed that contagious jaundice is transferred by a virus and human beings were desired for inoculation with germs which had been cultivated in animals. Grawitz advised that death of some of the experimental subjects must be expected. He wanted to know if Dr. Dohman would be permitted to carry out the experiments at the Sachsenhausen Concentration Camp, as desired by Dr. Karl Brandt.

4. Himmler wrote Grawitz that Dr. Dohman had his permission to conduct the experiments at Sachsenhausen and for that purpose he had Oswald Pohl allocate a number of prisoners to be used as experimental subjects. I know that these experiments were carried out and that some of the prisoners died as a result.

5. Dr. Eugene [sic] Haagen, Oberstabsarzt and consultant in hygiene for the Luftwaffe, had also been doing research work at the Natzweiler Concentration Camp in an effort to discover an effective inoculation against epidemic jaundice. As I recall, Dr. Dohman collaborated with Haagen in 1944 at Natzweiler and experiments on involuntary human beings were conducted which resulted in deaths.

6. These experiments were of course well known to Karl Brandt as he was personally furthering them. Handloser and Schroeder must also

117 Deposition of Rudolf Emil Brandt, Office of the U.S. Chief of Counsel, Document No-371, in *Trials NMT.*

> have known of them because Dohman and Haagen were doctors in the Medical Services of the Army and the Luftwaffe, respectively. Generalarzt Paul Rostock also was well informed on all research work of this nature.

Professor Eugen Haagen confirmed that the tests had occurred.

Extract from Haagen's Declaration, Document No-011

> The Military Tribunal of the Soviet Zone of Occupation, dealing with former commandants and administrative staff of the Sachsenhausen concentration camp, sat from the 31 October 1947 to the following day under the chairmanship of Colonel Mayorov. It sentenced Dr. Heinz Baumkotter, Senior Physician of the camp, to imprisonment for life with compulsory labour. Judgment mentioned among a number of experiments performed on prisoners by Baumkotter the infection with jaundice in 1944 of six girl prisoners between the ages of 8 and 14. The object was to test a new treatment of the disease.[118]

These are the only available clinical or experimental documents dealing with research on infectious hepatitis.

SURGICAL EXPERIMENTS

In the Second World War, the German military suffered heavy casualties, among them disabling injuries. The bone, muscle and nerve regeneration, and bone transplantation experiments conducted at the Ravensbrück concentration camp on female prisoners aimed at improving the rehabilitation rate among injured soldiers. So high was the importance of these experiments that they were directed personally by the head of the SS Medical Service, Dr. Ernst-Robert Grawitz.

The experimental procedures caused incredible suffering during surgery and the prolonged post-operative periods. Not only did they lead to the deaths of many research subjects, but also they left most of the survivors permanently disabled with experimentally induced illnesses and crippling injuries.

118 Mitscherlich and Mielke, eds., *The Death Doctors*, p. 167, citing *Documented Report of the Sachsenhausen Trial* (Berlin: SWA Verlag, 1948).

The following section presents affidavits and personal testimonies from survivors of the experiments, among them several former prisoner physicians, as well as testimonies of the expert witness at the Nuremberg Doctors' Trial.

Translation of Document No-871[119]
Office of Chief of Counsel

Extract
Deposition under oath of B. J. Zofia, female of 24 Av. de l'Yser, BRUSSELS,
Sworn before Major Arthur Keith Mant, R.R. M.C.
Of the Crime Investigation Unit at Brussels on 12 August 1946

I, Zofia Baj, 24 Avenue de l'Yser, Brussels, being duly sworn, depose and say:

Two experimental operations were carried out on me during my imprisonment in camp. The first on 3 November 1942 and the second on 23 February 1943.

...The operation lasted for 2 hours 45 minutes.

...I recovered consciousness later on in the evening, and I noticed that I could not move because my legs and hips were in a plaster-cast. I was suffering terribly and I screamed with pain, so that Fina came and gave me another glass with morphia.

...I did not leave the revier [sick-bay] between the first and the second operation.

After the first radiograph, which followed the first operation, Dr. Maczka told me that 5 centimeters of my left peroneus had been removed and about 5 or 6 of the right peroneus. About 10 centimeters of periosteum of both shinbones had been scraped and five holes had been made as deep as the marrow on the right shinbone and six on the left shinbone, also as deep as the marrow.

...My second operation was carried out on 23 February 1943... Maczka told me later during this second operation, my legs were opened up again and that the gaps between the two halves of the perones had closed by about 1 centimeter. During the operation, another piece was removed from the four ends of the peroneus, but nothing was done to the shinbones. After that my legs were sewn up again, but a curved nee-

119 Deposition of B. J. Zofia before the Nuremberg War Tribunal, 12 August 1946, in RG-30.001M.

dle and about 20 centimeters of silk thread were left in the wound of my left leg. This gave me horrible pain later on and was removed by Tzaite in February 1945.

...One week after the second operation, I was told that I could try to walk. As it was not possible, I was given two walking-sticks and only 6 months later could I walk without these walking-sticks.

At present, my legs hurt:

1. When I go downstairs,
2. I cannot run because my toes slip,
3. When I put my feet in hot water they contract and shake.

The following document offers a vivid description of the experimental process, and of the terrible suffering of the women who were made to serve as subjects. It also reveals a likely connection between these surgeries and the previously described phlegmone experiments.[120] The writer mentions that the attending prisoner doctors thought she had been infected with gas gangrene; gas gangrene, of course, is a form of phlegmone, a deep tissue infection with grave consequences for the victim.

Experimental Operations in Ravensbrück: A Reminiscence[121]

By Pelagia Mackowska
Former prisoner of Ravensbrück – Extract

As I wake up, I know that I am in the infirmary and that I have been submitted to an operation. There is a feeling of dull pain and numbness in my right leg. Dusk comes. I ask if it is still Wednesday. Jadwiga Kaminska, who has already been twice operated on with another group of women, bends over me. She hops about on one leg, very brave and kind to us, immobilized and helpless. She smiles at me and says, "No, dear, it is already Thursday." So I have slept for nearly two days and night without interruption... My temperature must be very high for all I know, for everything around me looks so blurred and unreal.

On the fourth day of the operation, we are being taken to something known as the "changing of dressings". We are taken to the operating room on the infirmary stretchers. There our faces are covered and a vivisection is performed.

120 For documents on the phlegmone experiments, see the discussion in this chapter.

121 In *Experimental Operations on Prisoners of Ravensbrück Concentration Camp* (Poznan and Warsaw: Wydawicho Zachodnie, 1960).

I don't know who is doing it. I only feel an indescribable pain surging from my leg and rising through my body up to the brain. I moan for one cannot help moaning. I bite into my own fingers and I think that I am unable to bear that infernal pain.

We begin to decay. We are rotting. From under some of the dressings we can hear gurgle of secreted pus which drips through the paper bandages. We are not allowed to touch anything. We must wait for the dressing.

The second dressing is now over. I overcame the suffering and I was able to notice to-day that they were putting some hard metal instruments into the wound, that a kidney-shaped dish was standing by the tray and that something extracted from the wound was being carefully put into the dish. I imagine that they are storing the pus secreted by my wound. For that matter there are several theories sprung from nowhere on this subject. The women doctors, our co-prisoners, although not initiated into these criminal secrets, put two and two together and draw their own conclusions from what we tell them and from their own observations. I am said to have been infected with gaseous gangrene.

I feel very much worse today. My leg is extremely painful. Temperature of nearly 41 °C. There is buzzing and roaring in my head. I beg for my bandages to be unwrapped for their pressure is unbearable, my leg is evidently swelling fast.

Although the prospect of having our dressings changed has always filled us with dread, I look forward to it today because I suppose they will help me, seeing that they still need me in my capacity as a guinea-pig. Indeed I was immediately given an anaesthetic, another incision has been made and a drain was introduced into the wound. I felt awful after waking from the anaesthetic. I had a long spell of nausea which utterly wore me out, but I realized at the same time that I had been saved from death – for the time at least.

I was anaesthetized again and another incision was made because the infection had not been checked. But after the third anaesthetic came relief and visible improvement.

The wounds, of course, do not show any intention of healing. They remain open, raw and purulent, but it is of no consequence at all to people whose attitude towards us is devoid of human feelings.

I was discharged from the infirmary at the end of November. On that day another numerous group of women from our transport was brought in to serve as new experimental subjects. As I was leaving the infirmary they were all ready for the operations. They lay on the beds, drugged by the initial injections waiting their turn. We parted not knowing if fate would allow us to meet again.

Every two or three days we now had to go to the infirmary (or rather to be carried there) for our dressings to be done in the usual way by some of our fellow-prisoners employed in the infirmary. Extraordinary things used to happen there sometimes, as for instance when an abscess formed on my leg outside the wound. When it was cut open, several splinters of glass and bits of cloth or some other fabric were extracted from the wound (exactly three splinters in two dressings). Sensational! Who had not seen it would not believe it. They said we were raving mad! Which of course might be true after all that we had been through and after all those narcotic drugs. It was not until the Nuremberg Trial that Dr. Fischer explained that they had deliberately put some foreign matter into our wounds to increase the infection process. So I was not quite mad after all!

Extract from the Affidavit of Fritz Ernst Fischer, 19 November 1945[122]

[Dr. Fritz Ernst Fischer was one of the SS doctors who performed the experiments.]

After the arrival of Doctor Stumpfegger from general headquarters in the fall of 1942, Professor Gebhardt declared before some of his coworkers that he had received orders to continue with the tests at Ravensbrück on a larger scale. In this connection, questions of plastic surgery which would be of interest after the end of the war should be clarified. Doctor Stumpfegger was supposed to test the free transplantation of bones. Since Professor Gebhardt knew that I had worked in preparation for my habilitation at the university on regeneration of tissues, he ordered me to prepare a surgical plan for these operations, which after it had been approved, he directed me to carry out immediately. Moreover, Doctor Keller and Doctor Heissmeyer were ordered to perform their own series of experiments. Professor Gebhardt was also considering a plan to form the basis of an operative technique of remobilization of joints. Besides the above, Doctors Schulze and Schulze-Hagen participated in this conference.

I had selected the regeneration of muscle for the sole reason because the incision necessary for this purpose was the slightest. The operation was carried out as follows:

122 Affidavit of Fritz Ernst Fischer, 19 November 1945, in RG-30.001M, pp. 9–12.

Evipan and ether were used as an anaesthetic, and a five centimeter longitudinal incision was made at the outer side of the upper leg. Subsequent to the cutting through the fascia, a piece of the muscle was removed which was the size of the cup of the little finger. The fascia and skin were closed in accordance with the normal technique of aseptic surgery. Afterwards a cast was applied. After one week the skin wound was split under the same narcotic conditions, and part of the muscle around the area cut out was removed. Afterwards the fascia and the sewed-up part of the skin were immobilized in a cast.

Since Professor Gebhardt did not ask me any longer for these operations, I discontinued them.

Dr. Zofia Maczka, a physician and former prisoner at Ravensbrück, made the following declaration about these experiments at the British Consulate in Stockholm, where she was residing at the time, on 16 April 1946.

Declaration of Zofia Maczka[123]

The aseptic, experimental operations consisted of:
Bone experiments
Muscle experiments
Nerve experiments

The bone experiments were checked by X-ray photographs. As ward attendant (Revierarbeiterin) I had to do all the X-ray photographs. In this way I was given the opportunity of gaining an insight in this matter. The following were carried: a) bone breaking, b) bone transplantation, c) bone grafting.

As to a): On the operation table, the bone of the lower part of both legs were broken into several pieces with a hammer, later they were joined with clips (for instance Janiga MARCZEWSKA) or without clips (for instance Leonarda BIEN) and were put into a plaster cast. This was removed after several days and the legs remained without plaster casts until they healed.

As to (b): The transplantations were carried out in the usual way, except that whole pieces of the fibula were cut out, sometimes with

123 Declaration of Zofia Maczka, 16 April 1946, Document No-861, in RG-30.001M, pp. 3–9.

periosteum, sometimes without periosteum. The most typical operation of this kind was carried out on Krystyna DABSKA.

As to (c) Bone grafting: These operations were with the school of Professor Gebhardt. During the preparatory operation two bone splints were put on the tibia of both legs; during the second operation such bone splints were cut out together with the attached bones and were taken to Hohenlychen. As a supplement to the bone splint operations such operations were also carried out on two protective prisoners who suffered from deformation of bones of the osteomyelitis type. These two were not Poles. One of them was a German from the Jehovah's Witness group (Bibleforscherverein), Maria KONWITSCHKA, and the other was a Ukrainian, Maria HRETSCHANA. It was interesting for Dr. Gebhardt to see how the diseased bones would react to such an operation.

The muscle experiments consisted of many operations, always on the same spot, the upper or lower part of the leg. On each further operation larger and larger pieces of muscles were cut out. Once a small piece of bone was planted into a muscle (this happened to BABINSKA). During nerve operations, parts of nerves were removed (for instance, Barbara PYTLEWSKA).

What problem did Prof. Gebhardt and his school wish to solve by these experiments? The problem of the regeneration of bones, muscles and nerves.

Was the thing carried out? No. It was not checked at all or only insufficiently. I do not know what was done at Hohenlychen, with those pieces of bone, muscle and nerves which were cut out and taken there.

What was the fate of the patients after they left the hospital? Almost all of the patients became cripples, and have suffered very much as a result of these operations. Even more severe was the moral torture inflicted on them as they lived under the conviction that they would all be shot in order that they should not be evidence of these murderous operations. The camp authorities – Commandant Suhren, Adjutant Braeuning and Oberaufseherin Binz – ensured through their orders that the victims should not forget that they were condemned to death. In the meantime, six of the patients were shot after surviving the operations.

If I am to give an opinion on these operations, I must say that the operations were carried out because it was the program of National-Socialist Germany to make experiments on protective prisoners in Concentration Camps, and that these experiments were carried out on the level on which medical science and morals were prevailing in Germany since 1933.

As a supplement to these operations I am submitting a description of "special operations" which were carried out at the same time.

A few abnormal protective prisoners (psychologically ill) were chosen and brought to the operating table and amputations of the whole leg (at the hip joint) were carried out, or on others, amputation of the whole arm (with the shoulder-blade) were carried out. Afterwards, the victims (if they still lived) were killed by means of Evipan injections and the leg or arm was taken to Hohenlychen and served the purposes known to Prof. Gebhardt. Ten such operations, approximately, were carried out.

During the whole time these operations were carried out, I was employed as a worker in the ward and investigated this matter risking my own life, with the idea that it was my duty, if I were saved, to tell the truth to the whole world. I conclude my statement with two questions: What kind of recompense can the world offer to those who were operated on in such a manner? What kind of justice has the world for those who carried out such operations?

(Signed) Dr. med. Zofia Maczka,
X-ray specialist from Krakow, former political protective prisoner,
No. 7403 at Ravensbrück, now at Stockholm,
serafirmerlasarettet Roentgen.

Stockholm, 16.4.46.

Translation of Document No-876[124]
Office of Chief of U.S. Counsel

Deposition of Jadwiga Kaminska

Deposition under oath of Jadwiga KAMINSKA
Born 14.4.14, female, of the Polish Red Cross, 24 Av. de l'Yser, Brussels, Belgium
Sworn before Major Arthur Keith MANT, RAMC of War Crimes Investigation Unit at Brussels on 12 August 1946

I, Jadwiga Kaminska, 24 Avenue de L'Yser, Brussels, make oath and state as follows.

I was arrested on 18 March 1941 and arrived in Ravensbrück on 27 September 1941 and left the camp on or about 16 April 1946.

124 Deposition of Jadwiga Kaminska at Crimes Investigation Unit, Brussels, Belgium, 12 August 1946, Office of Chief of Counsel, Translation of Document No-876, in RG-30.001M.

I was twice operated on during my stage in the camp. The first time was August 15, 1942.

I was in great pain after the operation.

About a week after the operation, I first saw my wound. It was about 10 cm long and 5 cm wide and full of green pus and very inflamed. (It is now 1 cm long and about 3 cm in width).

I was operated on the second time on 13 Sept. 1942.

After my second operation, I stayed in the Revier three months, during all that time with fever and felt very weak and I was given no care.

When I left the Revier, three months after that operation, my fever had almost gone but my wound was still open... In March 1943 my leg was still discharging pus.

In February 1945, the order came out that all of us who had been operated on were to remain in our blocks. We knew this meant we were to be liquidated.

...My leg is now healed but gets very tired, very quickly, and during the last three months I have had intermittent fevers which my doctor tells me is due to recurrence of infection in my leg and also the glands (ganglions) in my right groin have become swollen.

(Signed) Jadwiga KAMINSKA

Sworn by the said Deponent KAMINSKA Jadwiga, voluntarily in BRUSSELS on 12th August 1946 before me, Major Arthur Keith MANT, RAMC, Investigation Officer detailed by C.-in-C. British Army of the Rhine.

(Signed) A. K. MANT, Major
Investigating Officer

As in all cases, experiments on bone regeneration and bone transplant were performed with total disregard to the effects on the subject. Dr. Franz Stumpfegger's experiments are a good illustration of that.

Stumpfegger, Himmler's personal physician and protégé, who was on the surgical staff at the SS hospital Hohenlychen, was determined to turn that institution into an experimentation center for bone graft procedures. His plan was to have pieces of bone removed from inmates at Ravensbrück and transplanted into patients at Hohenlychen.

It happened that there was a German civilian at Hohenlychen on whom Dr. Gebhardt had performed surgery to remove a cancerous tumor. During the operation, the shoulder-blade, the site of the tumor, had to be sacrificed.

Stumpfegger proposed a graft. Gebhardt agreed and summoned Fischer, who regularly operated at Ravensbrück.

Gebhardt was responsible for finding a Polish woman in good health, a Ravensbrück inmate, of course, to serve as a graft donor. He had two SS men drag the unfortunate victim into the bunker where he anaesthetized her and Fischer proceeded with the surgery. The woman's shoulder blade was removed and immediately put into a container maintained at 100 °F. Fischer left for Hohenlychen where Gebhardt and Stumpfegger were waiting. Gebhardt performed the surgery; Stumpfegger merely inserted the shoulder-blade.

At Nuremberg, Gebhardt referred to the operation as a surgical success. He did not seem to be concerned about the fate of the Polish prisoner who involuntarily supplied the shoulder blade.

Stumpfegger, driven by experimental zeal, decided, with Gebhardt's approval and Fischer's cooperation, to expand the scope of this research. He chose two Polish women for a test. First, he broke their tibias. One of them was given a cast with an iron pin inside to support the bone, the other a plain plaster cast. Three weeks later, in Stumpfegger's presence, the casts were removed. The SS surgeon compared the two healing patterns, then removed the pin from the one subject's leg and left the broken bones to heal without casts.

One sixteen-year-old girl was operated on six times. The first time Stumpfegger cut the exterior surface of the two tibias. The second time, a few weeks later, he removed some bone fragments to take X-rays. He continued this way even though the subject was completely disabled as a consequence. Similar procedures were performed on other girls, so soon the infirmary was full of haggard young girls pulling themselves around on crutches. Herta Oberheuser and Gerhard Schiedlausky, the ward doctors, didn't hesitate to hit the girls if their moaning or weeping became annoying. The imperturbable Stumpfegger continued amassing data he considered highly interesting and valuable.

One day a Polish doctor, one of the rare prisoners to be employed according to his skills, received a visit from Dr. Oberheuser, who brought along a prisoner who was unable to stand on her feet. Her legs bore the signs of deep incisions. An X-ray showed that 1- to 2-inch fragments of the fibula had been removed from each leg. The periosteum on the right was still intact; that on the left had been removed. Horrified, the doctor asked Oberheuser how she hoped to obtain bone regeneration without the periosteum. Oberheuser replied, "That's exactly what we're trying to find out."

The words of Mrs. Zdenka, a survivor physician witness, bring alive the scene on the wards.

Translation of Document No-875, Prosecution Exhibit 230[125]

Affidavit of Mrs. Zdenka Nedvedova-Nejedla, M.D., of Prague, concerning Experimental Operations conducted on Fellow Inmates at Ravensbrück Concentration Camp

1. I, Zdenka Nedvedova-Nejedla, M.D., came to Ravensbrück concentration camp in a transport from Auschwitz on 19 August 1943, and I worked in the sick bay as a doctor prisoner from September 1943 until 30 May 1945. In the beginning I worked in the Department for Contagious Diseases at Station No. 1 and the Ambulatory. Besides this, I was in charge of Sucking Block from the fall of 1944 until May 1945.

2. Of the victims of experimental operations, I nursed personally Helena Piasecka, who was suffering from chronic osteomyelitis after completed operation of both shin bones. I knew that these operations were performed under Professor Gebhardt's supervision by Doctor Fischer, and a woman, Doctor Oberheuser, from the SS Hospital Hohenlychen, but I do not know which one of them had operated on Piasecka. The operation was performed in the "bunker", camp prison, where there were not even the most primitive sanitary installations and even fewer aseptic installations. Her general condition was good, but the defect in both bones made her an invalid for life. Before that operation Piasecka was completely healthy.

3. All women on whom experimental operations had been performed were placed in one block and they were generally known as "rabbits", so that I saw the effects of the operations on those women who had survived them. In each case of abbreviation of limbs, muscular atrophy of the highest degree set in, proving a grave injury of nerves during operations and deep indrawn scars where parts of muscles had festered away.

4. From lay reports of nursing personnel without any special training, I tried to construct the types of experimental operations:

a) Cultures of virulent germs (streptococci, staphylococci, maybe even tetanus and gas gangrene) were injected subcutaneously, intra-muscularly, and even directly into bones. These were the attempts to produce osteomyelitis experimentally. The resulting sepsis was checked by daily examination of the blood and urine to test the effectiveness of new medicaments of the sulfanilamide group.

125 Document No-875, Prosecution Exhibit 230, reprinted in Aziz, *Doctors of Death,* vol. 3, pp. 176–184.

b) Parts of long bones, as much as 5 centimeters (fibulae and tibiae), were removed and in some cases replaced by metal or left without connection. These operations were probably to prove the inability of bone to grow without periosteum.

c) High amputations were performed; for example, even whole arms with shoulder blade or legs with osiliaca were amputated. These operations were performed mostly on insane women who were immediately killed after the operation by a quick injection of Evipan. All specimens gained in operations were carefully wrapped up in sterile gauze and immediately transported to the SS hospital nearby (Hohenlychen presumably), where they were to be used in the attempt to heal the injured limbs of wounded German soldiers.

5. Operations were performed on 1 Yugoslav, 1 Czech, 2 Ukrainian, 2 German, and about 18 Polish women, of whom 6 were operated on by force in the bunker with the help of SS men. Two of them were shot after their operation wounds had healed. After operations, no one except SS nurses was admitted to the persons operated on, whole nights they lay without assistance and it was not permitted to administer sedatives even against the most intensive postoperational pains. From the persons operated on, 11 died or were killed, and 71 remained invalids for life.

6. The report mentioned in paragraph 3 to 5 was prepared on the basis of evidence given to me at Ravensbrück in the autumn of 1943 by these fellow prisoners: Zofia Maczka, M.D., Poland; Isa Siczynsak, medical student, Krakow, Poland; Jolay Krzyanowska, medical student; Krakow, Poland; Krisa Iwanska, medical student, Krakow, Poland; Emilie Skrbkova, medical student, Praha, Czechoslovakia; and Inka Katnarova, M.D., Hradec Kralove, Czechoslovakia.

Hohenlychen, identified above as the institution that supplied the doctors who took tissue from the involuntary experimental subjects at Ravensbrück, was an SS hospital during the war. It had been founded in 1902 as a sanitorium for women and children suffering from tuberculosis. In 1933, the institution was reorganized as part of the Nazification of medicine. First, the old board of directors was replaced by one consisting of Nazi officials and SS doctors, among them Reichsgesundheitsführer, Staatsrat und SS Brigadenführer Dr. Leonard Conti, Reichsärzteführer Dr. Gerhard Wagner, and, from 1936, Reichsführer der SS Heinrich Himmler, and Reichsartz der SS und der Polizei Dr. Ernst Grawitz. SS physician Dr. Karl Gebhardt was charged with the direction of the institution. The institution was transformed between 1933 and 1937 into a kind of sports medicine center, focusing on the rehabilitation of sports (and later also workplace) injuries. Facilities included a gymnasium, playing fields, swimming pools, and a boathouse. An on-grounds hospital building was outfitted with surgery and internal medicine wards; other buildings housed patients with knee and bone injuries or diseases. Although women and children with tuberculosis were still accepted for treatment, the number of beds for tuberculosis patients was starkly reduced.

After the war began, Hohenlychen was again transformed, this time into a military hospital for members of the armed forces and the SS. With the assistance of physicians Fritz Fischer and Herta Oberheuser, Gebhardt oversaw bone transplantation experiments with healthy tissue extracted from the female prisoners at Ravensbrück concentration camp.

An article printed in 1944 in the *German Surgical Journal* describes the results of the Hohenlychen transplantation experiments in clinical detail, but, of course, it fails to report that the tissue donations were involuntary, extracted from concentration camp inmates. Certainly the SS doctors knew the origins of the tissues they were using, for they were involved in extracting them too. But readers of the journal report learned only the results of the transplantation experiments; the sufferings of the involuntary donors were SS secrets revealed only later as Nazi physicians were brought to trial before international tribunals. Whatever the secrecy, one might reasonably have expected ethical physicians to wonder where so much human tissue was being obtained. The text of the journal article, reprinted below, is taken from published trial records.[126]

Translation of Gebhardt, Fischer, Oberheuser, Document No-6 Gebhardt, Fischer, Oberheuser Defense Exhibit 9

Extract from "Clinical and Practice Weekly" in *Journal for the Practicing Physician*
Re: Bone Transplantation
Editors: Dr. Herbert Volkmann and Dr. V. E. Mertens, Munich 2, Alfonsstrasse 1

126 The Hohenlychen description is adapted from the two-part web article by Hans Waltrich, "Zur Geschichte der Heilstalten vom Roten Kreuz in Hohenlychen…" The printed document is a translation of Gebhardt, Fischer, Oberheuser Document No-6, Gebhardt, Fischer, Oberheuser Defense, Exhibit 9, Stockholm, 16 April 1946. Originally published in the *German Surgical Journal,* 299, H.9-12 (1944), (Frankfurt-am-Main: H. Floercken-Frankfurt-am-Main).

Franz Stumpfegger – Hohenlychen: "The Five Autoplastic Bone Transplantations in the Restorative Surgery of Limbs – Experiences and Results"

During the past 10 years, 471 free autoplastic bone transplantations were carried out in Hohenlychen. Recent research results clearly showed that apart from the osteoplastic activity, a metaplastic formation of new bone occurs in the tissue. The newly formed bone trabeculae between transplant and old bone begin to connect with those formed in the osteoid tissue in the seventh week, and in this way constitute the bone connection between the graft and the original bone which have completely grown together in the ninth week. After the twelfth week no old bone can be detected in the entire region of the original graft, but only new bone trabecula. The question of the ever present hematoma can be answered in this way; a blood extravasation, lying in the gap between the transplant and the old bone, and not being subject to pressure, represents an adequate stimulation to the mesenchymal germinal tissue formation, while the large hemorrhage represents a negative stimulation and permits only a scarry connection of the transplant and the defective stump. The periosteum is no more important than the other layers, it is transplanted with the bone, because in connection with the bone it has osteogenic properties, but above all it effects a speedy supply from the surroundings.

A careful technique must be employed to spare the tissue layers, and bleeding must be stanched. Foreign bodies in the shape of wire slings to hold the transplant usually heal well into the body. Firm fixation in a plaster cast safeguards the result. When the graft has taken, a careful start with remedial exercises may be made in the third or fourth month. The clinical use of free bone transplantations is discussed with the help of numerous examples and many X-ray illustrations. The first task of the bone transplant to bridge over a gap in the bone is to provide sufficient support for the defective stump and, therefore, it has to be fairly strong. Bone splinters in the lower arm have roentgenologically completely taken after $1–1^1/_2$ years, those in the tibia after $1^1/_2–2$ years. The free bone transplant, some distance from the joints, has proved to be particularly valuable with the usual dislocations of the shoulder and the hip joints. The overlapping bone ridge prevents the bone from coming out of the articular cavity.

In the course of years, the piece lying in the soft parts is considerably reduced, so that only a small bone ridge remains. The graft effects a regeneration of the damaged edge of the articular cavity and in this way prevents further dislocation. Bone transplants in bone gaps after removal of growths are subject to special conditions of taking. Hyperemic phenomena in the zone of the tumor edge in the form of a mild inflammation, possibly also fermentation processes, accelerate the taking of the transplant compared with the process in healthy tissue. Increased local resorption processes, occasionally with spontaneous fractures, infrequently prevail, but they again are apt to heal well. In wounds which heal with difficulty owing to suppurative inflammations, there is a great danger of the transplant being pushed out. When the whole transplant region is inflamed, total sequestration cannot be stopped. If suppuration remains localized, partial sequestration of the transplantation must be awaited.

Several testimonies from the various post-war doctors' trials are printed below.

Extracts from the Testimony of Prosecution Witness, Miss Karolewska[127]

Q. Witness, you have told the Tribunal that you were operated on the second time on the 16th of September 1942. Is that right?
A. Yes.

Q. When did you leave the hospital after this second operation?
A. After the second operation I left the hospital on 6 October.

Q. Was your leg healed at the time?
A. My leg was swollen up, caused me great pain, and the pus drained from my leg.

Q. Were you able to work?
A. I was unable to work, and I had to stay in bed because I could not walk.

Q. Do you remember when you got up out of bed and were able to walk?
A. I stayed in bed several weeks, and then I got up and tried to walk.

Q. How long was it until your leg healed?
A. The pus was flowing from my leg till June 1943; and at that time my wound was healed.

127 Testimony of Prosecution Witness, Valdislava Karolewska, *The Doctors' Trial: The Medical Case of the Subsequent Nuremberg Proceedings,* United States National Archives, Record Group 238, M887. See also the National Holocaust Memorial Museum website.

Miss Karolewska had four (!) more operations on her legs, the last one on 15 September 1943. She stayed in the hospital for six months after the last surgery. At the Doctors' Trial she additionally testified:

> Q. Do you still suffer any effects from the operations?
> A. I am weak. I have no strength to work and my legs get swollen very easily.

Extract from the Testimony of Prosecution Expert Witness Dr. Leo Alexander[128]

> Direct Examination
>
> Q. Doctor, can you express any opinion as to the purpose of the type of operation to which she [Karolewska] was subjected, that is the bone removal?
> A. I think it must have been one of the bone transplantation experiments. Chances are that this tibial graft was either implanted in another person or grafts had been exchanged. Of course today, 3 years after the experiment, no trace of transplantation is left in this individual. Or if the object was, as alleged, in some statements I have seen, that tibial grafts were exchanged between the two legs, one must conclude that the experiment was negative because there is no evidence that a graft took. All we see now are the consequences of removal of a graft, and the graft had included the entire compact part of the bone, otherwise the repair would have been better. If some part of the compact had remained, the periosteum would have probably regenerated and today, 3 years after the operation, no X-ray would have shown the defect. So I feel that rather deep grafts were taken which went down into the spongiosa. Whether anything was replaced that later was destroyed, I do no know, except the patient stated that there was purulent discharge, indicating that the wound had become infected, and her statement of a subsequent operation, in fact, if I am not mistaken, two subsequent operations, indicates the probability that the grafts did not take and that they were removed after infection had become obvious.

128 Testimony of Prosecution Expert Witness, Dr. Leo Alexander, mimeographed transcript, 20 December 1947, pp. 838–847.

Extracts from the Testimony of Prosecution Witness Jadwiga Dzido[129]

Q. Witness, what is your full name?
A. Jadwiga Dzido.

Q. You are a citizen of Poland?
A. Yes.

Q. Have you come here to Nuremberg voluntarily to testify?
A. Yes...

Q. Were you ever operated on in the Ravensbrück concentration camp?
A. I was operated on in November 1942...

Q. When did you finally leave Ravensbrück?
A. On 27 April 1945.

Q. Have you ever received any treatment since you have left Ravensbrück in the last year?
A. Yes.

Q. Tell us what treatment you have received?
A. Dr. Gruzan in Warsaw transplanted tendons in my leg.

Q. When did he do that?
A. On 25 September 1945.

Q. Do you have to wear any special shoes now, Witness?
A. Yes, I should wear them, but I can't afford to buy them.

Extracts from the Testimony of Prosecution Expert Witness Dr. Leo Alexander[130]

Q. Dr. Alexander, have you examined Miss Dzido before today?
A. Yes, sir, I did on several occasions during the last 3 days.

Q. During your examination, did you have x-rays made of the patient's legs?
A. I did, sir.

129 Testimony of Prosecution Witness, Jadwiga Dzido, 20 December 1947, pp. 388–847.
130 From Testimony of the Prosecution Expert Witness, Leo Alexander, 20 December 1947, Mimeographed Transcript, pp. 848–855.

Q. Doctor, this x-ray you are referring to now is Document No-1092?
A. This is Document No-1091. The arrow points to the osteoporotic atrophy of the tibia. Document No-1092 is the X-ray of the leg. It shows the fibula which is the smaller of the two larger bones of the leg, about in the middle between the area just mentioned under the bracket called "B". On the side, looking toward the tibia is the osteoperiostitis of the periosteum. This group of marks is particularly severe in the smaller area which I have marked with the bracket "A", which indicates a smaller area of the shaft of the tibia within the larger area of the disturbance marked as "B". This alteration is indicative and consists of an ordinary inactive Coxa, which in view of the osteoperiostitis of the periosteum was probably an osteomyelitis process. However, there is no active osteomyelitis at the present examination of the right foot. In pictures 1093 and 1094, it shows arthritic changes of the cuneiform navicula joints with narrowing of the joint spaces and increased marginal sclerosis. This has been marked in the X-ray with an arrow pointing to the joint. The other prints are the same. The prints have come out too dark, but it shows the condition clearly in the film. This arthritis is due to the immobilization of the right foot. Secondary to the muscles and especially the paralysis of the perineal nerve. It is evidently arthritis of an immobilization nature which one sees also by inspection of the patient's foot.

Q. Doctor, can you determine from your examination –
A. (Interposing) 1094 – have I mentioned it? – shows the same as 1093 in a slightly different exposure. The marks are the same pointing to the most marked arthritis between the cuneiform navicular joints.

Q. Doctor, in your opinion, from your examination of this patient, can you determine what was the purpose of the experiment?
A. It appears that in this experiment a highly infectious agent was implanted, probably without the addition of a bacteria static agent such as sulfanilamide, and for that reason, the infection got out of hand and became very extensive.

The following is a legal document from the Commission for the Investigation of German Crimes in Poland, submitted to the International Military Tribunal in Nuremberg.

Translation of Document No-871[131]
Office of U.S. Chief of Counsel

Certificate

Under the participation of the president of the Chief Commission, Minister of Justice Harry Sventkovsko, Professor for Criminal Prosecution Dr. Stanislav Batavi, Dr. Stanislav Ploskov, the Justices of the Regional Court of Justice in Warsaw Nicholai Galfter, Dr. Alfred Fiderkevitsh, and the expert physicians: Prof. of forensic medicine, Dr. Victor Grshuvo-Dombrovski and Prof. Dr. Adam Groots, the Chief Commissioner for the Investigation of German Crimes in Poland, conducted the investigation of the conditions concerning the physiopathologic experiments on Polish women who were inmates of the concentration camp Ravensbrück-Mecklenburg.

The Commission interrogated 6 women who had been in this camp during the period of 1942–1945. As a result of this interrogation, the medical examination and legal expertise of those interrogated women, it was established: The concentration camp of Ravensbrück was an institution in which physiopathological experiments had been conducted by force on living human beings. Apart from the 6 women, experiments were conducted on 50 other Polish women. The number of female prisoners who served as "guinea pigs" was considerable.

When the prisoners saw which goal the German physicians had in mind, they tried to resist physically in order to escape in this manner the coming experiments. The resistence, which the women showed, was broken down by the Germans with brute force. The experiments were conducted by the physicians and the nursing personnel. We succeeded in establishing the names of the following criminals: Prof. Dr. Gebhardt, Dr. Fischer, Dr. Oberhauser, Dr. Rosenthal, Dr. Schiedlausky, Dr. Trommer. The experiments consisted in carrying out on women special surgical operations, experiments which were performed under anesthesia.

The resisting women were locked by force into a bunker and were operated there under primitive conditions without observing the hygienical conditions.

After the operation on the "sick persons", there appeared for several days, sometimes even for several weeks, high temperatures up to 41 °C, pains, swelling and bad discharge of pus.

131 Certificate by Commission for the Investigation of German Crimes in Poland, USSR-406, Office of the U.S. Chief of Counsel, Document No-871, in RG-30.001M.

The purpose of the healing of the sick persons was not to combat the sickness of the patients and to cure their disease, but only to keep up pathological conditions in the organism which served as motive for these experiments. The expert physicians concluded:

1. That the experiments conducted consisted of infusing dangerous bacteria into the organism of so far absolutely healthy women by means of injections and deep incisions which caused serious diseases and endangered the life of the operated women for many months. A certain percentage of the guinea pigs could not get over the artificially produced diseases and died even at the very beginning, as for instance, the prisoners Kraska and Freda Pruss.

2. That these experiments must be decried as very serious physical injuries, dangerous for the patients.

3. That even now during exercise, which is 2–3 years after the conducted experiments, as a result of these experimental operations, periods of fever and pains appear in the women.

4. Trouble in moving the legs and exterior deformations can be observed in the examined women as a remaining and unalterable result of the mentioned experiments.

Photographs of the women examined by the medical experts are included herewith.

Here are excerpts of the individuals' statement:

1. Maria Breel-Pechter, born in 1913, inhabitant of Warsaw, Grochawska Street, 171/9.

"On the morning of 20 November 42 I got an injection below the right knee. I awoke in the evening and felt a high temperature, pains, swelling of the right leg from toes to groin. For 3 days, every day, 100 cubic centimeters intravenous fluid."

After 3 days, the physicians conducted the operation. The prisoner remained unconscious for 3 days. On the right leg, two unhealing wounds, 15 to 20 cm long and 3 cm broad.

"Heavy, bad-smelling discharge of pus. Fever for 5 weeks. Dr. Oberheuser found weakness of the heart muscle."

2. Sofia Sas-Gaslowska, born on 2 January 1910, inhabitant of Warsaw, Pius Street, 11/24. On 30 November 42, experiment was conducted. Awoke with pains and swelling of the leg.

Groaning and cries of the individuals subject to the experiments. Remained unconscious for 4 weeks. Out of Group l0 experimental guinea pigs to which she belonged, two women died.

3. Maria Kismertchuk, 25 years old, Pius Street, 11/24.

"Operation 7 February '42. Bad pains. Fever up to 39 °C during 2–3 weeks."

4. Helen Heger, 29 years old, inhabitant of Warsaw, Grochowska Street 246. In November 1942, operation, fever above 39 °C.

Experiments were conducted every two weeks. Discharge of pus lasted 6 months. The wounds were opened up after the other and the physician infused irritable infectious substances.

According to the Polish law and to the Legal Sanction and on account of the decree of 10 November 1945 of the Chief Regional Commission for the Investigation of German Crimes in Poland (Journal of Laws of the Polish Republic, No. 51, afterwards, No. 293), this document is legal evidence and a supplement to the report of the Polish Government of 22 January 1946, submitted to the International Military Tribunal, in accordance with Charter 21.

Seal: (Signature) Kurovski
Grodno:

Investigation for German Crimes:

STEPHAN KUROVSKI
Plenipotentiary Member of the Polish Government and Member of the Presidency of the Cief Commission of the Investigation of German Crimes in Poland

Nuremberg, 1 February 1946

INCENDIARY BOMBS AND PHOSPHORUS BURNS

By the autumn of 1943, fighting was taking place in the heart of Germany. A massive Allied offensive aimed at destroying the Reich's economic and military potential had been mounted in early summer. In July, five successive phosphorus bomb raids had reduced Hamburg to a vast ruin.

The Allies were carrying out repeated bombing raids on the Schweinfurt factories, seriously threatening arms production. In many German towns, the incendiary, phosphorus bombs dropped by the Allies were causing such severe burns that copper sulphate, the usual remedy, was quite inadequate.

On 30 September 1943, SS Reichsarzt Ernst-Robert Grawitz drafted a secret note to Reichsführer Heinrich Himmler.

> Dr. Karl Brandt has asked me to try out a new ointment, at present at the research stage, and intended for the treatment of phosphorus burns. I think it would take too long to test it on civilians burned during air-raids.
>
> Moreover, I doubt animal experiments could resolve so great a problem. I, therefore, respectfully request your permission to experiment in the Sachsenhausen Concentration Camp Hospital on prisoners unfit for work.[132]

Exactly on 1 October 1943, Himmler's authorization arrived on Grawitz's desk.[133] The new series of experiments would not, however, take place at Sachsenhausen but at Buchenwald, under the direction of Sturmbannführer Dr. Erwin Ding.[134]

Before he started his work, Ding did some preliminary gathering of information and ideas. He visited a Dresden company where scientists had just discovered a new treatment for phosphorus burns that produced remarkable results in rabbits. Ding decided to test this remedy along with the already authorized ointment. He thus had two remedies to test and no lack of detainees on whom to experiment, an ideal situation for an ambitious SS doctor. On 9 November 1943, Ding began the testing.

Just one difficulty faced him: his detainee-subjects had not endured the bombings, so their phosphorous burns had to be artificially induced. Unperturbed, Ding asked to be sent the contents of a phosphorus bomb and received in response, a British bomb, found near Leipzig. On the first day of the testing, five German common-law criminals, who had survived other experiments, were taken to Block 50 in Buchenwald. They were given a mild anesthetic so that they could not defend themselves. When the anesthetic wore off, the poor wretches discovered that they had new, unbearably painful arm injuries. They had no idea what had happened. But Dr. Ding certainly knew. He had had marked off a skin area of about "$2^3/_4$ by $1^1/_4$ inches" to which he had applied a phosphorate rubber solution. He had then set the treated skin alight, letting the solution burn itself out. In most cases the flames lasted one minute, but in one instance the doctor had to wait twenty minutes for the flames to burn out.

After these burns had been created, treatment began. Ding chose a product to smear on the wounds, testing not only the remedies entrusted to him, but

132 Note from Grawitz to Himmler, 30 September 1943.
133 Aziz, *Doctors of Death*, vol. 3, pp. 117–119.
134 *Trials NMT*, vol. 6, pp. 309–310.

also copper sulphate, cod-liver oil – which merely irritated the wound – and even water.

The five prisoners suffered excruciating pain for two long months until February 1944. "In several cases", witness Eugen Kogon confirmed, "the healing could not possibly have been complete. The injuries were about one inch deep or more, and must have left bad scars". Another witness, former prisoner Alfred Balachowsky, gave similar testimony: "Phosphorus burns were inflicted in Block 50 on Russian prisoners for the following reason. Certain bombs dropped in Germany by the Allied aviators caused burns on the civilians and soldiers which were difficult to heal. Consequently, the Germans tried to find a whole series of drugs which would hasten the healing of the wounds caused by these burns. Thus, experiments were carried out in Block 50 on Russian prisoners who were artificially burned with phosphorus products and then treated with different drugs supplied by the German chemical industry."[135]

■

At the trial of war criminals before the Nuremberg military tribunal, the evidence of criminal activity included a lengthy, detailed report on the Buchenwald incendiary bomb experiments. One series of experiments, conducted 19–25 November 1943 sought to ascertain the effectiveness of the drug R 17 as well as echinacine ointment and liquid for the treatment of phosphorus burns. Five experimental persons were deliberately burned with ignited phosphorus taken from an incendiary bomb. The resulting burns were very severe, and the victims suffered excruciating pain and permanent injury. The drugs to be tested were manufactured at the Dr. Madaus Works in Dresden-Radebeul.

A description of the actual experimental procedure, again in cold clinical terms, follows.

Partial Translation of Document No-579,[136] Prosecution Exhibit 288

Report (Extract) on the Findings of 2 January 1944, on a Skin Ointment – R 17 – for Phosphorous Burns

135 Testimony of Witness Eugen Kogon, in Ibid.
136 Partial Translation of Document No-579, in *Trials NMT*, vol. 1, pp. 644–653.

EXPERIMENTS ON HUMAN BEINGS

A) Application of the phosphorus-caoutchouc mixture and immediate removal

1. With R 17, *19 November.* The mixture was dropped on a smooth spot of skin on the forearm and immediately thereafter wiped off with a tampon dipped in R 17. R 17 quickly dissolved the phosphorus and the caoutchouc. Subsequent checks showed a complete cessation of phosphorescence. The spot of skin showed an increased temperature until 14 December, as the testers ascertained by placing the backs of their hands against it.
2. With $CuSO_4$, *19 November.* The mixture, which had been applied to a smooth spot of skin on the forearm, was removed with a 2 percent solution of copper sulphate. There appeared a blackish-brownish, strongly viscous mass with a metallic sheen which, when rubbed off, spread over the entire experimentation area. After an initial formation of black smoke (phosphorus fumes) and a strong glow, the phosphorescence, because of the formation of a copper phosphate coating, ceased almost immediately. It seems to be possible that phosphorus, if it comes in contact with small skin wounds, is assimilated into the body by resorption. This spot of skin likewise showed an increase in temperature until 14 December.
3. With water, *19 November.* It was always possible to remove the mixture from the skin by water. However, in this case pronounced phosphorescence lasting several minutes and phosphorus fumes were observed.

B) Lighting of the phosphorus-caoutchouc mixture and treatment:

1. With R 17

   a) *Immediate ignition*

   25 November. The mixture was applied to a skin area of 6×3 cm and immediately ignited. After burning for 20 seconds, it was extinguished with water and then wiped off with R 17. A burn appeared, with a yellowish induration of the skin. Later a thin scab formed. After 3 days, the wound was treated with liquid echinacine. On 11 December the scab fell off; the surface of the wound was dry and rosy red. Epithelium formed very rapidly; on 21 December only 1/5 of the surface remained without epithelium. On 29 December this spot too was almost healed.

   25 November. The mixture was applied to a skin area of the same size (6×3 cm) and immediately ignited. It burned for 55 seconds until it went out by itself. The burned spot was wiped off with R 17. There appeared a yellowish-brown burn which exhibited a cavity at the proximal end and a blister at the distal end. An elastic scab formed. On the fourth day the wound was treated with *echinacine ointment.* Thereupon, on 3 December, the scab began to slough off; on 10 December the wound was dry and closed; on 13 December only the edge of the wound still showed a scab and the main part of the wound was covered with fine granulation. The wound continued to become smaller until 29 December without healing over.

b) *Ignition after 30 seconds*

19 November. The mixture was applied to 2 sq. cm of skin. After 30 seconds it was ignited and after burning for 40 seconds it was wiped off with R 17. A dry burn appeared. During the following days a small oedematous swelling developed. The wound was treated with *liquid echinacine.* Thereafter, the swelling subsided rapidly, so that on 1 December there remained a clear, dry wound without necrosis. Subsequently to this a broad zone of epithelization formed and by 29 December the wound had healed with the exception of 0.5 sq. cm still lacking epithelium.

19 November. The mixture was again applied to 2 sq. cm of skin, ignited after 30 seconds, but treated with R 17 only after burning 60 seconds. Here too a dry burn appeared, however with severe reddening and pain in the surrounding area. The wound formed a necrotic coating. On the third day it was treated with a 10 percent solution of cod-liver-oil ointment. On 19 December it was circumscribed and dry. A slow epithelization began. Later the wounded skin area became similar to the smooth surrounding area. On 29 December the wound had not yet healed over.

c) *Application to a piece of cloth covering the skin*

25 November. The phosphorus-caoutchouc mixture, applied to a piece of cloth covering the skin was ignited. Sixty-seven seconds elapsed before it had burned itself out. The piece of cloth, except for a small remainder, was carbonized. After it was wiped off with R 17 there appeared on a skin a burn with a central blister which later developed to a thin elastic scab. After 3 days the wound was treated with echinacine ointment. Until 3 December cleaning of the wound took place; at this date it was dry, rosy red and closed; a fine granulation covered it. Thereupon rapid epithelization began. On 29 December it was not yet healed.

2. With $CuSO_4$

a) *Immediate ignition*

25 November. The mixture was applied to a skin area of 6×3 cm and immediately ignited. After burning 20 seconds it was extinguished with water, and then wiped off with copper sulphate solution. During this operation the entire epidermis separated from the area of the wound. An oedematous swelling of the surrounding area, 12×13 cm, in extent and a thick scab formed. Treatment took place with liquid echinacine. On 7 December the necrosis began to slough off, and the gradual epithelization took place. On 21 December one-third of the area of the wound was still without epithelium (cf. II/1/a/aa). On 29 December the wound was healed over.

25 November. The mixture was again applied to a skin area of 6×3 cm and immediately ignited. After it had burned itself out in 60 seconds, the burned area was wiped off with copper sulphate solution. A brownish-grey burn with thickening of the skin reappeared. The thickening developed to a strong scab. It was treated with a 10 percent solution of cod-liver-oil ointment. The surrounding area remained very red and painful. On 10 December a subcutaneous suppuration appeared at the edge of the wound. Consequently the treatment with cod-liver oil was replaced by liquid echinacine. On 13 December the scab separated from the greater part of the wound, but the surrounding area remained more inflamed than in the corresponding experiment with R 17 (cf. II/1/a/bb). The granulation was coarse and uneven. On 29 December the wound was not yet healed over; epithelization advanced only slowly.

b) *Ignition after 30 seconds*

19 November. The phosphorus-caoutchouc mixture was applied to 2 sq. cm of skin and left there for 30 seconds; then it was ignited and after burning for 6 seconds wiped off with copper sulphate solution. A brownish-black vicious mass formed; the dry wound discolored to a blackish-grey. Thereupon a thick crust formed and a considerable oedematous swelling of the area surrounding the wound developed. Treatment took place with echinacine ointment. The swelling subsided more slowly than in the treatment with R 17 (cf. II/1/b/aa). On 5 December the wound was without necrosis, with a wide zone of epithelization. On 29

December it had healed over except for 1 sq. cm lacking in epithelium (cf. II/1/bb/aa).

c) *Application to a piece of cloth covering the skin*

25 November. The skin was covered with a piece of cloth 6×3 cm to which the mixture was applied and then ignited. After it had burned itself out in 57 seconds there remained of the piece of cloth only small carbonized remnants. After being wiped off with copper-sulphate solution a yellowish, rather strong thickening of the skin appeared. The wound was treated with a 10-percent solution of cod-liver oil. A few days later little blisters appeared, which then dried up on 5 December. On 9 December, thickened, shred-like necroses began to peel off, and a dark red surface with rough, uneven granulations developed. The epithelization progressed only slowly. On 29 December the wound was not yet healed over.

3. With water

19 November. The mixture was applied to a 2 sq. cm of skin and ignited 30 seconds later. After 45 seconds the fire was extinguished with a damp cloth and the burned spot washed off with water. A burn of parchment-like, dry, greenish-brownish appearance appeared. The wound was treated with *echinacine* ointment. On 3 December it was clean, dry, and without necrosis. On 5 December the epithelization began, which then made rapid strides, so that on 23 December the wound, in contrast to the treatment with a 10-percent solution of cod-liver oil, was considerably smaller. On 29 December it was not yet healed over, but was only half as large as the wound treated with a 10-percent solution of cod-liver oil.

At the Nuremberg trials, the witness Dr. Eugen Kogon testified further about the experiments performed in Buchenwald on the effects of and treatment for the injuries caused by incendiary bombs. The following is an extract from his testimony.[137]

137 Mimeographed transcription of the complete testimony, 6–8 January 1947, in *Trials NMT,* pp. 1150–1290.

Mr. McHaney: Witness, I had just asked you whether or not you know anything about experiments conducted at Buchenwald with the phosphorus content of incendiary bombs.

Witness Kogon: As far as I can recall, I was told by Dr. Ding in the spring of 1944 that he had been given orders by Professor Dr. Mrugowsky in collaboration with the firm Madaus & Co. at Dresden-Radebeul to carry out experiments on human beings regarding the effect of a drug against the contents of phosphorous-caoutchouc incendiary bombs. I had the impression that the idea for this experiment had come from Dr. Ding and had been given to Dr. Mrugowsky by him, and then he had obtained permission to carry out this experiment. On the part of the firm Madaus, negotiations were led by a certain Dr. Koch. He had a drug which he called R 17 and which was used by the German population after attacks in which incendiary bombs were dropped.

Q. Witness, did you see any of the experimental subjects who were burned with this phosphorus?
A. I personally saw all the experimental subjects. As far as I can recall the burns were very severe in three out of the four cases. During the first experiment at least, the subjects were given an anesthetic, and after about half an hour they regained consciousness and complained of very severe pains. You could see that they were really suffering very badly. I must confess that I personally, after having looked at the photographs, almost became sick.

Q. Do you know whether the injuries which they received are permanent?
A. In the case of some of the wounds, it is completely impossible that they will ever become completely healed; very deep scars must have remained because the wounds were big and were as deep as two or two and a half centimeters.

The following extract from the testimony of Professor Dr. Joachim Mrugowsky provides further information about the experiments aimed at finding the most effective therapy for phosphorus burns.[138]

138 Complete testimony is recorded in mimeographed transcript, 27, 28, 31 March and 2, 3 April 1947, in Ibid., pp. 5000–5244, 5334–5464.

Q. I am submitting to the Tribunal Mrugowsky 56, and it will be Mrugowsky Exhibit 50. I should like to read from page two:

"Treatment of phosphorus burns with 'R 17'

The dropping of phosphorus incendiary bombs made it necessary to find an adequate method of treatment. As the copper sulphate solution hitherto in use did not give satisfactory results, the firm of Dr. Madaus in Dresden looked for a different solvent and produced a liquid carbon tetrachloride which was called R 17. The efficacy of R 17 had been proved by means of experiments on rabbits carried out by the firm of Dr. Madaus.

After the completion of these rabbit tests, Dr. Madaus asked the Higher SS and Police Leader von Woyrsch, Dresden, to come and see the tests. As my emergency office was in the building of Gruppenführer von Woyrsch, he asked me to accompany him to the firm of Madaus in my capacity as a doctor and to watch these tests. That was in the autumn of 1943. At the request of Gruppenführer von Woyrsch and the firm of Madaus, I reported to the Reich Physician SS and Police the results achieved by the firm of Madaus in the treatment of phosphorus burns and suggested that the drug R 17 be made known to the air-raid precaution dispensaries. Grawitz promised to have another test made.

When, after a considerable time, I still had not heard from the Reich Physician whether the drug R 17 was to be made known to the air-raid precaution dispensaries, I asked the Reich Physician about it at a meeting. He then declared that the drug would not be introduced, as it only possessed phosphorus-dissolving properties, but did not directly contribute to the healing of burns. However, a drug was in preparation elsewhere that combined both qualities and this would be introduced."

MUSTARD GAS AND PHOSGENE EXPERIMENTS

On 1 March 1944, Hitler instructed Karl Brandt to prepare Germany for the possibility of gas warfare. Rumors had been circulating since the beginning of that February that the Russian Army was about to launch a massive offensive with poison gas against the Wehrmacht and certain densely populated German cities. In fact, these rumors had been started by KGB agents who had infiltrated the Abwehr and the Gestapo; the rumors were part of a psychological campaign to demoralize Germans, both soldiers and civilians. German Medical Corps officers such as Prof. Dr. Siegfried Handloser and SS Lt. General Hans Juettner, high government officials such as Martin Bormann, and even Himmler himself all fell victim to this propaganda. A veritable psychosis took hold of them.[139] At least this was the official line of the Nazis in the Nuremberg trials.

The prosecutor's opening statement at the Trials of the War Criminals before the Nuremberg Tribunal suggests a different motivation and cause. "Experiments concerning mustard gas were conducted at Sachsenhausen, Natzweiler, and other concentration camps and extended over the entire period of the war... The alleged purpose of these experiments was to discover an effective treatment for the burns caused by mustard gas. In 1944, the experiments were coordinated with a general program for research into gas warfare."[140] The KGB plot may simply have provided a convenient excuse for a program of research that was already occurring.

The following document is a sworn statement made by Rudolf Brandt about the *Lost* (mustard gas) experiments.

Translation of Document No-372[141]
Office of U.S. Chief of Counsel

Affidavit

I, Rudolf Emil Hermann BRANDT, being duly sworn, depose and state:
Experiments with LOST (mustard) gas

1. ...
2. ...
3. Towards the end of the year 1939 experiments were conducted at the Sachsenhausen concentration camp, on persons who were certainly not all volunteers, in order to ascertain the efficacy of the different treatments of wound inflicted by *Lost* gas. *Lost* is a poison gas which produces injurious effects on the epidermis. I think it is generally known as mustard gas. Since war had broken out it was deemed necessary to determine the best treatments for injuries caused by *Lost* gas in case this gas might be used against the Reich. Therefore experiments were conducted on inmates of concentration camps. As far as I understood the experiments consisted of inflicting wounds upon various parts of the bodies of the experimental subjects and infecting them thereafter with *Lost.* Various

139 Aziz, *Doctors of Death.*

140 "Opening Statement of the Prosecution by Brigadier General Telford Taylor, 9 December, 1946", in *Trials NMT,* vol. 1, p. 44.

141 Translation of Document No-372, Office of U.S. Chief of Counsel, in RG-30.001-M.

methods of treatment were applied in order to determine the most effective one.

4. SS Captain (SS-Hauptsturmführer) Dr. August HIRT, professor at the University of Strasbourg and collaborator in the "Ahnenerbe" had before 1942, undertaken experiments on Lost-injuries on the orders of the Wehrmacht. My attention was called to HIRT'S reports in HIMMLER'S office. In the second half of 1942 HIRT, together with First Lieutenant (med.) (Oberarzt) Dr. Karl Wimmer, who served in the Luftwaffe, initiated experiments on inmates of the Natzweiler concentration camp. The inmates for this as well as for other experiments were simply chosen by PHL's office, the Economic and Administrative Main Office (WVHI) in order to be employed for such purposes. The experiments on human subjects with *Lost* gas had been carried out during the year's 1943 and 1944 in the Sachsenhausen concentration camp as well as in the Natzweiler concentration camp. The result was that some of the inmates died.

5. In March 1944, the Führer ordered SS Brigadier General (SS Brigadeführer) Dr. Karl BRANDT, Commissioner for Health and Sanitation (Generalbevollmächtiger für Gesundheits- und Sanitätswesen) to encourage medical research in connection with gas attacks. BRANDT sent a copy of this decree to HIMMLER requesting him to distribute it to the competent persons in the SS and to induce them to enter into communication with BRANDT. Accordingly, since it was a question of experiments, I distributed copies of the Führer's decree to SS Major General (SS Gruppenführer) Dr. GRAWITZ, Reich SS Colonel (SS Standartenführer) Wolfram SIEVERS of the "Ahnenerbe" and SS-Lt General (SS Obergruppenführer) Hans JUETTNER, Chief of the SS Operational Main Office (Chef des SS Führungshauptamtes). SS-Lt. General (SS Obergruppenführer) POHL of the Economic and Administrative Main Office (WVHA) also received a copy of the decree of the Führer.

6. Thereupon SIEVERS informed Dr. BRANDT of the details of HIRT'S investigation with *Lost* on human subjects, although I think it possible that BRANDT, already in 1942, was generally speaking, acquainted with HIRT'S work, as BRANDT in that year was appointed Commissioner for Health and Sanitation (Generalbevollmächtigter für Gesundheits- und Sanitätswesen). HIRT carried on his experiments on human subjects with injuries caused by *Lost* gas during the year 1944. I remember that the experiments were made in the Sachsenhausen concentration camp.

7. Inmates who were subjected to experiments with *Lost* and other experiments were in many cases not of German nationality. Poles and Russians, as well as Gypsies and Jews were frequently employed. It is a fact that HIMMLER'S racial policy required the use of non-German nation-

als except in cases in which very serious political or criminal offenses had been committed.

8. Besides Karl BRANDT and the other above-mentioned persons, HANDLOSER and ROSTOCK also must have been aware of these experiments. Also Professor Kurt BLOME.

Deputy Reich Health Leader and Deputy Reich Leader of Physicians (stellvertretender Reichsgesundheitsführer und stellvertretender Reichsführer der Ärtze) under Dr. CONTI must have been informed of these experiments.

I have read the above affidavit in the German language, consisting of the three (3) pages and it is true and correct to the best of my knowledge and belief. I was given the opportunity to make changes and corrections in the above affidavit. This affidavit as given by me freely and voluntarily, without promise of reward, and I was subjected to no threat or duress of any kind.

(Signed) Rudolf BRANDT

Before me, Walter H. RAPP, D 415387, a U.S. civilian, appeared SS Standartenführer Rudolf Emil Hermann BRANDT, to me known, who in my presence signed the foregoing "Eidesstattliche Erklärung" (statement) consisting of three (3) pages in the German language and swore that the same was true. On the 14th day of October 1946.

(Signed) Walter H. Rapp

Selection from the Argumentation of the Prosecution at the Nuremberg Trial[142]

Extract from the Closing Brief against Defendant Karl Brandt
Lost (Mustard) Gas Experiments

An accurate and detailed description of the manner in which these experiments were carried out was given by a witness, Ferdinand Holl, a hospital attendant at Natzweiler and himself a political prisoner, who was charged with holding the prisoner's arm while Hirt placed liquid mustard gas a few inches above the forearm.

The first series of experiments was carried out by Hirt and an officer of the Luftwaffe in the following manner: One drop of the liquid was applied to the lower arm of the experimental subject. Approximately 10 hours later burns began to appear and spread over the whole body in

142 Closing Brief Against Defendant Karl Brandt, in *Trials NMT,* vol. 1, 318–323.

> every place where drops of the fluid contacted the skin. Some of the experimental subjects became partially blind. The victims of these experiments suffered terrible pain.
>
> Photographic pictures of the burns were taken daily. After the fifth or sixth day of the experiment, the first fatality occurred. The corpse of the victim was dissected and the autopsy showed that the greater parts of the lungs and other organs had been destroyed. On the following day, that is, on the seventh day of the experiment, another seven of the experimental subjects died. The remaining 22 were sent to another concentration camp after approximately 2 months when they had recovered sufficiently and became fit for transport.
>
> Other experiments on concentration camp inmates of the Natzweiler concentration camp were carried out in the gas chamber approximately 500 meters distant from the camp. The experimental subjects had to enter this gas chamber two by two. They had to smash small ampules which contained the liquid. This liquid evaporated and the experimental subject then had to inhale the resulting vapor. Usually they became unconscious and were returned to the Ahnenerbe station for further observation.
>
> Results were approximately the same as those observed in the first series. The respiratory systems were destroyed. Their lungs had been eaten away by the gas. About 150 concentration camp inmates were experimented upon in this manner... Approximately the same percentage as in the first series died as a result of this type of experimentation.

The external effects of *Lost* were not the only matter of interest to the Nazis; they also wanted evidence about internal effects. Consequently, some subjects were injected with *Lost,* in a special room adjoining the camp crematorium.[143] The victims of these experiments died without exception. Still other subjects had to take the liquid orally. On the results of this type of experiment, we have no information, as Holl, the attendant and prisoner whose testimony we have just cited, had been transferred before Christmas 1943 to an outside camp. He did, however, return once a month to the Natzweiler concentration camp and was at least able to observe that the *Lost* experiments continued until autumn 1944, when the Natzweiler camp was liberated by the Allies.

Holl's testimony paints a grim picture of the experimental wards. Approximately 220 inmates of Russian, Polish, Czech, and German nationalities were forced to serve as subjects. About fifty of them died. "The pain was increasingly sharp. The first night was hell. No one in the blocks surrounding the infirmary could sleep that night because of the heartrending cries from

143 See Mitscherlich and Mielke, eds., *The Death Doctors,* pp. 213–222.

their comrades."[144] The agony of the victims was so great that many of them welcomed death. For the hospital attendants, the scene was terrible too. Holl, who managed to save some of the prisoners, testified that the victims "were suffering terribly, unbearably. It was almost impossible to be around them."[145]

The first series of experiments was finished at the end of December 1943. Dr. Hirt informed Kommandant Kramer, "Keep the patients another week in the infirmary until they can walk. Afterwards they're all yours!" The SS men then decided that the patients should be transferred to another camp. When they left the infirmary, they could hardly stand but were made to walk with other prisoners down to the Rothau station. The convoy headed for an unknown destination. At the end of the war, not one survivor among these guinea pigs could be found.

After the completion of the experiments, Professor Hirt and Dr. Wimmer worked feverishly on their report. They sent copies to the Luftwaffe and to the Reich Chancellery. Labeled "top secret" it was sent to Himmler, to General Handloser and to Hans Lammers, three of the highest officials of the regime.

Hirt's report was favorably received. Sievers, the administrator of the Ahnenerbe, praised the "brilliant professor, the great scientist's research on gas is of vital interest to the protection of our troops and population".[146] And Himmler, obsessed as he was by the specter of chemical warfare, received the report with jubilation. He extolled the talents of the "excellent Dr. Hirt who devoted himself, mind and body, to the research of effective treatment in the event of gas warfare".[147]

Translation of Document No-099, Prosecution Exhibit 268[148]

Report by Hirt and Wimmer on the Proposed Treatment of Poisoning Caused by Lost *Gas*

TOP SECRET
[Handwritten] Enclosure of Top Secret Z. I. A. H. No. 36
From the Institute for Military Scientific Research Department H of the Research and Instruction Society Ahnenerbe (Reich Leader SS Personal Staff, Office "A") Strasbourg, Anatomical Institute.

144 Aziz, *Doctors of Death*, pp. 212–213.
145 Ibid.
146 Ibid., p. 223.
147 Ibid.
148 Report by Hirt and Wimmer on the Proposed Treatment of Poisoning Caused by *Lost* Gas, Document No-099, Prosecution Exhibit 268, in *Trials NMT*.

Proposed treatment of poisoning caused by *Lost* [Gas]
(By Professor Dr. A. Hirt, and Staff Surgeon of the Luftwaffe, Professor Dr. Wimmer, Strasbourg, 1944)

General Observations

The effect of *Lost* as a poison gas is immediate and by causing other pathological reactions within the cells and organs, it damages the entire efficiency of the individual cell as well as that of the organs. The organism stands the best chance of absorbing the damage caused by *Lost* if there is a large vitamin reserve in the body. In administering the vitamin treatment after *Lost* damage has been inflicted care must be taken that the medicaments are not administered indiscriminately. The vitamin combinations (A, B complex, C) taken orally or vitamin B administered intravenously in glucose suspension have proved most effective. Both methods aim at raising the resistance of the reticuloendothelial system, while simultaneously introducing therapeutic measures to protect the liver which can be further strengthened by food with a high carbohydrate and vitamin content. When definite damage to the organs (liver, cardiac muscles, kidneys) manifests itself, vitamin treatment has to be discontinued and injections of B. glucose substituted as the excretion of the surplus quantity of vitamins results in a temporary additional overstimulation of the cells of the excretory organs.

In addition the inter-connection between the effect of sulfanilamide and vitamin B_1 complex should be noted. In the case of pulmonary complications (bronchial pneumonia, pulmonary abscess) which are treated with sulfanilamides, the administration of yeast is definitely not indicated.

The general treatment, as set forth, especially the administration of vitamin B_1 glucose, also has a salutary effect on the healing of cutaneous necrosis. In average and serious cases, the length of the healing process can thereby be considerably decreased. Supporting measures to be taken are bandaging the affected limb in splints until the appearance of clean granulation or placing the patient in a suitable recumbent position as well as vigorous, systematic psychotherapy. The psychological influencing of the largely apathetic *Lost* patient constitutes an essential part of the treatment, due to the possibility of thereby influencing the parasympathetic system (circulation, circulatory system).

Outline of Treatment

Damp dressings with Rivanol (0.1–0.05 percent) and Trypaflavin (0.1 percent) have proved to be a successful treatment of the *skin symptoms* (reddening, swelling, blisters) of the first to fourth day. If necessary, ointment dressings (10 percent cod-liver oil, tannic ointment, boric acid ointment, etc.) may be applied.

General treatment of average and serious *Lost* damage begins with administering a vitamin mixture compounded as follows: Vitamin A (in the form of Vogane oil) increasing from 4 to 10 drops daily. Vitamin C (Cantan–Cebion tablets) 2 tablets 3 times daily. Yeast powder 3 teaspoonfuls daily.

One should consider whether a vitamin compound of similar preparation – if need be with the addition of glucose – should be produced for the combat troops. Such a powder mixture would have to be administered in increasing quantities as well. In all cases of absorbed *Lost* damage (liver damage indicated by increased secretion of urobilinogen in the urine, later icteric skin coloring, cardiac muscle damage with tachycardias, kidney damage with albumin secretion in the urine) treatment with vitamin mixtures is to be discontinued and to be substituted by injections of Vitamin B1, glucose (Betaxin–Betabion 2 cc. – also in larger doses – intravenously with 10 cc. 20 percent glucose solution).

Two more experiments were conducted in an attempt to find an effective prophylactic and therapy for mustard gas poisoning, as evidenced by the following official reports. The agents in question were called "F1001" and remedy "H" (Holzmann). Remedy "H" was ineffective. On "F1001", no follow-up report about effectiveness is available.

Translation of Document No-198[149]
Office of Chief of Counsel

VA-2 Berlin, 5 January 1940
From: Reichsführer SS, Reich Physician SS (Reichsarzt SS)
File No: Top Secret 5/40 Enclosures: Report
Top Secret (Handwritten) 11 January 1940
(Signature) H. H.

149 Cover memo Himmler and the attachment, Preliminary report from the Concentration Camp Sachsenhausen on the Application of the Holzmann "Lost Remedy", Document No-198, in RG-30.001M.

To the Personal Staff RFSS:
Berlin Sw 11
Prinz-Albrechtstrasse 9

A preliminary report from the concentration camp Sachsenhausen on the application of the Holzmann "*Lost* Remedy" submitted as enclosure

From this it is evident that no predominant importance is to be attached to the Holzmann remedy.

The Reich Physician SS
(Reichsarzt) (Signature Gravitz) [sic]
SS Brigradeführer

Stamp: Personal Staff RFSS
Received on January 8, 1940
Journal No. 672/39
Top Secret
To: RF (Reichsführer)

Summary of Preliminary Report:

1. Remedy "H" does not seem to be a specific remedy for cauterization caused by "Oil-0".

2. The application of remedy "H" does not seem to have a sufficient bactericidal effect. From two cases of induced infection, one case developed septic symptoms. The healing tendency is reduced in all cases.

3. The impression is given that the cauterized areas treated with Remedy "H" extended more than those treated according to the "F1001" dry method.

(Signature) Dr. Sonntag
Lt. SS (SS Untersturmführer)

Translation of Document No-199[150]
Office of Chief of Counsel for War Crimes

Reichsführer SS
Reich Physician SS (Reichsarzt SS)
File No: Top Secret 4/40 Enclosure: 1

150 Memo from Himmler containing the "Final Report of the Experimental Studies of Concentration Camp Sachsenhausen re: Remedy 'F1001'," Document No-199, in Ibid.

Top Secret
Dated: Berlin, 5 January 1940
(Signature) H. H.

To the Personal Staff RF SS:
Berlin Sw 11
Prinz-Albrechtstrasse 9

Enclosed please find the final report of the experimental studies of Concentration Camp Sachsenhausen re: Remedy "F1001".

Signed:

Reich Physician SS
(Signature) Gravitz [sic]
SS Brigadeführer

Personal Staff RF SS:
Date Received: 8 January 1940
Log No. 672/39
Top Secret
To: RF. Enclosures: 1

Final Report: Re: The 23 cases vaccinated with L. on 13 October 1939.

70 days after vaccinations, the areas of vaccination are, for the most part, healed up. Six of the cases treated still show scabs approximately the size of a 10-pfennig piece. The scabs formed about a fortnight ago and are fixed very firmly. Upon lifting them, healthy granulation tissue can be seen beneath. In the other cases, the skin over the vaccinated areas has turned bluish-red but is not sensitive to touch. Some cases evince considerable itching and smarting upon application of cold. The pigmentation around the vaccinated areas, which was very distinct in some cases, has given way to a striking lack of color. The general condition of the subject is not influenced by the vaccination.

(Signature) Dr. Sonntag
SS Untersturmführer

For the same reason that preparations were made to fight mustard gas warfare, experiments were also ordered on how to deal with possible phosgene gas attacks. Professor Otto Bickenbach conducted these experiments, and maintained, even at his Strasbourg trial, that he had succeeded in discovering a prophylactic against phosgen[e] poisoning: hexamethylentetramine(urotropin). He added that he had been ordered by Himmler in 1943 to test it on human beings. Bickenbach described the experiments to Brandt as follows.

Report from Bickenbach to Brandt[151]

Seventh Report
On the protective effect of hexamethylentetramine in phosgene poisoning.

Experiments were carried out on forty prisoners on the prophylactic effect of hexamethylentetramine in cases of phosgene poisoning. Twelve of those were protectively inoculated orally, twenty intravenously, and eight were used as controls… The experimental subjects were all persons of middle age, almost all in a weak and underfed condition. On principle, the healthier ones were used as controls, only control No. 39 (series J) and the orally protected experimental subject No. 37 (series A) had a localized cirrhotic productive tuberculosis of the lungs. With the others, no pulmonary disease could be found. In the first experiments up to 6 grams hexamethylentetramine were given orally, later, despite the much higher concentrations, 0.06 g · kg/body weight, orally as well as intravenously.

Experiment XV is characteristic of the test schedule and its results, and will therefore again be specially described. Of four test subjects, the first was protectively inoculated orally, the second intravenously, the third received an intravenous injection of hexamethylentetramine after the poisoning, in order once more to ascertain the effect of therapeutic treatment the fourth was not treated at all. The four subjects were placed in the chamber in which a phial containing 2–7 grams of phosgene was smashed. The test subjects remained under this concentration for twenty-five minutes. The phosgene content was measured three times during the inhalation. The readings showed an average concentration of 91 mg per cbm. The subject protected intravenously remained healthy, and did not show the least signs of difficulties or symptoms, the orally protected subject contracted a slight pulmonary oedema.

The official reports on both the mustard gas and phosgene gas experiments were misleading, at best. They downplayed the fact that subjects were suffering and even dying. They did note that the experiments were flawed by weaknesses in design and procedure, that certain potentially significant physical differences among the subjects had not been taken into account in either the selection of subjects or the analyses of results; but they went on to outline "decisive" findings. From the standpoint of professional methodology and ethics, however, these conclusions are inaccurate and useless; the suffering of these victims was for naught.

151 Document No-1852, printed in Aziz, *The Death Doctors*, p. 221.

Translation of Document No-1852[152] Prosecution Exhibit 456

Extract from Report on Medical Experiments Addressed to Karl Brandt

To the Führer's Plenipotentiary General For Health and Medical Services
Surgeon-General Professor Dr. Brandt,
Berlin Ziegelstrasse 5/9
Surgical Clinic at the University

Summary:

The conclusions of the experiment are impaired by the varying constitutions and the general poor state of nutrition and of physique of the experimental subjects, as well as by the different behavior and the different volume of respiration of the experimental subjects under gas. But the experiments gave the following decisive conclusions:

1. A previous intravenous injection of 3 grams of hexamethylentetramine completely prevents serious toxic and fatal phosgene poisoning from a c. t. of 2,275.
2. An endurable quantity of hexamethylentetramine taken prophylactically weakens a fatal poisoning to such an extent that it can be overcome without treatment, c. t. = 2,275.
3. Nonfatal but nevertheless oedema-producing poisonings are made positively ineffective by intravenous application, and are weakened by oral application, c. t. 250 to 1,980.
4. The oral application of hexamethylentetramine is no longer effective against phosgene poisoning of a c. t. = 5,400, the intravenous injection, however, weakens the effect to such an extent that the protected subject is able to overcome a lung oedema.
5. The *dosis letalis minima* (minimum lethal dose) based on these experiments cannot yet be determined with certainty. One c. t. of 2,275 resulted in the death of one experimental subject, and the second developed second degree oedema of the lungs which was cured.
6. Some of the protected experimental subjects who did not develop oedema of the lungs remained completely healthy, others suffered from slight bronchitis with a brief fever. In every case they recovered without treatment.

152 Document No-1852, in *Trials NMT,* pp. 341–348.

SULFONAMIDE EXPERIMENTS

Shortly after the outbreak of the war in 1939, the Nazis built a new concentration camp, in Mecklenburg, a town about fifty miles north of Berlin. The facility, which consisted of a main camp and several subsidiaries, all for women, became known as Ravensbrück. From its establishment until its liberation by the Russians, 123,000 prisoners were interned there.[153]

Among other medical experiments, tests on the efficacy of the drug sulfonamide were performed in Ravensbrück under the direction of Professor Dr. Karl Gebhardt, Consultant Surgeon of the Waffen SS and Head Physician of the Hohenlychen Orthopedic Hospital (located eight miles away). He began the tests after May 1942, having received an urgent order on the subject from Himmler. According to Gebhardt, three things happened in May 1942, which caused Himmler to sign the order.

First SS Gruppenführer Nebe, chief of the Reichskriminalpolizeiamt (Reich's Criminal Investigation Department), had reported at a conference that active duty troops were losing confidence in the Army surgeons, a serious problem for troop morale. The SS troops had experienced heavy casualties on the Eastern Front, owing both to "the destructive power of hostile armaments and the unalterably conservative methods of doctors in the field". Resentment and demoralization had increased notably in the wake of an Allied propaganda campaign aimed at highlighting the superiority of treatments available at the front to Allied soldiers; specifically, leaflets had been dropped behind German lines announcing that the Allied troops had access to two new miracle drugs, the life-saving antibiotics penicillin and sulfa.

It was also at this time that Himmler had informed Hitler of his first inspection, together with SS General Wolff, of a medical experiment by Rascher on a human subject. Hitler had then decided that "in principle, when the well-being of the nation is at stake, experiment on human subjects is permissible... and that the persons of those detained in concentration camps or prisons ought not to remain completely unaffected by the war while German soldiers are being subjected to almost unbearable strain and our native land, women and children are being engulfed under a rain of incendiary bombs".[154]

After Nebe's speech at the conference, Grawitz had given Himmler an exhaustive account of the positive results of research and therapy tests with human subjects at hospitals in Germany and abroad. He thus encouraged Himmler's constant search for expedients to bolster up his shaky position as

153 Hoedeman, *Hitler or Hippocrates*, p. 51.
154 Mitscherlich and Mielke, eds., *The Death Doctors*, p. 171.

"redeemer of the SS". Up until this point Gebhardt, who doubted that sulfonamides would be effective with war injuries, had opposed proposals to test them in hospitals. But having witnessed these conversations and realized that Hitler and Himmler wanted quick results, he changed his opinion; he decided that it was intolerable to withhold these drugs as therapies for wound treatment because of concern for possible side effects. He also recognized that the introduction of sulfonamides would likely compensate for the shortcoming of the doctors in the field.

There is no documentary evidence of this conference between Himmler, Grawitz, Nebe and Gebhardt. Gebhardt gave its date as between 22 and 25 May 1942. What is certain is that two days later, on 27 May, Reinhard Heydrich, SS Obergruppenführer, Chief of the Security Service and Deputy Protector of Bohemia and Moravia, was shot and died of the complications caused by infection of the wound. And this fact was of significance for Gebhardt's position. Heydrich had been hospitalized in Prague and Gebhardt had been flown in to treat him. As Heydrich's condition worsened, Hitler and Himmler pressured Gebhardt to call in two specialists, both of whom favored sulfonamide therapy in such cases, Professor Sauerbruch and Hitler's personal physician, Dr. Morell. Gebhardt refused and Heydrich died fourteen days after the shooting. Hitler summoned Gebhardt but then refused to see him, a clear sign of trouble. Himmler related Hitler's displeasure. Gebhardt's career and entire future seemed to be hanging on the sulfonamide question. His change of opinion may well have been a direct result of this event. Whatever the effect on Gebhardt, the influence of Heydrich's death on the subsequent performance of experiments on human beings at Ravensbrück can hardly be overestimated. It was resolved that tests on the efficacy of sulfonamides should be begun at once.[155]

The only available documents concerning the first series of experiments and naming the doctors directly participating are presented below.

Document No-2734, Prosecution Evidence[156]

To the Reich Leader SS H. Himmler
Berlin.

Reich Leader:

155 Ibid, p. 173.
156 Ibid, pp. 174–178.

Attached please find a provisional report by SS Brigadeführer Professor Dr. Gebhardt on his clinical-surgical experiments at Ravensbrück concentration camp, furthermore a concluding provisional report on experiments on the biochemical treatment of sepsis as performed at Dachau concentration camp

(Signature) GRAWITZ
(Handwritten)

Settled after conversation, with RF, SS Obersturmführer F. Fischer has been given new instructions for Ravensbrück and Dachau.

(Signature) Gebhardt

Document No-2734, Prosecution Evidence (cont.)[157]

From: Professor Dr. K. Gebhardt,
SS Brigadeführer and Brigadier General of the Waffen SS
To: The Reichsarzt SS Gruppenführer Grawitz

Provisional Report on Clinical Experiments at Ravensbrück Concentration Camp for Women
(From Gebhardt to Grawitz)

By order of the Reich Leader SS, I started on 20 July 1942 at Ravensbrück concentration camp for women a series of clinical experiments with the aim of analysing the sickness known as gas gangrene, which does not take a uniform course, and of testing the efficacy of the known therapeutic medicaments.

In addition, the simple infections of injuries which occur as concomitant symptoms in war surgery had also to be studied, and a new chemotherapeutic treatment apart from the known surgical measures had to be tried out.

I appointed SS Obersturmführer, Dr. Fischer as co-worker. SS Oberführer Dr. Blumenreuther put the complete surgical instruments and medications at my disposal. SS Standartenführer Mrugowsky put his laboratory and co-workers at my disposal. SS Obersturmführer Dr Lolling, Chief of Office HID at Oranienburg, assigned as co-workers: SS Obersturmführer Dr. Schiedlausky, SS Untersturmführer Dr. Rosenthal and Fraülein Dr. Oberheuser, all camp physicians at Ravensbrück.

157 Ibid.

The question was to define firstly, by way of a preliminary experiment, the mode of infection, making use of the known results from experiments upon animals. In these questions I was advised by SS leaders of the Hygienic Institute of the Waffen SS who had taken over the culture and dosage of the inoculation material.

The point was to implant the lymph cultures on the damaged muscle tissue, to isolate the latter from atmospheric and humoral oxygen supply, and to subject it to internal tissue pressure. The inoculation procedure was as follows: a longitudinal cut of ten centimetres over the musculus peroneus longus; after incision into the fascia the muscle was tied up with forceps in an area the size of a five-mark piece; an anaemic peripheral zone was created by injection of 3 cc adrenalin and in the area of the damaged muscle the inoculation material (a gauze strip titrated with bacteria) was imbedded under the fascia, subcutaneous adipose tissue, and skin sutured in layers.

In the first series of experiments (preliminary experiments) three selected prisoners of as much the same constitution as possible were used. They were inoculated as follows:

The first: Aerobic mixculture (staphylococci, streptococci, bact. comm. try. a 5 Mil).

The second: Para Oedema Malignum, sarc, flav. 4–5 mh [sic].

The third: Bact. Fraenkel and earth. Stimulus 4–5 mg.

The experiment was concluded after ten days. After an initial local swelling in the inoculation area and an increase in temperature up to 39°, the inflammation died down, the wound having broken open on the fourth day. There was no danger to the life of any of the prisoners. We succeeded in producing locally the symptoms of gas gangrene in the third prisoner.

After twenty days the prisoners were released again to their working blocks.

The course of the preliminary series of experiments had proved that we were not successful in producing the same symptoms of clinical gas gangrene. In a conference with the Hygiene Institute of the Waffen SS the nature of the infection and the conditions for the germs were not considered to be equivalent to the natural conditions in war surgery and consequently the experimental arrangements were changed.

Bacteria coli were added to the aerobe culture and the germ number was increased to twenty millions. Bacteria coli and dextrose were added to the mixture of para oedema malignum. Bacteria coli were added to the gas gangrene culture by Fraenkel, and while doubling the number of germs, earth was administered to produce a similar environment. Six selected youthful prisoners were inoculated two by two with the above mixture of bacteria in the subsequent first experimental series. One of them remained untreated for control purposes, the other one was powdered with Cataxyn wound powder immediately after the inoculation. The first change of dressing took place three days afterwards, the following each second day. Those who remained without treatment were covered with sterile layers, those treated with Cataxyn (indicated in the graphs as TK-cases) were continuously powdered with Cataxyn. The aerobe cultures in both cases showed local abscesses which could be easily treated surgically.

The para oedema malignum inoculation produced a local inflammation with central suppuration, small formation of necrosis in depth and moderate emphysema of the skin. The regional lymphatic glands were not affected.

Those prisoners who were infected with Fraenkel's gas gangrene, and who immediately received tetanus-antitoxin for the administered earth, produced by far the strongest inflammatory reaction: abscesses with deep necrosis in the area of the inoculation, emphysema of the skin with formation of blisters, and initial necrosis, with collateral oedema extending from above the joint of the knee to the lower third of the thigh and going as far as the back of the foot. The inflammatory appearances receded considerably after the opening of the injury on the first dressing day. The effect of the opening of the wound was particularly significant in the TK-cases which started inflammations in spite of simultaneous therapy. Greater pressure of the tissue due to oxygen, liberated by the medicament, was considered to be the reason for the accentuated local inflammation.

Comparing non-treated cases with the TK-cases (treated with Cataxyn), the final critical observation shows:

1. Immediate therapy does not prevent the occurrence of either an ordinary suppuration or of a "gangrene".

2. The cleaning of the wound is faster in TK-cases than in control cases.

3. The formation of fresh wound granulations occurs earlier in Cataxyn.

4. The part played by the paranchymatic organs (liver, kidneys) is less important under the influence of Cataxyn.

Since in this experiment definite gangrene could also be produced clinically speaking, though its picture did not in any way correspond to the one known in war surgery, after further consultation with the collaborators in the Hygiene Institute of Waffen SS, the vaccine was changed by adding wood shavings. It is known from bacteriological literature that the presence of the bacteria in the experimental animal can thereby considerably be increased.

The triple distribution was reserved for the second series of experiments now in progress. Three prisoners in each group were inoculated. One person was left without treatment as control, the second was treated with Cataxyn as before, and with the third the Marfanilprontablin powder manufactured by I. G. Farben was employed, since this was strongly recommended by the Army Medical Inspectorate. The powder was applied according to the Schmick procedure. This experiment is still in progress.

Even if as yet nothing definite can be said about this series of experiments it can already be stated that:

1. There is no decisive difference between cases which are treated and those which are not treated.

2. That opening the wound, in addition to immobilization, has proved the most effective means of controlling the inflammation.

3. The effect of the MP powder seems at least doubtful, since in the third TK-case the most definite gangrene observed up to now developed.

We are now investigating the problem as to why the gangrene in the present case did not fully develop. For this purpose, the injuring of the tissue and the exclusion of a muscle from the circulation of the blood were undertaken during a special operating session, and the large-scale necrosis resulting therefrom is to be inoculated with bacteria strain which has already had one human passage. For it is only when the really definite clinical picture of gas gangrene has appeared that conclusions may be drawn on therapy with chemotherapeutics in connection with surgical operations.

(Signature) Gerhardt, SS Brigadeführer

Himmler was of the opinion that since the experiments proceeded "quite harmlessly", they represented "an excellent chance of reprieve and therefore should be open to the Polish women who are under sentence of death".[158]

Gebhardt ordered Fischer to continue the experiments. Thirty-six women were selected for this trial. Dr. Fischer described the organization of the experiment as follows.

158 Prosecution Protocol 4077, in Ibid., p. 179.

Prosecution Protocol 4345

> This group was divided into three sections of twelve persons each so as to afford comparison of results. Two in each section were given no sulphonamide [sic]. The other ten were given it after inoculation, at different times. In all three groups the only uniform result was that inflammation did not occur when the sulphonamide was administered to the wound at the same time as the bacterial cultures. In the other cases local inflammation appeared which at times reached the dimensions of a boil about the size of a walnut. The swelling, accordingly, was absolutely restricted to a certain spot and did not affect the rest of the body. But as stated above, two in each section, that is to say six subjects, who had been injected with sulphonamide at the same time as with the bacterial cultures, developed no inflammation at all. In the first of these series, only bacteria, in the second, bacteria and tiny splinters of wood, and in the third, bacteria, splinters and glass were introduced into the wounds.[159]

In a third experimental series, Gebhardt and Fischer took steps to aggravate the conditions by applying ligatures to vessels in the areas of the leg to be inoculated. The ligatures decreased the blood supply to the leg, thus making healing much more difficult and more closely approximating wartime conditions. There were twenty-four subjects in this series, of whom twelve were exposed to mixed infection with gangrenous septic material. Fischer described the progress of the infection as follows:

> ...The symptoms of inflammation were definitely more severe. But they did not affect all the twenty-four subjects. At first there was no inflammation in the case of the four who had received, as before, the specific in combination with the cultures. Moreover, so far as I remember, and I can in fact recall a curve we showed, symptoms of inflammation were relatively insignificant in the case of the other eight. They were again boils of about the size of a walnut. In twelve of the subjects, however, inflammation was more severe, closely resembling gas gangrene. At any rate the slightest of them was highly intensive. Of those who were inoculated in isolation with agents which could live without air three subjects died in consequence of a spread of inflammation which we could not control even by surgical methods.[160]

159 Prosecution Protocol 4345, in Ibid.
160 Affidavit of Dr. Gebhardt, in Ibid., pp. 179–181.

Gebhardt provided further details:

> All the recommended sulphonamide preparations were classified by their local and internal effects in differently composed doses, which were changed from time to time. Comparisons were made through the so-called "Check Cases", in which sulphonamide was not given but every therapeutic prophylactic measure was taken. The data obtained showed unmistakably the fact, extremely important for the care of wounded persons, that the sulphonamides are not suitable specifics for the prevention of the infection of wounds. In addition, we determined by clinical analogy what is still generally accepted today, viz. that the sulphonamides, like all other remedies, penicillin for instance, cannot be carried along the blood-vessels in an abscess, owing to the latter's capsular membrane.[161]

In spite of the above results, on 10 September 1942, Gebhardt decided to continue the tests, this time in a bunker which had formerly served as a prison. The bunker was filthy; not a single aseptic installation, not even a sanitary one! That was no obstacle, for the experimenters were seeking to approximate the conditions on the front. Gebhardt did not hesitate to infect the sores of his subjects with bits of dirt or glass particles. He achieved speedy results. Within a few days, the infections took on frightful proportions. The sick wards became an inferno.

A seventeen-year-old girl, newly arrived at Ravensbrück, died four days after she had been infected, in terrible pain. The experiment assistant, Dr. Rosenthal, had been advised to save her from gangrene by amputating her leg, but he refused. The procedure could have saved her life. After her death, Rosenthal performed a complete autopsy. Interestingly, two days later, when three prisoners were putting the body in a coffin, they discovered that one leg had been amputated *after* her death.

Fate was on Gebhardt's side. At the beginning of 1943 the sulfonamide experiments had already been going on for a number of months without yielding the slightest positive result. This finding would give Gebhardt the upper hand over Morell, the tireless advocate of sulfa drugs. He would finally prove to the entire German medical corps that Morell's theories had no scientific value and that he, Gebhardt, couldn't have prevented Heydrich's death. And by another twist of fate, he would do so from within the comfortable surroundings of Hohenlychen, his home institution. The SS Reichsführer had suggested that

161 Ibid., pp. 182–183. Also see Aziz, *Doctors of Death,* pp. 172–173.

Gebhardt give a report to the Military Academy Assembly in Berlin, but the repeated allied bombings of the capital, required a change of venue for the conference. When Gebhardt proposed Hohenlychen, the offer was accepted: not only was the clinic sheltered from bombings, but also there would be no problem housing the two or three hundred participants.

On 9 May 1943, Gebhardt and Dr. Fritz Fischer took the floor to deliver his report "Special Experiments on the Effect of Sulfonamides" before an audience of some one hundred people:

> Orders were given to carry out experiments on prisoner[s] condemned to death who were, in turn, given a chance for survival. The legal aspect of the matter did not come into consideration. I received and carried out these orders and assume responsibility for their scientific value as well as for the involvement of human beings.
>
> All the doctors present understood perfectly that he [Gebhardt] was talking about experiments performed on prisoners. Not one of them raised the slightest objection. Gebhardt and Fischer avoided saying that the guinea pigs had been women.
>
> Fischer gave his account of the research; he didn't hide the fact that seventy-five people were submitted to the experiments, although he limited the number of deaths to three. In documents for army distribution printed after the congress, Gebhardt and Fischer's report was entitled, "Special Experiments". Gebhardt had seen to it that the effectiveness of sulfa be considerably depreciated. Fischer's conclusions were a masterpiece of duplicity:
>
> 1. The immediate utilization of sulfa drugs locally or internally, in no way prevents bacteria-caused suppuration of sores.
>
> 2. In order to treat inflammation with success, surgical measures are indispensable.[162]

Gebhardt was categorical: sulfa drugs serve almost no purpose whatsoever. The pain and death of the "little test rabbits" of Ravensbrück had served merely to reinforce Gebhardt's position, called into doubt for a moment in the aftermath of Heydrich's assassination.

The prisoners of Ravensbrück had not, unfortunately, seen the end of their suffering. Gebhardt would continue his experiments, as already mentioned, right up until August 1943.

It is worth mentioning that at the May 1943 conference, the following officials were present: Dr. Paul Rostock, chairman of the conference; Dr. Siegfried

162 Aziz, *Doctors of Death*, pp. 174–176.

Handloser, then Chief of the Armed Forces Medical Services; Prof. Karl Brandt; Reich Health Leader Dr. Leonardo Conti; Prof. Sauerbruch; Dr. Frey; and Prof. Heubner. The Air Force Medical Service was represented by Dr. Hippke, its Chief, and by Dr. Oskar Schroeder. The Medical Service of the Waffen SS was represented by its Chief, Dr. Karl Genzken. In addition, Dr. Helmut Poppendick (Chief of Staff for Reichsarzt SS und Polizei Dr. Ernst-Robert Grawitz) was present. None of these physicians found any fault with the experiments. Dr. Frey and the world-famous surgeon Prof. Sauerbruch participated in the discussion that followed, also without raising any objections about the procedures or the findings.[163]

■

On the matter of the sulfonamide experiments, one of the surgeons at Ravensbrück, Dr. Rolf Rosenthal, gave the following deposition on 10 October 1946 to the War Crimes Investigation Unit. The most noteworthy part of the deposition is the description of the kind of "post-operative" care the doctors gave to the severely ill patients.

Excerpts from the Deposition of Dr. Rolf Rosenthal, Given at the War Crimes Investigation Unit, Minden[164]

> Deposition under oath of Dr. Rolf Rosenthal, male, of BEVERN KREIS HOLZMINDEN, born on 22 January 1911 at BRAUNSCHWEIG, sworn before Major A. K. Mant, RAMC, of War Crimes Investigation Unit, at Minden on the 10th October 1946.
>
> ...The first experimental operations were carried out in summer 1942 at RAVENSBRÜCK... My duty was to assist during these operations.
>
> After these operations the patients were accommodated in separate rooms in other departments of the infirmary. Sulphonamide-preparates were administered to them, and as far as I know these patients were nursed exactly in the same way as ordinary patients. Gas gangrene cultures (Gasbrandkulturen) were instilled into the artificially caused wounds. These cultures were delivered by the Hygieneinstitut of the

163 Mitscherlich and Mielke, eds., *The Death Doctors*, pp. 65–66.
164 Deposition Given at War Crimes Investigation Unit, Minden, 10 October 1946.

Waffen SS in Berlin, where they had been cultivated. These cultures were implanted into the wounds with or without foreign matter. I believe that the foreign matter which was either cloth or splinters of wood or perhaps even glass, was also delivered by the Hygieneinstitut of the Waffen SS at Berlin.

Sometimes I have seen that Dr OBERHAUSER administered petrol injections to the prisoners. She used a syringe for 10 cubic centimeters and the injection was administered into the vein of the arm. The injection gave the impression of an acute apoplexy. The patient reared up and then suddenly collapsed. It lasted between 3 and 5 minutes from the time the injection was administered until they were dead. The patients were entirely conscious until the last moment. It took approximately 15 to 30 seconds to administer the injections. Dr. OBERHAUSER told me that the prisoners who received petrol injections were severely ill and could not be cured.

I have administered the overdose of morphine to about 20–30 severely ill patients to ease their death.

Extract from the Closing Brief Against Defendant Gebhardt, Nuremberg trial[165]

The witness Kusmierczuk was one of the subjects in the sulfanilamide experiments. She was a Polish national who arrived in the Ravensbrück concentration camp in the fall of 1941. She was operated on in October 1942 and developed a severe infection. She remained in the hospital until April 1943, but her wound was still not healed at the time she was discharged. Readmitted on 1 September 1943, she had her second surgery by Dr. Treite for deep-seated infection and left the hospital the second time in February 1944. Her wound did not heal completely until June 1944.

Kusmierczuk suffered permanent injuries as a result of the experiment and her condition was described for the Court by expert witness, Dr. Leo Alexander. Kusmierczuk was operated on by Dr. Treite in an effort to cure deep-seated infection.

Dr. Maczka, a prisoner physician, who worked as an x-ray technician in the Ravensbrück concentration camp during the course of the experiments, testified concerning the death of five Polish experimental subjects resulting from the sulfanilamide experiments. Wronica Kraska devel-

165 Closing Brief Against Defendant Gebhardt, in *Trials NMT.*

oped typical tetanus symptoms a few days after the experimental operation and died. Kazimiera Kurowska was artificially infected with gangrene bacillus. She was a healthy Polish girl, 23 years old. From day to day her leg became more black and more swollen. She was given some care for only the first few days. After that she was taken to Room 4 in the hospital where she lay for days in unbelievable pain and finally died.

Vniela Lafanowicz was infected with oedema malignum. Her leg kept bleeding. Maczka testified that the blood vessels should have been tied off and an amputation carried out in order to save her life. She was completely neglected after the first 2–3 days.

Zofia Kiecol died under similar circumstances.

Alfreda Prus was infected with oedema malignum the same day as the witnesses Kusmiercuzk, Kiecol and Lefanowicz. She was a beautiful, young 21 year old girl, a university student. She proved to be stronger than Kiecol and Lefanowicz and lived a few days longer. She suffered terrible pain and finally died of hemorrhage. Kusmiercuzk was the only subject to survive the series of experiments.

It is hardly necessary to point out that all of the experimental subjects *suffered severe pain and torture* [italics in original]. The Tribunal was able to observe for itself the mutilations to which the Polish witnesses were subjected and pictures of their scars were introduced to form a permanent part of the record.

The post-operative care of the experimental subjects was entirely inadequate. Many of the subjects were given neither medicine nor morphine by order of defendant Oberheuser. They were given bandages from time to time when the doctors felt like it. Sometimes they waited 3 days, sometimes 4 days. There was a terrible odor of pus in the rooms. The girls were forced to help each other. Post-operative care, such as it was, was administered by the camp doctors. The witness Broel-Plater testified that: "My leg pained me. Blood flowed from my leg. At night we were all alone without any care. I heard only the screaming of my fellow prisoners, and I heard also that they asked for water. There was nobody to give us any water or bed pans."

Many human lives were sacrificed in the sulfanilamide experiments, and all of the surviving victims suffered terrible pains and were crippled for life. The experiments were not even scientifically successful. The results, as reported by Gebhardt and Fischer, at the Third Conference of the Consulting Physicians of the Wehrmacht at the Military Medical Academy in Berlin in May 1943 were not adopted. The sulfanilamide experiments were entirely unnecessary since similar results could have been achieved by treatment of wound infections of German soldiers normally contracted during the course of the war.

> At least six of the experimental subjects were executed after having survived the experiments. The names of the Polish girls who were shot were Pajaczkowska, Gans, Zielonka, Rakowska, Sobolewska and Gutek. It was not a question of experimentation or execution, but experimentation *and* execution.

After the war, at the request of the Polish Ministry of Health, an investigative board made up of professors of medicine examined fifty-one women who had served as "guinea pigs" at Ravensbrück:

> The criminal experiments consisted in the deliberate cutting out and infection of bones and muscles of the legs with virulent bacteria, the cutting out of nerves, the introducing into the tissues of virulent substances and the causing of artificial bone fractures.
>
> The experiments were conducted in conditions of utter disrespect for the basic principles of asepsis. After an operation, the victim was left to her own fate and was in most cases exposed to harmful factors hampering self-defence by the organism.
>
> Some victims died in consequence of the operation itself or of the resulting complications and several were shot, while the survivors suffered major and extensive injuries to their organs of movement.
>
> The changes in the organs of movement consisted in extensive crippling scars, defects, cicatrization of muscles, prolapse of the injured nerves, prolonged suppurative infections of the bone tissues, deformations of legs, defective positioning of individual joints, limitation of movement ability and various statical disturbances.
>
> A characteristic feature of the injuries was the high degree of deformation of legs, which, together with the fact that the experiments were made on young women, endows the criminal actions with even more sinister meaning.
>
> The changes in the organs resulting from the experiments being irreversible and the resulting neuroses, frequently even bordering on the psychopathological, have deepened with time.
>
> In consequence of these criminal operations, most of their victims became invalids, while the others have had their ability of active life and work permanently impaired.[166]

166 "Experimental Operations on Prisoners of Ravenbruck Concentration Camp", *Studies and Monographs* (Poznan and Warsawa, Poland: Wydawnictivo Zachodnie, December 1960).

TUBERCULOSIS (TBC) EXPERIMENTS

The Nazis made the eradication of tuberculosis, or "tbc", one of their chief medical hygiene goals. Initially, cases in the concentration camps were "treated" with death. According to Dr. Wladyslaw Tondos, a Polish prisoner physician who testified about the conditions in Auschwitz, patients were simply being killed in 1941 by means of intravenous phenol injections; later, on the orders of SS camp physicians Entress and Jung, these injections were given directly into the heart. Approximately two hundred tuberculosis sufferers were murdered this way in Block 20.[167]

It was only in the first month of 1943 that permission was given to set up a center for the treatment of tuberculosis in Block 20. But this change did not bring the medical murders to an end; certain patients were still sent to the gas chambers or killed with phenol injections. The reports sent out of the camp by the International Resistance Movement Group confirm that the murders continued. For instance, a letter of 24 November 1942, mentions among other things that "tbc is being ruthlessly eliminated". Additionally a report on the gypsy camp in Auschwitz notes that "seriously ill people (tbc) – with general utter exhaustion are being killed with phenol injections into the heart". And a report of April 1943 notes, "In the case of open tbc nothing can be done, even the Reichsdeutsch have to go."[168]

■

Hohenlychen, established in 1902, was originally a Red Cross sanitorium serving women and children. Prior to the discovery of antibiotics, treatment for tuberculosis and other respiratory ailments consisted of rest and relaxation in healthful surroundings such as the Swiss Alps or the Mediterranean lands, or, as at Hohenlychen, on the shores of a lovely lake. Thus Hohenlychen was a sort of health spa with all the facilities and grounds associated with such institutions. In the Nazi era, parts of the institution and its grounds were transformed into a training and rehabilitation center for athletes; the number of beds reserved for tuberculosis sufferers was starkly reduced. The place soon became a favorite retreat for SS leaders in need of a rest. Top SS offi-

167 Dr. Tondos, a prisoner physician who participated in the research at Auschwitz, left extensive notes and numerous case histories. Fellow prisoner Wolkowitz, a lawyer from Warsaw, saved the notes and case histories, which provided evidence in the hearings before the International Military Tribunal in Nuremberg.

168 All quotations come from IAC, *Inhuman Medicine,* vol. 1, pt. 2, pp. 163–184.

cers met there with politicians from Berlin, for Hohenlychen was a quiet, secluded place, safe from Allied bombs. Rudolf Hess, Hitler's deputy, went there often, as did the Nazi architect, Albert Speer; the Propaganda Minister, Josef Goebels; Oswald Pohl, Obergruppenführer and General for the Waffen SS; and, above all, Heinrich Himmler, Reichsführer of the SS. Even Hitler visited a few times.

In the spring of 1941, Reich Minister Dr. Leonardo Conti, and Dr. Ernst-R. Grawitz, Chief Physician of the SS and Police, happened to be staying there, and Dr. Kurt Heissmeyer, the ambitious, thirty-eight-year-old assistant director of the spa, seized the opportunity brought by their visit to present a research proposal for their consideration. Heissmeyer had been working as a physician at Hohenlychen for ten years, and he hoped one day to become a Professor of Medicine. His proposal, to investigate the efficacy of the Kutschera-Aichbergen tuberculosis treatment, was designed with that personal goal in mind. The experiment was to be undertaken not on animals but on people.

A. and H. Kutschera-Aichbergen were Austrian researchers, father and son, who had proposed "combating severe tuberculosis of the lungs by artificially inducing tuberculosis of the skin". In a number of publications between 1929 and 1939, they had suggested that the "immunity of a patient with active tuberculosis of the lungs" could be improved by "implanting" an additional tubercular node. Heissmeyer, who was a general practitioner, seems not to have known that most eminent tuberculosis specialists did not accept the Kutschera-Aichbergen theory.

Heissmeyer's interest in doing the experiments with human subjects may, however, also have been motivated by his commitment to Nazi racist views. His published writing suggest that he regarded the Nazi teachings on race as legitimate science; certainly the design of his experiments fit with Nazified racial hygiene theories. In 1943, for example, he submitted a paper entitled "Principles of Present and Future Problems of TB Sanatoriums", which argued that "racially inferior" patients have lower resistance than racially superior ones to illnesses such as tuberculosis. For this reason, he believed, doctors should base their decisions about appropriate therapeutic intervention not only on the "condition of the organ itself", but also on the race of the patient. By the phrase "condition of the organ" Heissmeyer meant what physicians the world over mean by "diagnosis". But to him, considerations of race came first. Another paper, "The Theory of Exhaustion", in which Heissmeyer argued that only "exhausted" and "inferior" organisms could be infected with tubercle bacilli *[mycobacterium tuberculosis]*, was rejected by experts as inadequate. But Heissmeyer had good professional and political connections, and eventually received Himmler's permission to start his experiment.

In early June 1944, the experiments began at Neuengamme concentration camp, with adults and in absolute secrecy. No one was permitted to enter the "Heissmeyer Barracks" except the experimental subjects, a German orderly named Herbert Kirst, and the French inmate doctors Professors Florence and Quenouille.

Every Wednesday for several weeks Heissmeyer traveled from Hohenlychen to Neuengamme, 165 miles away. On the first visit he took with him a glass bottle containing a strain of live, virulent tubercle bacilli, obtained from the laboratory of Professor Meinicke, a bacteriologist from Berlin. Heissmeyer later testified at his interrogation:

> When I received the serum, I was cautioned by Meinicke to be absolutely sure to test it on animals first in order to determine its effects. This, in fact, is what I did. However, during the whole course of the testing, I injected only twelve animals with the serum, even though I knew that this number was totally insufficient. Besides, the animal testing ran parallel to the testing of the inmates. Meinicke had advised me to observe the injected guinea pigs for at least three to four months, because only then could the effect of the serum be determined.
>
> But I did not do this. I wanted to have the results of the use of serum on humans in as short a time as possible. Therefore, soon after receiving the serum, I injected a number of adult prisoners at Neuengamme (I no longer remember how many); in other words, I did not await the results of the animal testing.
>
> Being a doctor, I knew, of course, that I was not allowed to do this, for it was after all a virulent serum that I was injecting. Thus I was knowingly exposing human subjects to the danger of contracting tbc and probably endangering their lives.[169]

The experiment went like this. The inmate-experimental subject had to sit on a stool, while Heissmeyer inserted a rubber tube down the subject's trachea into his lungs. This, of course, was very painful and caused a strong fit of coughing. At times, Heissmeyer injured the windpipe and caused bleeding. Most patients would scream during the procedure.

Next the person was required to step behind an X-ray screen. Heissmeyer checked the position of the tube, took an initial X-ray and then injected the tubercle solution into the lung. He also injected tubercle suspension under the skin or rubbed tubercle sputum into scratches made in the skin.

169 See Schwarzberg, *The Murders at Bullenhuserdamm: The SS Doctors and the Children*, pp. 3–7, 18–29, and 37–49.

Heissmeyer used four different test groups for the experiment. He began with a group of inmates suffering from extensive bilateral tuberculosis of the lungs, then turned to a group whose disease was confined to only one lobe. A third group was free of tbc of the lungs but had it in other organs. Finally Heissmeyer gathered together at random a number of healthy prisoners, free of tbc, to serve as the "control group".

At his postwar hearings, when asked what he told his test subjects about the nature of the experiments, Heissmeyer replied: "In answering this question I must admit that I did not tell them anything about the character and purpose of the experiments, nor the dangers connected with them. This was, in any case, not necessary, because as inmates of the concentration camp they had no rights whatsoever, and given the existing conditions in the camp, they were more or less forced to be at my disposal if I felt they were suitable for the experiments."[170]

Heissmeyer saw the results of his testing when the autopsies were performed. After observing for four weeks how the patients first developed a high fever and how the tubercular nodes spread in the lungs, he declared that the experiments were completed. The following day – "Heissmeyer Day" – the freshly hanged corpses of his patients were in the morgue, ready for autopsy. Heissmeyer had ordered all of the experimental subjects murdered!

At his interrogation, Heissmeyer further testified:

> After determining in the fall of 1944 that my plan to heal tbc patients with the aforementioned serum had failed, and that the condition of most of the inmates had worsened and not improved (I no longer know how many inmates were involved), I discontinued the experiments. I then ordered twenty children to be brought in, on whom I used the same serum to see if they were inherently immune to tbc as well as to see if I could immunize them against the disease.[171]

The experiments had failed, at least with respect to their stated purpose, but Heissmeyer went on with them just the same. He wanted to complete his research, and one experimental group had yet to be tested: children. Thus, in November 1944 twenty-five children from Auschwitz arrived at Neuengamme. Dr. Heissmeyer had personally selected them to participate in additional testing "for the benefit of progress in medicine". They appeared to be healthy.[172]

170 Ibid.
171 Ibid.
172 See IAC, *Inhuman Medicine*, vol. 1, pt. 2, pp. 163–184; and Schwarzberg, *The Murders at Bullenhuser Damm*, pp. 2–7, 18–29, and 37–49.

Two or three weeks after the children's arrival medical experiments were started with them. Dr. Heissmeyer made incisions in the skin of their arms and rubbed the incisions with cultures of tubercle bacilli. After a few days, the children began to experience both general as well as local signs of infection: redness and a slight swelling around the area where the bacilli had been rubbed in and a fever that intensified for several days before breaking.

A week later, procedures began to extract tubercle bacilli from the children. From each child one enlarged lymph node was excised and sent to Berlin where it was used to grow new tubercle bacilli cultures. From these cultures, emulsions were made and given to the children as inoculations. For each child, the inoculation consisted of bacilli grown uniquely from his or her lymphatic node. Heissmeyer wanted to see whether such specific inoculations might improve resistance. That he had to infect the children with the disease in order to protect them was of no concern!

The results were as follows. After receiving bi-weekly inoculations, after four to five months, the majority of the children were running a temperature. In the third month eighty percent of the "inoculated" children had enlarged lymph nodes. In the fourth month changes appeared in the lungs (foci and bilateral lesions), and in the sixth month cavities had formed in the lungs.

On 18 April 1945, as the Allies were about to arrive at the gates of Neuengamme, General Pohl, following Dr. Heissmeyer's advice, ordered the children transferred to the sub-camp Bullenhuserdamm, there to be murdered so that all traces of the experiments might be erased.

The children in Bullenhuserdamm were taken to a basement, undressed, given morphine injections, and hanged. In the words of Johann Frahm, who put the rope around each victim's neck, "they were like pictures hung upon on a wall on hooks".

This criminal experiment with children was observed by the two prisoner-physicians of the Neuengamme camp, Drs. Marcel Prenant and Kaufmann. In his testimony given before the English military court, Dr. Prenant (Prisoner No. 34190), a professor of comparative anatomy at the Sorbonne, stated that all Heissmeyer's experiments with children were kept strictly secret. The other prisoner-physicians working in the camp, Drs. Florence, Quenouille and Billiet, had been warned that giving away the secret would be punished with death by hanging.

The following are quotes from the trial of the Bullenhuserdamm murderers.

Interrogation[173]

Presiding judge: "Who brought each of the children into the room where they were to be injected?"
Frahm: "They were called in."

Presiding judge: "And every child came?"
Frahm: "Yes. Some of them were also brought in."

Presiding judge: "Who brought them in?"
Frahm: "I brought them in."

Presiding judge: "Were the children naked?"
Frahm: "They were undressed."

Presiding judge: "And one child after another were hanged or a few at a time?"
Frahm: "Two at a time."

Presiding judge: "So you mean to say two of them were pulled up over the pipe at one time?"
Frahm: "The grown-ups were pulled up over the pipes. The children were hanged on the hooks."

Presiding judge: "How many children were hanged at one time on these hooks?"
Frahm: "One."

Presiding judge: "Not two?"
Frahm: "There were two hooks there."

The bodies were taken by truck from Bullenhuserdamm to Neuengamme, where, on the night of 21 April 1945, they were cremated.

Drugs for Tuberculosis

German pharmaceutical companies had several experimental drugs, which they hoped might prove useful in the fight against tuberculosis. They were happy to support testing by SS physicians on human subjects in concentration camps. The SS doctors sent their findings to I. G. Farbenindustrie and also to the Bayer firm in Leverkusen. The fact that human beings were being infected

173 See Schwarzberg, *The Murders at Bullenhuser Damm,* pp. 42–43.

with a killer disease in order to test the efficacy of experimental drugs was never a concern for the directors of these firms.

The following document will illustrate the moral and ethical standard of the Bayer pharmaceutical firm.

Memo from Bayer[174]

Bayer Gruppe WIII
Leverkusen Nr 326 15.12.43
Dr. W./T/Nr 118423. Dez. 1943
Präparat 3582
Rutenol/ruthenol preparation

> With interest we have heard about Dr. Vetter's findings and have first of all given instructions that the 250 × 100 g – 3582 granulated preparation, is sent to him, according to wishes.
>
> In regard to these findings, it should be emphasized that 3582 is a strongly polyvalent nitro-acridine preparation. Its chemotherapeutic effect is relatively far-reaching; however in the fight against tubercle bacilli 3582 is not particularly effective. Therefore, the findings of Dr. Vetter can either be explained in such a way that there may have been a beneficial effect in the case of secondary infection for people suffering from tuberculosis, or maybe matters are, after all, different with human beings than they are with animals. We are at the time not in a position to start with corresponding experiments with animals. Though we have always adopted a very reserved attitude in regard to reports about the chemotherapeutic effectiveness of preparations in the fight against tuberculosis, this does not mean that Dr. Vetter should give up his work, conducted so far and that he should not continue to gather experience.

Two hundred and fifty new packages of 100 g granulated B-1034, 3582 were in fact received.

Who was Dr. Vetter? Dr. Helmut Vetter joined the SS in 1933, and from 1938 on was also an employee of the I. G. Farbenindustrie. He served as a camp physician in Oranienburg, Dachau, Auschwitz and Mauthausen-Gusen. Three Polish physicians who had been prisoners in Auschwitz and Mauthausen,

174 From Dr. Stanislaw Klodzinski, "Criminal Experiments with Tuberculosis carried out in the Nazi Concentration Camps", in International Auschwitz Committee, *Inhuman Medicine,* vol. 1, pt. 2, pp. 173–174.

Professor Wladyslaw Fejkiel, Dr. Wladyslaw Tondos, and Dr. Stanislaw Klodzinski, testified against Vetter for the tribunal in Nuremberg. They had observed Vetter's experiments with Ruthenol, preparation B-1034 and 3582 in the Auschwitz I camp. Evaluation had showed that both B-1034 and 3582 in cases of tuberculosis of the lungs were ineffective. They did, however, cause serious side effects such as persistent vomiting of bile, loss of appetite and loss of weight. Of the seventy-five people subjected to these experiments, forty died.[175] But once the drug experiment was deemed a success, the survivors were of no further use. After all, they had tuberculosis! Albert Haas narrates what then transpired:

> At 5:00 A.M. on an unusually bitter February morning, the Blockältester [prisoner head of the block] roughly woke all of my patients and tore off their nightgowns. Easily reverting to the brutality that had been so blissfully absent, he kicked the terrified herd of naked inmates into the subzero cold. I watched the Blockältester and the Stubendienst [prisoner assistant to the Blockältester] bring out some garden hoses, as innocent-looking as the ones you would use for watering your flowers. They opened the nozzles and began to spray the naked men, continuing until the last of my special patients had frozen to death.[176]

EXPERIMENTS WITH POISONING

Towards the end of 1943, Nazi physicians working in the concentration camps received instructions to begin experiments with various poisons, administered by mouth or in bullets. Whether the motivation for these experiments was, as some witnesses claimed at Nuremberg, the fear of a Soviet offensive with poison, or simply the desire to find another means of mass extermination, is not known. What is known is that the experiments were conducted at Sachsenhausen, Buchenwald and Dachau concentration camps, in the utmost secrecy. Results were reported only orally, leaving only the war-trials testimonies of physicians and laboratory personnel as evidence. Witnesses tes-

175 The autopsies showed kidney failure and severe liver damage. At this point the prisoner doctors secretly stopped giving the drugs to the patients. After awhile, the survivors began to look close to normal. Dr. Vetter happily noted the "favorable response".

176 Albert Haas, *The Doctors and the Damned* (New York: St. Martins Press, 1984), pp. 273–275.

tified that defendant Dr. Joachim Mrugowsky, Chief of the Hygiene Institute of the Waffen SS, ordered the experiments, at least at Sachsenhausen and Buchenwald.

Argumentation of the Prosecution at Nuremberg[177]

Extract from the Closing Brief against Defendant Mrugowsky

Poison experiments were carried out in the Buchenwald and Sachsenhausen concentration camps by order of the defendant Mrugowsky. The first series of the experiments was carried out in December 1943 in order to determine the fatal dosage of poisons of the *alkaloid group.* Four Russian prisoners of war were experimented upon by Dr. Ding. The poison was administered to the experimental subjects in their food without their knowledge. All four survived, but were strangled in a crematorium of the concentration camp in order that autopsies could be performed.

On 11 September 1944 Mrugowsky and Ding carried out an experiment with *aconitine nitrate projectiles* in the Sachsenhausen concentration camp. The projectiles were filled with crystallized poison and five experimental subjects were shot in the upper part of the left thigh with these projectiles. In two cases, no effect of the poison could be observed. In the other three cases, the suffering of the experimental subjects was terrible. All three died after approximately two hours of agony. The poison bullets used in the experiments were allegedly of Russian origin. (No-201, Pros. Ex. 290)

On 26 October 1944 still another poison experiment was carried out by Ding in Buchenwald. The entry in the Ding diary for that date states: "Special experiment on 6 persons according to instructions of SS Oberführer Lecturer Dr. Mrugowsky and RKPA. (Report on this orally.)" The Russian prisoners were later autopsied and burned. Ding reported to Mrugowsky orally. These experiments were connected with the poison bullet experiments in the Sachsenhausen concentration camp.

Depositions were taken at Buchenwald shortly after it was liberated.

177 Extracts from Argumentation and Defense of Prosecution and Defense, in *Trials NMT,* vol. 1.

Translation of Document No-508[178]
Deposition of Gerhard Schiedlausky, Freising, 7 August 1945

> Another experiment of SS Sturmbannführer Dr. SCHULER was with a poison which the Russians supposedly used against Germans in Russian territory when they wanted to get rid of them. SS Sturmbannführer Dr. SCHULER, as far as I know, had orders from the chief SS hygienist, SS Oberführer Prof. Dr. Joachim MRUGOWSKI, to study how this poison takes effect and to use prisoners for the experiment. I don't know how prisoners were chosen for this nor upon whose orders. One day he asked me to visit the crematorium where the experiment was to take place. There were, as far as I remember, 4 to 6 prisoners. When I got there the poison had already begun to take effect on some. This was visible because the victims threw up, had stomach cramps, and their faces had begun to discolor. One was unconscious.

Despite the secrecy surrounding the experiments, Dr. Mrugowsky did report to the Criminology Institute that the experiments had been performed, allegedly on patients already condemned to die.

Partial Translation of Document No-201[179]
Prosecution Exhibit 290

Report from Mrugowsky to the Criminology Institute, 12 September 1944, on Experiments with Aconitine Nitrate Projectiles

Reich Physician SS and Police	Berlin-Zehlendorf 6
The Chief Hygienist	12 September 1944
Journal No.: Secret 364/44 Dr. Mru./Eb.	Spanische Allee 10-12

Top Secret
Subject: Experiments with aconitine nitrate projectiles
To the Criminological Institute (Stamp)
Attn: Dr. Widmann

178 Excerpt from Declaration of Gerhald Schiedlausky, Freising, 7 August 1945, Translation of Document No-508, in RG-30.001M, pp. 10–11.
179 Partial Translation of Document No-201, Prosecution Exhibit 290, in RG-30.001M.

Berlin

Criminological Institute
Department: Chemistry
Received: 13 Sep 1944
Journal No. g53/44
In charge:

In the presence of SS Sturmbannführer Dr. Ding, Dr. Widmann, and the undersigned, experiments with aconitine nitrate projectiles were conducted on 11 September 1944 on 5 persons who had been condemned to death. The projectiles in question were of a 7.65 mm caliber, filled with crystallized poison. The experimental subjects, in a lying position, were each shot in the upper part of the left thigh. The thighs of the two of them were cleanly shot through. Even afterwards, no effect of the poison was to be observed. These two experimental subjects were therefore exempted.

The entrance of the projectile did not show any peculiarities. Evidently the arteria femoralis of one of the subjects were injured. A slight stream of blood issued from the wound. But the bleeding stopped after a short time. The loss of blood was estimated as having been at the most $^{3}/_{4}$ of a liter, and consequently was on no account fatal.

The symptoms of the condemned three showed a surprising similarity. At first no peculiarities appeared. After 20 to 25 minutes a motor agitation and a slight ptyalism set in, but stopped again. After 40 to 45 minutes a stronger salivation set in. It could not even be overcome by swallowing. Foamy saliva flowed from their mouths. Then choking and vomiting set in.

After 58 minutes the pulse of two of them could no longer be felt. The third had a pulse rate of 76. After 65 minutes his blood pressure was 90/60. The sounds were extremely low. A drop of blood pressure was evident.

During the first hour of the experiment the pupils did not show any changes. After 78 minutes the pupils of all three showed a medium dilation together with a retarded light reaction. Simultaneously, maximum respiration with heavy breathing inhalations set in. This subsided after a few minutes. The pupils contracted again and their reaction improved. After 65 minutes the patellar and Achilles tendon reflexes of the poisoned subjects were negative. The upper abdominal reflexes of the two of them were also negative. The upper abdominal reflexes of the third were still positive, while the lower abdominal reflexes were negative. After approximately 90 minutes, one of the subjects again started breathing heavily. This was accompanied by an increasing motor unrest. Then the heavy breathing changed into a flat, accelerated respiration, accompanied by extreme nausea. One of the poisoned persons tried in vain to vomit. To do so he introduced four fingers of his hand up to the knuckles into his throat, but nevertheless could not vomit. His face was flushed.

The faces of the other two experimental subjects became pale early on. The other symptoms were the same. The motor unrest increased so much that the persons flung themselves up, and down, rolled their eyes, and made meaningless motions with their hands and arms. Finally the agitation subsided, the pupils dilated to the maximum, and the condemned lay motionless. Masseter spasms and urination were observed in one case. Death occurred 121, 123, and 129 minutes after entry of the projectile.

Summary. The projectiles filled with approximately 38 mg. of aconitine nitrate in solid form had, in spite of only insignificant injuries, a deadly effect after two hours. Poisoning showed 20 to 25 minutes after injury. The main reactions were salivation, alteration of the pupils, negative tendon reflexes, motor unrest, and extreme nausea.

(Signature) MRUGOWSKY SS Lecturer Oberführer and Office Chief

Prosecution witness Dr. Eugen Kogon, on direct examination, provided details of the scene at Buchenwald during the experiments. He highlights the fact that these experiments, which ended in murder, were ordered by the SS courts.

Extract from Testimony by Dr. Eugen Kogon, Given on Direct Examination 6–8 January 1947[180]

Mr. MCHANEY: Do you know anything about the experiments with poisons in the Buchenwald concentration camp?

Witness KOGON: I know of two such cases. The one case was about the turn of the year 1943-44 or in the late fall of 1943, and the second case was probably in the summer of 1944. In each case Russian prisoners of war were used for these experiments. In the first case various preparations of the so-called alkaloid series were put into noodle soup and administered to 4 of these prisoners of war who were in Block 46. They, of course, had no idea what was going on. Two of these prisoners became

180 Complete testimony is recorded in a mimeographed transcript dated 6, 7, 8 Jan. 1947, in *Trials NMT,* vol. 1, pp. 1150–1290. See also testimony of defendant Mrugowsky, in Ibid., vol. 2, sec. VIII–G.

> so sick that they vomited, one was unconscious, the fourth showed no symptoms at all. Thereupon, all four were strangled in the crematorium. They were autopsied and the contents of their stomachs and other effects were analysed. The experiment was ordered by the SS Court, by the SS investigating judge, Sturmbannführer Dr. Morgen. It was carried out in the presence of Dr. Ding, Dr. Morgen, Dr. Wehner, SS Hauptsturmführer and SS judges, and one of the three camp leaders, I do not know whether it was SS Sturmbannführer Schubert or SS leader Florstedt.
>
> Q. Now, will you explain to the Tribunal about his second poison experiment?
> A. In the summer of 1944 – I am not quite sure of the exact date – Dr. Ding, who was already called Schuler, came from Berlin at the time and told me that he had a very unpleasant task to perform. He said it was extremely secret and a few hours later, without my having asked, he told me details about it in his room.
>
> He said, "...I am supposed to test a poison here on Russian prisoners of war. I have to report on it immediately."
>
> ...The Russian prisoners of war, again, four of them, had been taken into the cellar with the 46 hooks on the walls on which the people were strangled. These four Russians were given this poison. I do not know how it was administered. As Ding-Schuler told me later, they died in a very short time. Then they were autopsied and cremated. Dr. Ding did not send a written report on this matter to Berlin. He told me he had to report on it to Mrugowsky orally.

Dr. Albert Aidman, head of the Chemical Department of the Criminal Technical Institute of the Security Police of the Reich Criminal Police Bureau also conducted experiments with poisoned bullets in Sachsenhausen. Portions of his testimony, as reprinted in Philippe Aziz, *Doctors of Death,* appear below.

> Five Russian prisoners of war were lying on stretchers in a small room adjoining the crematorium of Sachsenhausen. Three doctors were present – Professor Mrugowsky, Dr. Ding, and Dr. Widmann, a chemical expert form the Kripo, the criminal police.
>
> Five gunshots went off. The five men were hit in the thigh with poison bullets of aconitine nitrate. These experiments were carried out at the request of Dr. Widmann. Just two weeks before, a high Nazi official had been grazed by a bullet in a murder attempt in Poland. He died a few hours later, showing the symptoms of having been poisoned. The assassin had in his possession hollow bullets containing a poison in crystal form, which turned out to be aconitine. The weapon was of Russian ori-

> gin, and they had to find out whether this was the beginning of an all-out poison warfare. How would Germany counteract?... Dr. Ding noted carefully the victims' reactions.[181]

Dr. Sigmund Rascher oversaw the experiments in Dachau. He was already conducting a series of experiments on the effects of cold and high altitude, when he received instructions to carry out tests with poisons. Daily, he prepared some sixty to eighty cyanide tablets. He would then take prisoners into the crematory barracks and make them swallow his pills. None came out alive.

No one knows how many men died in this manner. "We often used to say among ourselves that they were experimenting with drugs to take themselves when things went badly."[182]

LIVER BIOPSY

Biopsy of the liver is an accepted and frequently used diagnostic procedure, which provides information unattainable by any other diagnostic means. It should only be performed when definite indications exist and other diagnostic methods fail, and then only by a physician experienced with its technique. It is a relatively simple procedure, but in inexperienced hands, it can cause very severe, even life-threatening injury.

As proven by official documents and personal testimonies, physicians at Dachau performed many liver biopsies. The procedure was relatively new and in need of further testing to verify its efficacy and accuracy. But the Dachau biopsies violated professional and ethical standards, since they were being conducted in the absence of genuine medical indication. One must conclude that some physicians at Dachau subjected patients to this procedure simply to gain experience with its techniques. Once again the ethical demands of the Hippocratic oath proved weaker than those of physicians' self-interest.

181 Aziz, *Doctors of Death*, vol. 3, pp. 123–135.

182 Ibid., p. 78, quoting prisoner Walter Neff. The cyanide experiment is also described by Leo Alexander, M.D., "Medical Science and Dictatorship", *New England Journal of Medicine* 241: 2 (14 July 1949), p. 2.

Translation of Document No-3249-PS Extract from Affidavit of Dr. Franz Blaha, Given in Dachau, 24 November 1945[183]

> Liver Biopsy
> (Note: In the translation from German "liver puncture" is used instead of "liver biopsy".)
>
> Liver puncture experiments were performed by Dr. Rudolf Brachtl on healthy people and on people who had diseases of the stomach and gall-bladder. For this purpose a needle was inserted into the liver of a person and a small piece of the liver was extracted. No anaesthetic was used. The procedure was very painful and often had serious complications as the stomach or large blood vessels were often accidentally punctured, resulting in hemorrhage. Many persons died of these tests for which Polish, Russian, Czech, and German prisoners were employed. Altogether these experiments were conducted on about 175 people.

The following paragraph, part of a report on the Dachau concentration camp, can be found in the Yad Vashem Archives.

> In 1942–1943 the SS doctors at Dachau were experimenting with liver biopsy as a diagnostic method. Again without their consent, healthy and sick prisoners were subjected to this procedure. Since the doctors were apparently completely inept, several cases of death resulted from perforation of the intestines, and those who did not die suffered great pain, intra-abdominal hemorrhage being a fairly common complication.[184]

From the following document, a record of the direct examination by the Military Government Court of Dr. Franz Blaha, we see that the doctor was aware of the dangers associated with liver biopsy.

183 Translation of Document No-3249-PS, YVA, JM/10046, p. 2.

184 *Report of the Atrocities Committed at the Dachau Concentration Camp,* vol. 1, YVA, JM/10046, p. 19.

Direct Examination of Dr. Franz Blaha, by the Military Government Court[185]

Q. Would you describe the nature of the liver puncture (biopsy) experiments?
Blaha: That was done by Doctor Brachtl. He made a series of liver punctures on ill people, on healthy people, people who had stomach diseases and people who had gall bladder disease.

Q. How were these liver punctures performed?
Blaha: By means of a puncturing needle in the vicinity of the liver.

Q. Were the people upon whom these experiments were performed alive at the time?
Blaha: Yes.

Q. Were they given any kind of anaesthesia?
Blaha: Without anesthesia.

Q. Do you know whether or not this type of experiment is painful to the subject undergoing it?
Blaha: Yes, because they were done in a series of several punctures and they also died as a result of that.

Q. Were these people prisoners in Camp Dachau at that time?
Blaha: Yes.

Q. Will you tell the court how these persons were selected?
Blaha: Doctor Drashal did that with the hospital capo [cameraden Polizei, prisoners assigned to police fellow prisoners]. They selected the people and took the people into the hospital.

Q. From where did they select those people?
Blaha: From work blocks.

Q. Was the nature of those liver puncture experiments one that was dangerous?
Blaha: Yes.

185 Military Government, Dachau, Germany, 2 November 1945, Direct Examination of Dr. Franz Blaha, YVA, JM/10049, pp. 11–12.

NUTRITION EXPERIMENTS[186]

On 12 August 1942 Himmler instructed Oswald Pohl, Director of the SS Wirtschafts-Verwaltunghauptamt (WVHA), to organize experiments on nutrition in the concentration camps. The goal was to identify the cheapest method of supplying the minimal nutrition needed by active laborers in the camps. Several diets, with and without nutritional supplements were eventually tested. The physician and chemist Ernst-Günther Schenk was appointed Nutrition Inspector and directed to assess the status of nutrition in the camps; Schenk spent the period of November 1942–January 1943 visiting eight concentration and penal camps. He reported that the quality of food was good, including excellent vegetables, but that 20–30 percent of the prisoners seemed, nevertheless, to be suffering from malnutrition.

Some sort of dietary supplement, cheap and readily available, was needed. Schenk suggested brewer's yeast, which could be provided without taxing the civilian food supply. The WVHA favored another supplement, a mold-infused egg white available under the trade name Biosyn.

In 1943 Biosyn was incorporated into a vegetable sausage that resembled common liverwurst in smell and taste, and the product was sent to the camps for initial tests on 100 prisoners. The sausages were alleged to have come from the cellulose and paper factory in Lenz, but camp lore had it that they were actually made out of sewage sludge; even dogs would not touch them! The undernourished experimental subjects suffered from intestinal problems after ingesting the sausages, and 70–80 percent of them became seriously ill. These dire results did not deter Pohl from continuing the experiments; he actually expanded their scope for three months (January–March 1944) to include 100,000 prisoners in Dachau, Buchenwald and Sachsenhausen.

The results of these tests were among the reports given on 27 January 1944, at a conference in Berlin of leaders in the bio-nutrition field. The participants included the 1938 Nobel Prize winner for chemistry, Professor Richard Kuhn; Otto Flossner, Director of the Nutrition Physiology Department of the Reich's Health Department; and Wilhelm Nonnenbruch, Professor of Medicine; among others. The vote was unanimous in favor of continuing the experiments.

186 For the material in this chapter, I am indebted to Ernst Klee's excellent volume *Auschwitz die NS-Medizin und Ihre Opfer*, pp. 179–189.

Report on Nutrition Experiments Conducted 1 December 1943 to 31 March 1944 in the Infirmary at the Mauthausen Concentration Camp[187]

The objective of the experiments was to discover the most beneficial form of nutrition for concentration camp inmates.

For the sake of comparison, three basic types of diet were established:
Type A: so-called "Eastern Diet"
Type B: Normal diet + nutritive yeast
Type C: Normal diet

Type A (Eastern Diet) consisted of vegetables and farinaceous food served exclusively in the form of a thick soup without any meat or bread.

Type B consisted of the normal diet, which was without any hard-labor rations but with an added 30.0 g of nutritive yeast per person. The yeast was evenly mixed into the midday diet.

Type C was the normal diet of a prisoner at the concentration camp, who was not subjected to hard labor.

The majority of the prisoners sought out for experiments consisted of invalids, cripples and those who were over 55 years old. Only 30 percent comprised strong, young individuals. Therefore, it is obvious that weakness was a common characteristic, which made the prisoners more susceptible to different types of illnesses mainly affecting the digestive tract and the circulatory system.

The prisoners selected for the experiments worked in the weaving mill, which was located near the infirmary block. This work was done while seated most of the time and was in general less exhausting, so that the caloric need was much less than that necessary for those subjected to hard labor.

The clinical and laboratory experiments, which were conducted in conjunction with nutrition tests, were expected to give as objective a picture as possible of the influence of the respective forms of diet on the human body, especially on hematopoiesis (production of blood cells) and on the circulatory and excretory systems. The experiments were also expected to cover the pathological changes, which surfaced as a result of various, accidental disease-causing factors. In addition, they were also expected to enable one to differentiate between the changes that could be attributed to the diet and those that could be attributed to pathogenic causes. Naturally, one encountered many practical difficulties. For

187 Ibid.

example, the frequent emergence of acute enterocolitis had a significant influence on the weight curve; body weight was increased due to edema that was frequently present. One encountered problems while doing hematological work since furuncolosis and certain illnesses influenced the leukocyte count and the leftward shift of the blood picture, while causing irregular appearance of white blood cells.

The tests were conducted during three periods. At the time various diet-experiments began, during the nutrition experiments, and during the two months after the conclusion of the experiments.

The nutrition experiments started on 12/01/1943 ended completely on 05/31/1944, after which further comparative experiments were conducted until 07/31/1944, at which time a normal diet was prescribed to all prisoners.

The numbers initially selected for the experiments were as follows:

For Group A (Eastern Diet)	150 prisoners
For Group B (Normal Diet + yeast)	110 prisoners
For Group C (Normal Diet)	110 prisoners
	370 prisoners

At the end, 7/31/1944:

Total Deaths:

Due to:

Colitis	62
Myodegeneratic cordis	19
Tbc pulmonem/Tbc lungs	12
Pneumonia	8
Cachexia universalis	3
Septicopyaemia	2
Erysipelas	2
Phlegmona gangraenosa	2
Pleuritis exsudativa	1
Glomerulonephritis	1
Uremia	1
Septicaemia	1
Meningitis epidemica	1
Carcinoma hepatic	1
Total	*116*

The number of survivors consisted of:

In Group B	67%
In Group A	54%
In Group C	48%

Through the examinations and the evidence that was obtained while conducting them, be it in hematology, electrocardiography, clinical diseases, it was concluded that the most suitable diet was that of Group B: i.e., normal diet plus yeast, and the most unsuitable diet was the diet of Group C: i.e., normal diet. As mentioned before, this was the diet provided to all prisoners in the concentration camps.

ALLOPATHIC AND HOMEOPATHIC EXPERIMENTS

Experiments at Ravensbrück, Dachau and Auschwitz during the years 1942–43, on various therapeutic agents, were designed not only to test potential remedies but also to compare the effectiveness of allopathic and homeopathic medicine. Dachau was the site of experiments with the treatment of cellulitis by homeopathic means.[188]

During the Nuremberg trials, the witness Heinrich Stohr, a political prisoner who had worked as a male nurse at Dachau testified about these experiments. The first tests comparing the two concepts of therapy were conducted on patients with spontaneously developed cellulitis, the "typical camp complaint". Upon their completion, tests were begun on individuals in whom cellulitis had been induced by artifical means. The first subjects selected by Chief Surgeon Waldemar Wolter were German prisoners, ten of them. Next in turn were Catholic priests and monks, selected from the camp's clerical block. Infection was induced in each subject in the operating room of the camp hospital. Stohr observed, as did SS Major Schutz and the homeopath Dr. Rudolf Kiesewetter, while Dr. Hermann Pape, a camp physician, performed the procedures.

Stohr testified about the experiments with both spontaneous and artificially induced infections. Here he speaks of his observations in the spontaneous cases.

188 For the experiments at Ravensbrück, see *Experimental Operations on Prisoners of Ravensbrück Concentration Camp* (Poznan and Warsaw, Poland: Wydawich Zachodwie, 1960).

Testimony of Witness Heinrich Stohr[189]

> Three identical or similar cases [spontaneous infection] were observed. One of these cases was treated allopathically, another homeopathically, while the third received only ordinary wound treatment, i.e. no medication of any kind. The limb bearing the wound was immobilized, treated with compresses and the like, as the case might be. The patients frequently recovered faster without any medication, i.e. without tablets, injections, etc. Experiments of this character were conducted for several weeks, and if I as a layman am permitted any judgment, I must say that to my observation the physicians were not satisfied with such experiments.
>
> I must emphasize, by the way, that not merely wounds were treated by these methods but also internal diseases. The chief aim was to find out whether the homeopathic drugs were also useful in combating dropsy, which was very common in camp. It developed that the homeopathic drugs had no effect whatever on the course of the disease.

The infections placed experimental subjects in grave danger, as further testimony reveals:[190]

> Q. Now, you have told us that they had one group, the first group, consisting of ten Germans. How many died in this group?
> A. ...Of these, as far as I recall, seven died.
>
> Q. Now, you have told us of a second group, of forty clergymen. How many died in that group?
> A. I saw a list of the survivors, and according to this list about twelve priests or monks died.
>
> Part of these test persons was treated with sulfonamides, the other with homeopathic preparations.

A report by Reich Physician SS Dr. Grawitz to Himmler, which formed part of the prosecution exhibit at the Nuremberg proceedings, gives an excellent and detailed description of these experiments.

189 Mitscherlich and Mielke, eds., *Doctors of Infamy*, pp. 66–67.
190 Ibid., pp. 68–71.

Translation of Document No-409[191]
Prosecution Exhibit 249

Report from Grawitz to Himmler, 29 August 1942, concerning Experiments with Biochemical Remedies Conducted at the Dachau and Auschwitz Concentration Camps

[Note: The term "biochemical" here refers to natural homeopathic remedies]

The Reich Leader SS
Reich Physician SS and Police
Telephone: 924249.924351.924373
924406
Az: 738/IV/42

Berlin W 15 29 August 1942
Knesebeckst. 50/51
(Stamp)
Personal Staff
Reich Leader SS
G 213

Subject: Biochemical treatment of sepsis etc., with biochemical remedies.

To the Reich Leader SS H. Himmler
Berlin SW 11 Prinz Albrechtstrasse 8

Reich Leader!

I take the liberty of submitting the following intermediate report of results obtained so far with the homeopathic treatment of sepsis and other complaints:

In the SS Hospital at Dachau, during the period covered by the report, the following forty cases were treated by homeopathic means. In addition to septic infections, other complaints were treated in which homeopathic treatment had shown promises of improvement.

Cellulitis	17
Sepsis	8
Furunculosis and abscesses	2
Infected operative wounds	1
Malaria	5
Pleural empyema	3
Septic endocarditis	1

191 Report from Grawitz to Himmler, 29 August 1942, Concerning Experiments with Biochemical Remedies Conducted at the Dachau and Auschwitz Concentration Camps, Document No-409, Prosecution Exhibit 249, in *Trials NMT*, vol. 1, 657–669.

Nephrosis	1
Chronic sciatica	1
Gallstones	1

In accordance with therapeutical directions provided by homeopathy, the following preparations were administered, according to the case:

Kalium phosphoricum (potassium phosphate)	D6
Ferrum phosphoricum (ferric phosphate)	D6, D12
Silicium (silicon)	D6
Natrium muriaticum (sodium chloride)	D6
Calcium phosphoricum (calcium phosphate)	D6
Natrium sulfuricum (sodium sulphate)	D6
Magnesium phosphoricum (magnesium phosphate)	D6
Natrium phosphoricum (sodium phosphate)	D6
Calcium fluoraticum (calcium fluoride)	D6

In the majority of cases septic infection was artificially administered. Results so far indicate that the unfavorable course of these severe complaints is scarcely affected by homeopathic means in even a single instance. All cases of sepsis ended fatally. The malaria cases remained completely unaffected.

The cases of extensive cellulitis with abscess formation, empyema septic endocarditis, chronic sciatica, nephrosis, and gallstones afforded not the slightest degree of certainty as to the effect of homeopathic treatment. Insofar as they showed a favorable course, medical experience shows it to be no different from what would have ordinarily occurred with absolute immobilization in bed and no other special measures.

Only in five cases was the impression offered that the complaints were favorably influenced by homeopathic means. Of these, four cases were comparatively light. The fifth case was that of a seventeen-day-old child with severe furunculosis. Here a turn for the better was experienced only a few days after the onset of the treatment. It must be mentioned, however, that there was an error in the experimental arrangements on this case, since at the beginning of treatment, Alvucid, a sulfonamide preparation, was also administered.

The stronger pus formation plainly observed in some cases may also perhaps be attributable to the effect of the homeopathic preparations. Perhaps this is the result of the frequent dosage with sugar, since the homeopathic tablets consist almost entirely of lactose. Experiments to clear up this point have been scheduled.

In one case of joint surgery potassium phosphate was given as a prophylactic antiseptic, since the operative incision was particularly exposed to infection. Nevertheless, the next day a temperature of 102.2 degrees F was measured. Homeopathic treatment thus proved incapable of preventing the onset or outbreak of infection, though potassium phosphate D6 was at once administered intensively. It is also noteworthy that after a short time all the severe cases vigorously rejected the homeopathic tablets, since it meant torture for them to take the medicine every five minutes, even at night.

In summary, it is stated that of a total of forty cases, one is evaluated as positive, and four as positive with reservations, as opposed to thirty-five failures, including ten deaths.

The tests at Dachau are being continued.

In addition to the present program, we are especially on the look-out for twin cases of the greatest possible similarity, the one to be treated allopathically, the other homeopathically.

At the Auschwitz concentration camp, these three typical cases of septic infection, developing from tissue inflammation, were treated with potassium phosphate D4 according to directions. In none of these cases was a therapeutic effect on the course of the complaint observed.

All three cases ended fatally. The tests are being continued.

(Signed) Grawitz

THE AHNENERBE

The Ahnenerbe e. V.–Studiengesellschaft für Geistesurgeschichte (Ancestral Heritage Society), which was founded by Himmler in Berlin on 1 July 1935, played significant supporting roles, financial and ideological, in the conduct of experiments in concentration camps.[192] Originally established to assist in the implementation of Nazi racial policies by determining the origins, spirit, exploits and heritage of the Aryan race, the Ahnenerbe metamorphosed into a scientific research center particularly involved with medical research. It financed experiments and supplied necessary materials, or arranged their supply. No discussion of the Nazi atrocities committed in the name of medicine would be complete without at least a brief mention of this organization.

The guidance of the Ahnenerbe was entrusted to a former bookdealer named Wolfram Sievers, who later testified at the Nuremberg proceedings.

192 Hoedeman, *Hitler or Hippocrates,* pp. 48–50.

Sievers would have had the court believe that the organization played but a trivial role in the matter of the camp experiments, despite its size (no less than forty-six scientific departments and fifteen research commissions) and its intimate association with the Nazi racial ideology and policies. All the Ahnenerbe archives were destroyed by the Germans shortly before they capitulated to the Allies, so the prosecutors at Nuremberg had to turn to other sources for evidence. Fortunately, Himmler's private files yielded some incontestable clues. But they did not reveal the names of the thirty professors who Sievers claimed had been working for the society; their names have never been exposed.

It has been established that the part the Ahnenerbe played in the experimentation was hardly as trivial as Sievers would have liked the Nuremberg judges to believe. In fact, on orders from Himmler himself, the Ahnenerbe directed doctors in the camps to perform experiments on humans. Consequently, it was with the collaboration of the Ahnenerbe that thousands of defenseless concentration camp prisoners were murdered.[193] And "the tests were not only criminal but also, from the scientific point of view, incompetent"![194]

The Ahnenerbe was one of the institutions that provided special opportunities and privileges for doctors willing both to embrace Nazi racial theory and to apply their talents towards implementing it. The experiments authorized by the society offered unprecedented opportunities for medical experimentation otherwise unthinkable. And participating doctors, if troubled by qualms of conscience, could comfort themselves with the knowledge that they were working for the greater good of the Reich.

That ethical boundaries were being crossed in this program, Himmler dismissed as nothing more than a logical consequence of a wholly justifiable philosophy. The ends – the purification of the Aryan race through the conquest of troubling diseases and abnormalities, and the elimination of unwanted marginal groups – would wholly justify the shocking means. In a famous speech in Posen, Himmler undescored his conviction with these chilling words: "We must remember our principle: blood, selection, austerity..."[195] Heinrich Himmler, we can see, was a man of disquieting intellectual and moral mediocrity and of equally disquieting contrasts. And a man whose importance was no less disquieting.

Among the allegedly trivial activities directed by the Ahnenerbe were the experiments with *Lost* (mustard gas) and the collection of Jewish skeletons and

193 Desoille and Lafitte, *Psychologie criminelle des Hitleriens* (Paris, 1972), p. 4.
194 Telford Taylor, "Opening Address", in *Trials NMT,* vol. 1, p. 72.
195 Quoted in Hoedeman, *Hitler or Hippocrates,* p. 50.

skeletal parts, described respectively in the previous sections of this chapter. The involvement of the Ahnenerbe in these programs came to light with the recovery of Himmler's personal files from their subterranean hiding place.

Translation of Document No-422[196]
Office of U.S. Chief of Counsel

Sample of the Orders given by Himmler to the Ahnenerbe

The Reichführer SS Operational Headquarters
7 July 1942
AR 48/6/42
Stamp:
Personal Staff Reich Leader SS
Archives
File No. AR/22/21

Secret!

To the Reichsmanager of the "Ahnenerbe" SS Obersturmbannführer Sievers
Berlin–Dahlem

I request the "Ahnenerbe"

1. To establish an Institute for Military Scientific Research,
2. To support in every possible way the research carried out by SS Hauptsturmführer Prof. Dr. Hirt and to promote all corresponding research and undertakings,
3. To make available the required apparatus, equipment, accessories and assistants, or to procure them,
4. To make use of the facilities available in Dachau,
5. To contact the Chief of the SS Economic and Administrative Main Office (Wirtschafts- und Verwaltungshauptamt) with regards to the costs which can be borne by the Waffen SS.

(Signature) H. H.

196 Document No-422, Office of the U.S. Chief of Counsel, in *Trials NMT,* vol. 1, RG-30.001M.

Copy mailed to the Chief of the Economic and Administrative Main
Office (Wirtschafts- und Verwaltungshauptamt)
SS Obergruppenführer Pohl
Berlin–Lichtenfelde-West
With the request to take note.
By order,
(sig) Brandt
SS Obersturmführer N.7/7.
True Copy:
(signature)
SS Obersturmbannführer 7.7.

THE RAJSKO INSTITUTE

A few miles from Auschwitz, at Rajsko, after the Polish inhabitants had been deported, the Nazis established a satellite camp dedicated primarily to agricultural research. The camp contained facilities for growing the plant sources needed to manufacture latex; conveniently, an I. G. Farben latex-producing factory stood nearby in Monowitz.

Rajsko, however, contained other facilities involved in less benign activities, most notoriously, one of the hygienic institutes operated by the SS. There, clinical research using Auschwitz inmates as subjects, and as workers, was designed and implemented. As was true in most of the SS research organizations, the stated reason for setting up the program – the need to find effective vaccines against and treatments for typhus – masked another goal – the desire to secure a reliable, steady supply of test sera for the blood-typing of SS members. Even more important, the absence of direct administrative relations between the camp at Auschwitz and the research institute at Rajsko obfuscated the fact that institute doctors were actually assisting with an extermination program.

Hans Muench was one of the SS doctors who conducted experiments at Rajsko. The following extract has been taken from his written testimony, given after the war.

Post-war Testimony Given by SS physician Hans Muench[197]

QUESTION 16: You write that the Institute of Hygiene came to Auschwitz because the spotted fever epidemic of 1942 could not be stopped with the means Hoess applied extermination of lice together with the sick. What was the contribution of the Institute of Hygiene in fighting this epidemic? What was the main task of the Institute?

Dr. MUENCH: Typhus epidemic had already broken out in 1941 and was spreading all over the camp, which mainly brought the Institute of Hygiene to Auschwitz. The Institute of Hygiene had five to seven so-called field laboratories. Every military establishment has these installations, a bacteriological and also a modest serological laboratory, which under conditions of field hospitals, can perform examinations. The Rajsko Institute started out as such a field laboratory.

Mrugowsky, Chief of the Hygienisches Institute of the Waffen SS, was happy to send a laboratory to Auschwitz because he needed far less personnel there since the laboratory technicians could be replaced by prisoners.

Dr. Weber, the head researcher there, was an excellent organizer. He enjoyed the chance of building an institute for scientific research. He was actually not interested in basic scientific investigation but rather in the production of test sera for blood groups. Test sera for blood groups can only be obtained from human blood and are very perishable. It was in demand for the SS because all members of the SS had their blood group tattooed under their arm, so they all had to have their type determined. For this purpose they required vast amounts of test sera of blood types in a form which could be kept for a long time without refrigeration or other conservation. This was very difficult and was one of the major task[s] of the Institute in Rajsko.

That was the background... but the actual cause for the opening of the Institute was the typhus epidemic...

Spotted fever did, of course, play a large role in Auschwitz, but to combat it one did not necessarily need a laboratory. One had to take general hygienic measures. This was not possible in camps. One could not continue to use the same method the camp administration had employed, i.e., gassing the lice together with the people, because the spotted fever spread even faster this way. We were supposed to devise measures against it, but the camp administration did not allow us to do so.

197 Correspondence with former SS-Physician Dr. Hans Muench, in Shelley, ed., *Criminal Experiments on Human Beings*, pp. 288–302.

QUESTION 25: Dr. Mark Klein (formerly a professor at Strasbourg University) often asked what actually was the purpose of the South-Eastern Institute of Hygiene. He later asserted that all investigations were lacking a plan and originality. What is your opinion?
Dr. MUENCH: Mark Klein is absolutely right. There was no coordination and no original planning, exactly as Prof. Klein stated.

Question 26: Klein further asserted that there was a lot of sabotage which was not discovered by the SS. Do you agree?...

QUESTION 27: Did you know about all this?
Dr. MUENCH: Histological and bacteriological diagnoses were often forged in order not to jeopardize prisoners by positive results (in the cases of Koch bacilli for tuberculosis, malaria, typhus, etc.). By the way, Langbein reports how Mrs. Rohde, the wife of an SS physician, forced inmate physician Dr. Andre Lettich to declare her diphtheria slide as negative because she wanted to get rid of the bothersome quarantine. ...He who knows conditions in Auschwitz would realize that certain quid pro quo diagnoses and certificates were unavoidable... that was inherent in the omnipresent corruption. A case in point was the false diphtheria result for Mrs. Rohde to shorten her quarantine. This was the order of the day and could not be controlled. The possibilities for manipulation were always available and not difficult to realize.

QUESTION 28: Did you ever have any scruples about using human flesh as a culture medium for bacteria in your laboratory?
Dr. MUENCH: I must confirm that this happened twice and I want to give an explanation. Once, during the time of the Hungarian transports, we needed a large quantity of cultural media because a typhus epidemic had broken out in the military hospital in Cracow. We have always been in short supply of culture medium because the deliveries from the slaughterhouse were meager and much of the meat from these sparse deliveries disappeared for "business".

Unterscharführer Zabel knew the SDGs (SS hospital orderlies) of the camp Revier [sick-bay] well. He needed their assistance, when he had to take blood from prisoners for the serological laboratory, doing the research on blood group test sera. Bread and sausages were distributed and volunteers could donate blood to "make themselves useful", as the saying went. Thus, Zabel complained about the shortage to the SDGs and they persuaded him to simply take the meat which was lying around in large quantities in front of the crematoria. Zabel listened and cut out human flesh from the corpses. He told me about it and said that the same had been done earlier, before he joined the Institute. He had heard this from the prisoners. It simply had been an emergency... and that had been dealt with properly. However, I know that he did the same thing a second time, shortly after the first occurrence. The prisoners of the culture medium kitchen informed me.

You will probably ask what I did with Zabel, who did not follow my orders. Well, I have to admit that for reasons of prudence, I did not do anything because I knew it would only backfire. The prisoners would have been in trouble. He would have denied it if I had confronted him and I did not have any proof except to refer to prisoners. Zabel would surely have found ways and means to make them suffer. And I decided to check better in the future and as far as I know it did not happen again...

Dr. MUENCH further stated this:

In our laboratory we had examined the nutrition provided to prisoners by contents and by calories, and it had been established that the average prisoner would vegetate on 1500 calories. It followed that one could stand this as nutrition for a limited time only. Now I had the time and opportunity to check the figures statistically.

I searched for the notes which showed diagnoses of people who did not have long to live, i.e., who were already in the "Muselmann" stage. There were those suffering from diarrhea without any bacteriological cause or disease, simply due to the shortage of albumin. The prison number was also listed on those notes and from the prison number I knew how long the prisoner had been in camp. In this way, I arrived at my statistics. With 1500 calories one obtained a life expectancy curve of four months, i.e., somewhere between three and five months. The span is so large because there are different types, good and bad food utilizers. Anyway, the curve that can be drawn coincides completely with the statistics.

In my description of "Muselmann", I did not restrict myself to the purely physical symptoms but also discussed the mental state which characterizes this stage, for example, this indifference to the environment. This state of resignation did not actually alleviate the lot of these poor people or improve their chances for survival, just the contrary. But it made them bear the end more easily.

The SS men at Rajsko, needless to say, preferred the stability, comfort and security of jobs at the Institute to the dangers of the battlefield. To keep the employees busy, the SS had samples of blood, urine, fecal matter, sputum, and mucous secretions taken from prisoners, even those who, in a matter of days, would be sent to the gas chamber. Obviously, the taking of these samples had no connection to any goal of healing the patient. The doctors, who were aware of the futility of these exercises, were nevertheless compelled to analyze the samples. They sometimes faked results to protect their patients and yet meet the demands of the SS.

Dr. Lettich, a bacteriologist who had been transferred to Rajsko from the hospital at Birkenau, described the situation.

> The SS pushed cynicism to extremes... During the last months of 1944, when the Russian Front came near to Auschwitz, our SS chiefs invented a new test. With a long-handled swab, normally used for taking samples of mucous at the back of the throat, they took numerous samples of fecal matter from the rectum. This became a special distraction for certain SS men – Rottenführers Kapmayer, Sender and others – who amused themselves at the women's camp by having the prisoners file past to take these samples. We used to receive two to three thousand samples of this kind a day for examination, in the hope of finding some typhus germ-carriers.
>
> It would have been totally unthinkable to accomplish such a gigantic task in a day, if we had not adopted a straight-forward method. We took Petri dishes divided up into twelve or sixteen squares; and in each square we passed the same swab. All the rest were destroyed, for we had no intention of discovering germ-carriers.[198]

■

Dora Kleinova, a former prisoner assigned to the Institute, testified about Dr. Bruno Weber, the director of the Rajsko programs, and his scientific work.[199]

> His research was mainly concerned with the preparation of dehydrated serum: to obtain it, he ordered the bleeding of victims. This was carried out by Unterscharführer Zabel, who used to make as many as fifty blood tests a day. He took 55 cc at a time, which, in our condition, brought on death quickly. Dr. Weber boasted of these exploits to Mrugowsky, his superior, when he received his visit.
>
> Generally speaking, these experiments had no scientific basis, and it was my impression that their main interest for those who were carrying them out was to give the illusion of important activity to Berlin, to keep the courageous researchers at a restful job far from the front.

198 Dr. Lettich quoted in Aziz, *Doctors of Death*, vol. 2, pp. 186–191.
199 Doris Kleinova quoted in Ibid., vol. 2, pp. 189–190.

Dr. Mark Klein, formerly Professor at Strasbourg University and employed at the Rajsko Institute, recounted:

> It is my opinion that this laboratory, like those in other concentration camps was probably part of an SS plan to obtain scientific material, thoroughly imbibed in the ideological system and the SS hierarchy, and independent of already existing university and scientific institutions. SS men employed there had relatively stable jobs, and an easy life sheltered from the dangers of battle at a time when there was tremendous activity on every front.[200]

■

Imrich Goenczi, who worked as a cook at the Institute, added disturbing details to the story of the Institute's work.

> I was brought to the Rajsko Institute as a cook for bacteriological culture medium. My task was to prepare bouillon from beef or horsemeat. The SS man Franz Fugger, an Austrian, brought the material in a suitcase. ...When the SS man noticed that we used the cooked meat as food, they kept the meat supply for themselves and brought us a substitute. From then on, the SS man Fugger brought small bloody pieces of meat in earth-ware pots. With the help of Prof. Tomasek, former bacteriologist at the Masaryk University in Bruenn, we found out that the new deliveries were human flesh. We had microscopes in our lab. Using them Prof. Tomasek conducted histological examinations. There were also small pieces of skin on the supplied flesh, which indicated clearly and without any doubt the source of the meat. Fugger delivered this meat weekly, continuously for half a year.[201]

An excellent summary description of the work and research done at the Rajsko Institute of Hygiene was provided in the testimony of Abraham Treger, a former prisoner worker at the facility.

200 Mark Klein quoted in Ibid.

201 Excerpt from Declaration of Imrich Goenczi, Office of the U.S. Chief of Counsel, in *Trials NMT*, vol. 1, 0.33/4334, pp. 2–4.

Testimony of [Abraham] Treger[202]
Office of U.S. Chief of Counsel

Extract

On 2 February 1943, I came with a transport from Ghetto Pruzany to Birkenau, (Auschwitz II)... I got a number (98130) tattooed on my arm.

...On March 24, 1943, the SS Hauptsturmführer Dr. B. Weber told me briefly that I was to work in his Institute for Hygiene. The Institute for Hygiene had been built a short time before in Rajsko which was 3 kilometers from the Main Camp Auschwitz. I worked in this Institute from the very beginning, until the evacuation of Auschwitz on January 18, 1945.

The *Kommando* (work unit) which worked for the Rajsko laboratory resided in Auschwitz and walked every day to the Institute. The number of the members was about 120 – all of them qualified specialists: physicians, biologists, serologists, bacteriologists, chemists. They came from various countries: Czechs, Frenchmen, Jews, Poles, Hungarians, Dutchmen, etc. Beside the specialists, hard-laborers aged from 25 to 65 were also employed.

In this "international" laboratory there were the following departments: bacteriology, serology (experiments and research), histology, chemistry and bacterial cultures. Each department was personally supervised by the laboratory director, B. Weber who in early 1943 had the rank of an SS Hauptscharführer (a low-ranking officer). And by 1945, had advanced to the rank of an SS Hauptsturmführer (a captain), his deputy, Dr. Muench, their colleague Dr. Del of Belgian nationality.

The work in the institute was done in two stages:

1. Bacteriological, serological and chemical analyses of the material which was being sent in.

2. Research work.

The material for examination was received from concentration camps affiliated with Auschwitz.

Dr. Weber's research work concerned initially the problem of artificially raising the titer of hemoagglutination in men. For this purpose, he made intravenous injections of 5 cc of human blood of incompatible blood groups. The patients reacted with strong anaphylactic tremor, headaches and fever. They never knew what the purpose of these injections was. Soon afterwards, blood was taken from these patients for

202 Testimony of Abraham Treger, in Ibid., vol. 1, 0.33/4334, M-1/E 817/686.

experiments and research concerning the titer of hemoagglutination. It was difficult to know what the consequences of these experiments for the health of the patients were because after having left the hospital, they were sent to an unknown destination. The second "scientific" domain of Dr. Weber's research work which he conducted for 1 $^1/_2$ years was to produce a so-called dry serum, like agglutination test serum of high quality, or possible a dissoluble dry product of serum, for transfusion purposes. During the aforementioned period, approximately 20,000 liters were used which had been extracted from various camp inmates. The minimal quantity of blood at one extraction was 250 cc. He (Dr. Weber) often took a number of liters of blood taken at one extraction. One can easily imagine the looks of a prisoner, exhausted by hard work and starved, from whom, in addition, a liter of blood had been taken. Dr Weber derived particular pleasure from taking blood from women.

Large quantities of blood were taken from typhus- and TBC-patients. Dr. Weber would make direct experimental injections (without previous experiments on animals) of serum samples containing drastically changed quantities of aluminum salt. For him human beings served as experimental rabbits. He frequently "borrowed" for this purpose women from the infamous Block No. 10 in Auschwitz. That Block held 300 women who were especially designated for experiments.

Dr. Weber would say: "Today, in Germany rabbits have more value than people." It is impossible to state the number of people who died as a result of these experiments.

It is well known that the normal nourishing substance for bacteria is a broth of beef or horsemeat. There were rumors that the SS-man Zabel supplied the department where the nourishing substance for the bacteria was prepared with meat of suspect origin. People whispered that that meat which came packed in wood cases was human flesh. I managed to steal some pieces of that meat. Even with the bare eye one could see what the origin of this meat was. The skin alone was sufficient evidence. But I did not yet quite trust my eyes. I washed the meat, cut it into pieces, extracted some drops of blood from the inner layers and made an analysis of the blood group. It was human blood, group B.

There was no doubt that the broth obtained from this boiled meat was human broth. I have seen dozens of liters of this substance. For a while, the dogs were being fed with the meat, which remained from the broth; later on, the meat was being buried.

THE JEWISH SKELETON COLLECTION

Nazi racial theory rested on the principle of a hierarchy of races, marked by the continuous struggle of the presumed superior race (the Aryans) against the degenerative influences of the allegedly inferior races (Jews, Gypsies, Negroes, and Slavs). This racist ideology infiltrated in Germany, not only the entire society, but also all scientific fields, particularly medicine.

Protecting the Aryan race by preventing contact with the inferior races assumed paramount importance in the Nazi program. The ghettoes, the various prohibitions against intermarriage, the murderous experiments, and, in the end, the gas chambers all functioned to accomplish this overarching Nazi goal. But the whole program rested on the shaky proposition that the races can be reliably and validly distinguished one from the other. Nazi theorists needed to be able to point to definitive traits that distinguish the Jew, or other *Untermenschen,* from the Aryan. To this end they sponsored, under the aegis of the Ahnenerbe, several experimental programs as well as the notorious project of categorizing individuals according to their racial blood lines. Several "scientists" sought to differentiate the races according to specific variances in one or another physical trait. One of these scientists was Dr. August Hirt, Professor of Anatomy at the University of Strasbourg, who wanted to prove that the structures of the human skull vary consistently and reliably according to race, so that by measuring skulls and observing other features the members of the inferior races could be differentiated from Aryans.

For his research Hirt needed a collection of human skulls, and he was particularly interested in obtaining Jewish specimens. Accordingly, he turned to the Ahnenerbe Society, the organization charged with assisting any and all research that supported Nazi ideology, for help getting study subjects. His research proposal was forwarded by Wolfram Sievers (head of the Ahnenerbe Society) to Himmler in February 1942.

Translation of Document No-085[203]

Opening Statement of the Prosecution, 9 December 1946

We have a nearly complete collection of skulls of all races and peoples at our disposal. Only very few specimens of skulls of the Jewish race, how-

203 Document No-085, "Opening Statement of the Prosecution", 9 Dec. 1946, in *Trials NMT,* vol. 1, pp. 54–56.

> ever, are available with the result that it is impossible to arrive at precise conclusions from examining them. The war in the East now presents us with the opportunity to overcome this deficiency. By procuring the skulls of the Jewish-Bolshevik Commissars, who represent the prototype of the repulsive, but characteristic subhuman, we have the chance now to obtain a palpable, scientific document. The best, practical method for obtaining and collecting this skull material could be handled by directing the Wehrmacht to turn over alive all captured Jewish-Bolshevik Commissars to the Field Police.
>
> They in turn are to be given special directives to inform a certain office at regular intervals of the number and place of detention of these captured Jews and to give them special close attention and care until a special delegate arrives. This special delegate, who will be in charge of securing the "material" has the job of taking a series of previously established photographs, anthropological measurements, and in addition has to determine, as far as possible, the background, date of birth, and other personal data of the prisoner. Following the subsequently induced death of the Jew, whose head should not be damaged, the delegate will separate the head from the body and will forward it to its proper point of destination in a hermetically sealed tin can, especially produced for this purpose and filled with a conserving fluid.
>
> Having arrived at the laboratory, the comparison tests and anatomical research on the skull, as well as determination of the race membership of pathological features of the skull form the form and size of the brain, etc., can proceed. The basis of these studies will be the photos, measurements, and other data supplied on the head, and finally the tests of the skull itself.

Himmler expressed interest in Hirt's proposal and gave Sievers the job of contacting Hirt to develop a plan of action. Sievers immediately left for Strasbourg where he and Hirt, who was ill at the time, discussed the horrible plan. Hirt proposed that they begin with a collection of 150 skeletons. Sievers thought that there was only one place that could meet that demand: Auschwitz. He contacted the Reichssicherheitshauptamt (Reich Security Main Office), Department 4 B-IV, and asked SS Obersturmbannführer Adolf Eichmann to arrange the transportation of the subjects from Auschwitz to Natzweiler. But before that could happen, a selection, of course, had to be made; and for this purpose, the philosopher-physician, Dr. Bruno Beger, who was working for the Ahnenerbe, made his way to Auschwitz. Beger was given the honor of selecting from this reservoir of "*Untermenschen,* seventy-nine Jews, thirty Jewesses, two

Poles and four Asians. These were the chosen few whose skulls might adorn the Aryan museum galleries of the University of Strasbourg [sic]."[204]

The following correspondence outlines the process by which the arrangements were made for Professor Hirt's "scientific study".

Document No-090[205]
Office of U.S. Chief of Counsel
Subsequent Proceedings Division, ap 124-a, U.S. Army

Staff Evidence Analysis, Criminal Organizations
By: Henry Sachs
Date: 8 August 1946

Doc. No. or other description: No-090
Title and/or general nature: Skeleton collection at the Anatomical Institute of Strassburg.
Date: 27 February 1942.
Source: (Location of Original, etc.): Berlin Document Center
Language of original: German
Translation in English
Persons or organizations implicated:
Ostbf. Wolfram SIEVERS
Ahnenerbe Society
Prof. August HIRT
Stbf. Dr. Rudolf BRANDT
To be filed under these reference headings: Same as above.

Summary (Indicate page nos. of original or translation):

This is a one page letter by Brandt to Sievers. He states that Himmler is very much interested in Hirt's work and is willing to place everything necessary at his disposal so he can continue his experiments. Sievers is to see Hirt and provide for everything that will speed up his recovery. As soon as Hirt is well enough a discussion with Himmler is to take place. Sievers is to report again on the progress made in Hirt's work.

See: No-085, No-086, No-087, No-088, No-089, No-091, No-092, No-116.

204 Hoedeman, *Hitler or Hippocrates*, pp. 140–149.
205 Ibid.

Translation of Document No-090/a[206]
Office of U.S. Chief of Counsel

The Reichsführer SS
Führer Headquarters
27 February 1942
Personal Staff

Journal No. AR/493/37
Bra/H.

Re: Your letter of 9 February 1942 – G/R/2 S. 1.

To the Reich Business Manager (Reichsgeschaeftsführer)
of "Ahnenerbe," SS Obersturmbannführer SIEVERS
Berlin–Dahlem
Pücklerstr. 17

Dear Comrade Sievers:

I was able to inform the Reichsführer SS of the reports of Prof. Dr. HIRT. As I have told you before, the Reichsführer is very much interested in Prof. Dr. HIRT'S work. Perhaps you could call on HIRT sometime soon and tell him again that the Reichsführer SS will place at his disposal everything he needs.

First of all, we for our part ought to do everything that would aid Prof. Dr. HIRT in regaining his health. Please make some suggestions as to how you and we could be helpful in this respect. Perhaps a small shipment of fruit would also contribute essentially to his recovery.

After Dr. HIRT'S recovery, it would be best if a conference with the Reichsführer SS took place.

On your next visit, which probably will take place in the near future, you could report once more on Dr. HIRT'S work.

Best wishes
Heil Hitler!

always yours
(Signature) R B
SS Sturmbannführer

206 Ibid.

Translation of Document No-086[207]
Office of U.S. Chief of Counsel

Letter from Wolfram Sievers to Rudolf Brandt, 2 November 1942

The Ahnenerbe
Berlin
2 November 1942

The Reich Business Manager (Stamp)
(Reichsgeschaeftsführer)
Personal Staff RF SS
Registration of Files
Secret 5/116

SECRET
To: SS-Obersturmbannführer Dr. BRANDT
Berlin

Dear Comrade BRANDT!

The Reichsführer SS once ordered, as you know, that SS Haptsturmführer Prof. Dr. HIRT should be provided with all necessary material for his research work. I have already reported to the Reichsführer SS that for some anthropological studies 150 skeletons of inmates or Jews are needed and should be provided by the concentration camp Auschwitz. It is only necessary that the Reich Main Security Office (Reichssicherheitshauptamt) will now be furnished with an official directive by the Reichsführer SS; by order of the Reichsführer SS, however, you could advise so yourself.

Sincerely yours
Heil Hitler
Your
(Signature) SIEVERS

1 enclosure
Draft of a letter to the Reich Main Security Office (Reichssicherheitshauptamt)

207 Letter of Wolfram Sievers to Rudolf Brandt, 2 November 1942, Nuremberg Document No-086, in Mendelsohn, ed., *The Holocaust: Selected Documents,* vol. 9, p. 217.

Document No-089[208]
Office of U.S. Chief of Counsel
Subsequent Proceedings Division, ap 124-a, U.S. Army

Letter from Rudolf Brandt to Adolf Eichmann, 6 November 1942
Staff Evidence Analysis, Criminal Organizations
By: Henry Sachs
Date: 8 August 1946
Doc. No. or other description: No-089
Title and/or general nature: Organization of a skeleton collection at the Anatomical Institute of Strasbourg.
Date: 6 November 1942.
Source: (Location of Original, etc.): Berlin Document Center
Language of original: German
Translation in English
Persons or organizations implicated:
Ostbf. Wolfram SIEVERS
Prof. Dr. August HIRT
Ostbf. Rudolf BRANDT
Ahnenerbe Society
Prof. August HIRT
Ostbf. Dr. Rudolf BRANDT
To be filed under these reference headings: Same as above.

Summary (Indicate page nos. of original or translation):
This document, marked secret, is a directive originating with Himmler and passed on to Eichmann by Brandt. It states that Dr. Hirt is to be furnished with everything he needs for his research work. Eichmann is to make possible the establishment of the planned collection. Sievers is to see Eichmann to make arrangements for necessary details.

A copy of this directive was sent to the Ahnenerbe society.
See: No-085, No-086, No-087, No-088, No-089, No-091, No-092, No-116.

208 Letter from Rudolf Brandt to Adolf Eichmann, 6 November 1942, Nuremberg Document No-089, in Ibid., vol. 9, p. 219.

Document No-087[209]
Office of U.S. Chief of Counsel
Subsequent Proceedings Division, ap 124-a, U.S. Army

Staff Evidence Analysis, Criminal Organizations
By: Henry Sachs
Date: 8 August 1946
Doc. No. or other description: NO-087
Title and/or general nature: Establishment of a collection of skeletons
Date: 21 June 1943.
Source: (Location of Original, etc.): Berlin Document Center
Language of original: German (Translation in English)
Persons or organizations implicated:
Ostbf. EICHMANN
Hstf. Dr. BERGER
Prof. Dr. August HIRT
Ostbf Dr. Rudolf BRANDT
Ahnenerbe Society
Wolfram SIEVERS
To be filed under these reference headings:
Same as above.
PW Affairs
Deportation, Jews, Persecution of,
Atrocities against Military Personnel

Summary (Indicate page nos. of original or translation):

This document termed "Top Secret" is a letter of Sievers to Eichmann. After referring to a letter of 25 Sept 42 and several personal conversations Sievers informs Eichmann that the latters' associate Dr. Beger who had been in charge of the project had concluded his experiments at Auschwitz on 15 June 43 because of the danger of epidemics. He then gives figures on the concluded undertaking: 115 persons were experimented on (79 Jews, 30 Jewesses, 2 Poles, 4 Asiatics). The prisoners are being kept under quarantine and segregated by sex in two hospital buildings at the Auschwitz concentration camp.

For further experimentation the above mentioned prisoners are to be transferred to the concentration camp Natzweiler. The transfer should be carried out speedily as to prevent the outbreak of an epidemic at Auschwitz. Eichmann is to give the necessary directives. Immune and

209 Staff Evidence Analysis of Nuremberg Document No-087, in Ibid., p. 224.

clean prisoner suits for 80 men and 30 women are to be sent to Auschwitz immediately. Lodgings for the women are to be prepared at Natzweiler.

The letter mentions a list of the 115 prisoners, which is not attached to the document. Copies of the letter were sent to:
Hstf. Dr. Berger
Prof. Dr. August Hirt
Ostbf. Dr. Rudolf Brandt

See: No-085, No-086, No-088, No-089, No-090, No-091, No-092, No-116.

Translation of Document No-087[210]
Office of the U.S. Chief Counsel for War Crimes

Letter from Wolfram Sievers to Adolf Eichmann
(Handwritten) XI a 56

Office "Ahnenerbe" Institute for Military Scientific Research
Berlin-Dahlem,
Puecklerstrasse 16
G/H/6, S2/He.
21 June 1943

Top Secret
G.E.Z.I. A.H. Sk. No. 10
5 copies, 2nd copy
No enclosures

To:
Reich Main Security Office
Office IV B 4
Attention: SS-Obersturmbannführer EICHMANN,
Berlin SW 11
Prinz-Albrechtstrasse 8

Subject: Assembling of a collection of skeletons.

With reference to your letter of 25 September 1942 IV B 4 3576/43 g 1488 and the personal talks which have taken place in the meantime on

210 Letter from Wolfram Sievers to Adolf Eichmann, 21 June 1943, in Ibid., vol. 9, p. 224.

the above matter, you are informed that the co-worker in this office who was charged with the execution of the above-mentioned special task, SS Hauptsturmführer Dr. Bruno BEGER, ended his work in the Auschwitz concentration camp on 15 June 1943 because of the existing danger of infectious diseases.

A total of 115 persons were worked on, 79 of whom were Jews, 2 Poles, 4 Asiatics and 30 Jewesses. At present, these prisoners are separated according to sex and each group is accommodated in a hospital building of the Auschwitz concentration camp and are in quarantine.

For further processing of the selected persons an *immediate transfer* to the Natzweiler concentration camp *is now imperative,* which must be accelerated in view of the *danger of* infectious *diseases in Auschwitz.* Enclosed is a list containing the names of the selected persons.

It is requested that the necessary directives be issued.

Since with the transfer of the prisoners to Natzweiler the danger of spreading diseases exist, it is requested that an immediate shipment of *disease-free* and *clean prisoners' clothing* for 80 men and 30 women be ordered sent from Natzweiler to Auschwitz.

At the same time one must provide for the accommodation of the *30 women* in the Natzweiler concentration camp for a short period.

(Signature) SIEVERS
SS Standartenführer

Carbon copies to:
a) SS Hauptsturmführer Dr. BEGER
b) SS Hauptsturmführer Prof. Dr HIRT
c) SS Obersturmbannführer Dr. BRANDT

(stamp)
Personal Staff Reichsführer SS
Remitted 22 June 1943
Journal No. 1657 43 Secret
RF (Reichsführer)

Testimony of the following eyewitnesses vividly describes the practical details of Hirt's experiment.

Translation of Document No-807[211]
Office of Chief of Counsel for War Crimes

Document from the French Republic Permanent Military Tribunal of the Tenth Military Region in Strasbourg

In the year 1945 on July twenty-sixth at fifteen hours, appeared before me, Major Jadin, Military Judge at the Military Tribunal of the Tenth Region, assisted by Lieutenant Jr., HERTZOG, stenographer at the same Military Tribunal, also functioning as interpreter of German and who was under oath according to the Article 332 of the Criminal Investigation Code, in my office which had been taken to Colle, according to my verbal summons, the witness named hereafter, which has outside the presence of the other witnesses, in the presence of the Major G. Dill SMITH of the English Service of War Crimes, after having shown the summons which was given to him, after having sworn to say the entire truth and nothing but the truth, and interrogated by us on his surname, given name, age, status, profession and calling, if he is domestically related or allied to the parties at which degree.

He answered that he was named KRAMER Josef, Haupsturmführer SS, thirty-nine years old, living in Bergen-Belsen.

I used to be a bookkeeper in Augsburg before 1932, year in which I have volunteered in the SS and I have been asked to guard the inmates of concentration camps.

Before the hostilities I have been as a Lieutenant in various concentration camps, especially in Estervegen, Sachsenhausen, Dachau, Mauthausen and Auschwitz.

In April 1941 I have been sent by the superior SS authorities to the Natzweiler-Struthof as a lieutenant, Adjutant to HUTTIG, Commander-in-Chief of the camp.

In October 1942 I have been named commander of the camp in replacement of the Commander ZILL who had succeed HUTTIG. I have commanded the camp until April 1944, date on which I have been sent to Auschwitz and in December 1944 to Belsen...

During the month of August 1943, I received from the Orangeburg camp, or rather from the Supreme SS Command in Berlin who sent it to me, the order to receive about eight inmates coming from Auschwitz. In the letter which went with this order, it was stated that I had to get in touch immediately with Professor Hirt of the Medical Faculty of Strasbourg.

211 Document from the French Republic: "Permanent Military Tribunal of the Tenth Military Region in Strasbourg", Translation of Document No-807, Office of Chief of Counsel for War Crimes.

I went to the Anatomical Institute of Strasbourg where Hirt was. The letter told me that he knows of an inmate convoy of Auschwitz for Struthof. He told me that these persons were to be executed in the gas chamber of the Struthof Camp with asphyxiating gases and that their bodies were to be driven to the Anatomical Institute so that he could dispose of them.

After this conversation he gave me a bottle of one-fourth of a liter containing salts which I think were cyanhydrique salts...

The professor told me about the approximate dose that I had to use to asphyxiate myself the inmates coming from Auschwitz of which I have spoken to you.

In the beginning of August 1943 I received the eighty inmates who had to be killed with the gases that had been given to me by Hirt and I started to take to the gas chamber, on a certain evening, at about nine o'clock, with a small van, the first time, about fifteen women. I told these women that they had to go to the disinfection chamber and I did not tell them they were going to be asphyxiated.

Helped by a few SS I undressed them completely and I pushed them into the gas chamber when they were completely naked.

When I closed the door, they started to howl. I introduced, after having closed the door, a certain amount of salt in a funnel that was placed above and to the right of the observation window. Then I closed the opening of the funnel with a tap which was adapted at the bottom of this funnel with a metal tube on it. This metal tube drew the salt and water into the inside opening of the chamber of which I have spoken. I lit the inside of the chamber with a switch placed near the funnel and I observed through the observation window which what was going on inside of the chamber. I have seen that these women have continued to breathe about half a minute, then they fell on to the floor. When I opened the door after having made at the same time function the ventilation inside of the chimney, I found out that these women laid without life and that they were full of excrements.

I have told to make the nurses of the SS to put these bodies in a small van the next morning, about five-thirty, so that they could be taken to the Anatomical Institute as Professor Hirt had asked me to...

A few days later, in the same above-mentioned condition, I have taken again to the gas chamber a certain quantity of women who were asphyxiated in the same way; then again a few days later I have taken to the gas chamber, in two or three times, about fifty men, maybe fifty-five, who were killed always with the salts Hirts had given me.

(S) E. Hertzog
Joseph Kramer
Gadin

The following extract comes from the testimony of Henri Henripierre, a French citizen who was arrested by the Germans in Paris. Taken to Strasbourg, he was assigned to work in Professor Hirt's institute with the principal of the "preparatory", Otto Bong.

Testimony of Henri Henripierre at the Nuremberg Trial[212] 18 December 1946

HENRIPIERRE: ...In the month of July 1943, Professor Hirt received a visit from a senior officer of the SS...

A few days later, Mr. Bong told me that he would have to prepare the tanks to receive a hundred and twenty corpses. We prepared the tanks. In these tanks there were synthetic spirits of 55 degrees.

The first convoy which we received was a convoy of thirty women. It was supposed to arrive at five o'clock in the morning, but it only arrived at seven. After having interrogated the driver about the delay, the driver gave answer, "They gave us a lot of trouble." These thirty corpses of women were unloaded by the driver and two assistants, also helped by Mr. Bong and myself.

The preservation of these corpses started straight away. The corpses arrived when they were still warm. The eyes were wide open and brilliant; they seemed congested and red, and they were popping out of the orbits. There were traces of blood at the nose and at the mouth, and there was evidence of fecal matter coming out. There was no rigor mortis apparent. At that moment I judged for myself that it was a case of victims who, in my opinion, had been poisoned or asphyxiated, because in the case of no victim of any previous preservation were there presented the symptoms and signs that these victims showed when they arrived. That is why I made a note of the serial numbers that the women had tattooed in their left forearm. I made a note of them on a piece of paper, and I kept them in secret in my house. The serial numbers consisted of five digits.

A few days later we received a second convoy of thirty men. These arrived exactly in the same state as the first, that is, still warm, with wide open eyes, congested, eyes brilliant, bleeding at the mouth and bleeding at the nose, and also losing their fecal matter.

212 Testimony by Henri Henripierre, Document from the French Republic: Permanent Military Tribunal of the Tenth Military region in Strasbourg (Nuremberg Trial Transcript, U.S.A. v. Karl Brandt), December 18, 1946, pp. 708–718, reprinted in Mendelsohn, ed., *The Holocaust: Selected Documents*, vol. 9, pp. 187–198.

The preservation of these thirty men was also proceeded with immediately, with one slight difference. The left testicle in each case was removed, which was sent to the Laboratory for Anatomy Number 2. That was a private laboratory run by Professor Hirt.

Some time later, thereupon, we received a third and last convoy, namely, of twenty-six men. They also arrived in the same state as the two previous ones.

I should like to make it clear once more – and I say this knowing it be true. After the first convoy of women's bodies that we received, Professor Hirt, having met me at the door of an Anatomical Department, told me laterally, "Peter, if you don't hold your mouth, you won't get out of this..."

A. [HENRIPIERRE]: Once they were preserved, the corpses were placed in the tanks, about fifteen to each tank. These bodies were all superb. The bodies of the prisoners which I had previously seen were all emaciated, whereas these eighty-six corpses that I am talking of were magnificent; finely muscled, and did not show any signs of neglect. The only thing that was remarkable was that there were a certain numbers of peculiar wrinkles in the back.

Q. Do you know, witness, whether or not the people who were killed and delivered to you were Jews?
A. At the time that I saw these bodies I did not know whether they were Jews or not. I merely questioned Mr. Bong and I asked him what he thought those people were. It was Mr. Bong who said, "Da sind alles Juden," "They are all Jews."...

A. [HENRIPIERRE]: Once the bodies had been prepared, they were put into the tanks. They remained in the tanks an entire year without anybody touching them. In the month of September 1944, the Allies were advancing and therefore, at that time, Professor Hirt ordered Mr. Bong and Mr. Meier, the laboratory assistants to cut up these eighty-six bodies and to have them cremated in the Strasbourg City Crematorium. The work having been accomplished by Mr. Bong and Mr. Meier in the actual room where these tanks were. I asked Mr. Bong the following morning if he had cut up all of the bodies. He replied, "We couldn't cut them all up, it was far too much work. We left some of the bodies at the bottom of the tanks." I then asked Bong, "Were all the corpses buried with their gold teeth?" At that moment, Bong replied, "The gold teeth that were already found on the Jews were handed over to Professor Hirt by Mr. Meier."

Photos taken by the French authorities after the liberation of Strasbourg tell the story of this mass murder more vividly than a witness or a document could. Presented here are the captions of the three pictures.

Translation of Document No-807[213]
Office of Chief of Counsel for War Crimes

Regional Services of Legal Strasbourg Police

I, the undersigned, HELFFER Eugene, principal Commissary, Chief of the Sixteenth Mobile Brigade of the legal Police of Strasbourg, certify that the documents herein affixed on eight pages, including photos No. 1 to 21 of bodies, and No. 1a to 8d of documents, are photographs of bodies, and of French and German authenticated documents which have been taken by the French Police immediately after the liberation of Strasbourg in the Anatomical Institute of the University of Strasbourg...

Translation of Captions of Photographs

Picture No. 1.

Alcohol containers for the bodies which were used for anatomic preparations. A few bodies of the eighty-six people assassinated in August 1943 in the Struthof gas chamber: sixteen of these bodies have been found whole.

Picture No. 13.

Bodies defleshed at the end of 1944 on order of the German Professor Hirt, Director of the Anatomic Institute from 1941 to 1944. The number of each body, tattooed on the left forearm, has been removed by order when the bodies were defleshed. The vital organs and the heads have been incinerated in the Crematorium of Strasbourg – actions which were meant to prevent identification of the bodies and to obstruct the French Medico-Legal research.

Picture No. 17.

Body of a young girl, healthy and robust, taken at the time of the autopsy. Notice in the incisions done on the body the layer of grease which shows execution shortly after the arrest.

213 Ibid.

As the fortunes of the war turned against Germany and the Allies began moving eastward through France, the Nazis began making plans to destroy any evidence that might reveal their criminal activities.

Document No-088[214]
Office of U.S. Chief of Counsel
Subsequent Proceedings Division, ap 124-a, U.S. Army

Staff Evidence Analysis, Criminal Organizations
By: Henry Sachs
Date: 8 August 1946
Doc. No. or other description: No-088
Title and/or general nature: Collection of Jewish Skeletons at Strasbourg
Date: 5 September 1944
Source: (Location of Original, etc.): Berlin Document Center
Language of original: German
Translated in English
Persons or organizations implicated:
Stbf. Wolfram SIEVERS
Stbf. Dr. Rudolf BRANDT
Prof. Dr. August HIRT
Ahnenerbe Society
To be filed under reference headings:
Same as above.
Atrocities against Russian military personnel
Jews, Persecution of,

Summary (Indicate page nos. of original or translation):

This teletyped one-page letter, marked "Top Secret" is by SIEVERS and addressed to BRANDT. SIEVERS asks for direction as to what to do with the collection in case Strassburg should be endangered. The collection had been assembled by HIRT according to the proposal of 9 Feb 42 and BRANDT'S approval of 23 Feb 42 AR/493/37. Because of the vast amount of work connected with the research activities defleshing of the corpses has not been completed. If the corpses were defleshed immediately important scientific data could not be obtained and part of the work

214 Staff Evidence Analysis of Nuremberg Document No-088, in Mendelsohn, ed., *The Holocaust: Selected Documents*, vol. 9, p. 226.

would have been done for nothing. On the other hand this procedure would make the corpses unidentifiable and the remaining flesh parts could be declared as having been left by the French when the Germans took over the Anatomical Institute. SIEVERS asks for advice as to which of the following proposals should be carried out:

1. Preserve the collection as a whole.
2. Dissolve part of the collection.
3. Dissolve the whole of the collection.

There are marginal notes in shorthand on the document.

See: No-085, No-086, No-087, No-089, No-090, No-091, No-092, No-116.

Document No-091[215]
Office of U.S. Chief of Counsel
Subsequent Proceedings Division, ap 124-a, U.S. Army

Staff Evidence Analysis, Criminal Organizations
By: Henry Sachs
Date: 8 August 1946
Doc. No. or other description: No-091
Title and/or general nature: 2 Notes re skeleton collection in the Strasbourg Anatomical Institute
Date: 15 Oct 1944 and 25 Oct 1944
Source: (Location of Original, etc.): Berlin Document Center
Language of original: German
Translated in English
Persons or organizations implicated:
Hstf. BERG
Stbf. Wolfram SIEVERS
Stbf BAUMERT
Prof. Dr. August HIRT
Stbf. Dr. Rudolf BRANDT
Ahnenerbe Society
To be filed under these reference headings:
Same as above.
Atrocities against civilians
Jews, Persecution of

215 Staff Evidence Analysis of Nuremberg Document No-091, in Ibid., vol. 9, pp. 228, 231.

Summary (Indicate page nos. of original or translation):

This document consists of 2 notes by BERG. The first note refers to a telephone conversation with SIEVERS in which SIEVERS was asked to preserve a certain part of the collection in case the dissolution had not been completed yet. However, if the military situation of Strassburg should be endangered, the complete dissolution of the collection was to be carried out. SIEVERS promised to inquire and report.

The second is directed to Dr. BRANDT, informing him that upon an earlier order the complete dissolution had been carried through already. SIEVERS who had given this information to BERG has the view that in consideration of the situation, this arrangements is the best.

See: No-085, No-086, No-087, No-088, No-089, No-090, No-091, No-092, No-116.

Berg's Second Note
Translation of Document No-091
Office of U.S. Chief of Counsel

Note:
(shorthand notation:)
"Completely broken up according to information from Standartenführer SIEVERS"

On 12 October 1944 I talked to SS Standartenführer SIEVERS on the telephone and asked him whether the skeleton collection at Strassburg had already been completely broken up in accordance with instructions given by SS Standartenführer BAUMERT. SS Standartenführer SIEVERS could not tell me anything about that, since he had not yet received any detailed news from Professor HIRT. I told him that, if the dissolution had not yet taken place, some part of the collection should still be preserved. It had to be certain however that the complete dissolution could be accomplished promptly if Strassburg should be endangered because of the military situation. Standartenführer SIEVERS promised to have the appropriate investigations made and to report about them.

(Signature) BERG
15 October 1944
SS Hauptsturmführer
Bg., /Wm

(page 2 of original)
(handwritten notation Z XI a-156, Ab Bg 1/11

Note for Standartenführer BRANDT:

During his presence at the Field Command Post (Feldkommandostelle) on 21 October 1944, Standartenführer SIEVERS informed me that the dissolution of the collection in Strassburg, had already been completed in compliance with the orders given formerly. Considering the whole situation he thinks that this procedure was the best one.

(Signature) BERG
26 October 1944
SS-Hauptsturmführer
Bg.,/Wm

STERILIZATION EXPERIMENTS

In their zeal to create an Aryan Germany, shorn of its racially undesirable, "unfit" members, the Nazis resorted to a range of strategies, of which the gas chambers represented unambiguous efficiency. Other methods, among them compulsive sterilization, were less direct, and chilling in their adaptation of utilitarianism to murderous ends. Compulsory sterilization for individuals with certain hereditary conditions was instituted in Nazi Germany on 7 July 1933. The program expanded during World War II to become one prong of the "final solution" to the problem of the millions of Slavs and Jews who had fallen into German hands. Party officials debated whether it would be preferable to exterminate them on racial grounds, or to preserve them as a source of slave labor.

It was decided that these prisoners would indeed be useful to the Reich as laborers: Yes, they would work – they would be worked to death – but they would not be allowed to reproduce. Thus both practical and ideological goals would be satisfied. Dr. Adolf Pokorny, a skin and venereal disease specialist writing to Himmler in October 1941, laid bare the appeal of this logic: "The thought alone that the 3,000,000 Bolsheviks presently in German hands could be sterilized, making them available as workers while excluding them from procreation, opens vast perspectives."[216] Viktor Brack argued similarly, saying, "Out of a total of some 10,000,000 Jews, there are in my opinion 2,000,000 to 3,000,000 men and women well able to work. In view of the extraordinary

216 Letter from Dr. Adolf Pokorny to Heinrich Himmler, October 1941, quoted in Mitscherlich and Mielke, eds., *The Death Doctors*, p. 132.

difficulties facing us in the manpower question, I am in favor of selecting and maintaining these at all costs. True, this will be possible only if they are at the same time rendered incapable of procreation."[217]

Thus research into mass sterilization techniques became a priority for Nazi medical scientists. Three alternatives to surgery, all of which were eventually judged impractical, were considered: X-ray, a procedure that had first been used as early as 1940; intrauterine injection of a variety of chemicals; and ingestion or injection of the plant extract caladium seguinum.

■

Experiments with caladium seguinum were the first to be tried. Related documents follow.

Translation of Document No-035[218]
Office of U.S. Chief of Counsel

To the Reich Commissioner for the Consolidation of German Folkdom,
SS Himmler,
Chief of Police, Berlin.

...Led by the idea that the enemy must not only be conquered but destroyed, I feel obliged to present to you, as the Reich Commissioner for the Consolidation of German Folkdom the following:

Dr. Madaus published the result of his research on a *medicinal sterilization* (both articles are enclosed). Reading these articles, the immense importance of this drug in the present fight of our people occurred to me. If, on the basis of this research, it were possible to produce a drug which after a relatively short time, effects an imperceptible sterilization on human beings, then we would have a new powerful weapon at our disposal. The thought alone that the 3 million Bolsheviks, at present German prisoners, could be sterilized so that they could be used as laborers but be prevented from reproduction, opens the most far reaching perspectives.

217 Letter from Brack to Himmler, in Ibid. p. 137.

218 Translation of Document No-035, Office of U.S. Chief of Counsel, in RG-30.001M. The term *caladium seguinum,* a botanical term, has been italicized by the editors, following customary practice, even though the italics were missing in the original documents.

Madaus found that the sap of the Schweigrehr *(Caladium seguinum)* when taken by mouth or given as injection to male but also to female animals, after a certain time produces permanent sterility. The illustrations accompanying the scientific article are convincing. If my ideas meet your approval the following course should be taken:

1. Dr. Madaus must not publish any more such articles (The enemy listens!)
2. Multiplying the plant (easily cultivated in greenhouses!)
3. Immediate research on human beings (criminals!) in order to determine the dose and length of the treatment.
4. Quick research of the constitutional formula of the effective chemical substance in order to
5. Produce it synthetically if possible.

As German physician and Chief physician of the reserves of the German Wehrmacht, retired, (d.R.a.D.), I undertake to keep secret the purposes as suggested by me in this letter.

Heil Hitler!
Signed: Dr. Pokorny
Specialist for skin and venereal diseases
M.U.Dr.
Komotau, October, 1941

Ad) Pokorny
Komotau
Graben 33

Translation of Document No-3963[219]
Prosecution Exhibit 528

Extracts from the Affidavit of Karl Wilhelm Friedrich Tauboeck, 18 June 1947, concerning the Development of, and Experiments with Sterilization Drugs

I, Karl Wilhelm Friedrich Tauboeck, swear, depose, and state:

1. I was born on 21 September 1904 in Josefstadt, Czechoslovakia. I have been an Austrian citizen all my life… In December 1927 I was made Doctor of Philosophy with special distinction. My thesis

219 Affidavit of Karl Wilhelm Friedrich Tauboeck, Prosecution Documents, in Ibid., p. 710–719.

dealt with a problem concerning vegetable chemistry – urea in the plant world.

2. From 1928 to 1929 I was assistant in the Institute of Plant Physiology of the University of Vienna, Austria.
3. From 1930 to 1945 I was employed as a biochemist and botanist in the biological laboratory of the I. G. Farbenindustrie A. G. at Ludwigshafen/Rhine. I specialized there in drugs with particular effects on the animal and human organisms, respectively...
4. In the fall of 1942, I was instructed by the director of my laboratory, Dr. Mueller-Cunradi, to devote my time to research on the effective substance from the plant *caladium seguinum* (Schweigrohr). At the beginning of November 1942, I was sent to Dr. Schamberger of the Research Institute Grunewald-Berlin for the purpose of obtaining further information. The Research Institute Grunewald was a cover name for a camouflaged SS office. There I was told that this plant was to be used for sterilizing mental patients. In order to obtain further information about the progress of experiments with *caladium seguinum* which had already taken place, I had to visit the firm Madaus in Dresden-Radebeul, together with Dr. Schamberger and another SS man. While visiting the firm Madaus, I checked all the equipment and experiments in the course of one day. By careful examination of sections of mice and rats and of the histological preparations, I was convinced that the publications of the firm Madaus were perfectly true. By this examination I, as a specialist in this field, gained the conviction that sterilization with *caladium seguinum* is no Utopia, but something which is quite within the bounds of possibility.

   On the return journey from Dresden to Berlin, the SS men revealed to me that this research was being carried out on the express order of Reich Leader SS Himmler in order to suppress births among the eastern nations. After this fact had been revealed to me I was sworn to secrecy. I was furthermore informed at the Research Institute Grunewald-Berlin that the first preparations were to be supplied as soon as possible, as the Reich Leader SS had ordered the testing of the new method on inmates of concentration camps to take place at once.
5. I would like to add that *caladium seguinum* is not considered a sterilization drug in the ordinary sense of the word, but a castration drug. This is evident from the fact that the experiments carried out by the firm Madaus have clearly shown that a destruction of the sexual glands of the experimental animals occurred which is equivalent to the surgical removal of such glands. *Caladium seguinum* is a plant which comes from Brazil. As I know from the

literature and the publications made by the firm Madaus, this plant has already been used by Brazilian natives as a means of sterilization of their enemies. It was administered either in food or in arrow wounds. By this method of injection by arrows, only relatively small portions of poison gained from *caladium seguinum* could have been administered, as the wound produced by arrows may be compared with a large intramuscular injection. From this fact, as learned from literature, results the conclusion that this poison, if obtained by the correct process, is effective even in very small doses.

6. As a result of all examples and explanations mentioned, I am of the opinion that mass production of a castrating preparation from *caladium seguinum* in Germany or in the German occupied countries is no dream, but could easily have been put into practice. The SS took a great interest in this matter. I received my orders as an employee of the I. G. Farbenindustrie from the Chief of the Security Police, first through the camouflaged office of the Research Institute Grunewald-Berlin and later direct.

Nuremberg, 18 June 1947 (Signature) Dr. Karl TAUBOECK

Translation of Document No-036[220]
Office of U.S. Chief of Counsel

The Reichsführer SS
Führer Headquarters
10 March 1942
Journal No. 752/5
RF/H.
2) *W 1.5.*

1. Dear Pohl,

I read Dr. Pokorny's very interesting memorandum and Dr. Madaus's publications on medicinal sterilization. I would ask you to get in touch with *Dr. Madaus* and to inform him, on my behalf, that he should not publish anything else on these questions of medicinal sterilization, and offer him possibilities of doing research – in co-operation with the Reich Physician SS, in criminals, who would have to be sterilized in any case.

220 Document No-036, in RG-30.001M.

The intended plan of research is, however, to be submitted to me by the office engaged on the subject.

Heil Hitler!
Yours
sgd. H. HIMMLER

2. A copy is forwarded to the Reich Physician SS, SS Gruppenführer *Dr. Grawitz* with a request to take cognizance.

by order
Initial: Br.
SS Sturmbannführer

The following letters show the frustrating difficulties that faced the experimenters.

Document No-046a[221]
Office of U.S. Chief of Counsel

Chief of SS Main Office for Economics and Administration
Ch.P./Ha
Berlin. 3 June 1942.

Subject: Sterilization by means of Drugs
Re: Your letter of 3 October 1942. Journal No. AR.752/5, RF/H

To the Reichsführer SS
BERLIN SW 11
Prinz-Albrechtstrasse 8

Dear Reichsführer:

In reference to the above matter I had a conversation today with the director of the Biological Institute of Dr. MADAUS & Co., at Radebeul/Dresden, Dr. phil. et med. Dr. E. KOCH.

I advised him of your desire to have publications on this subject discontinued for the time being. Dr. KOCH will comply with your request.

Furthermore, experiments have reached a dead point because the "Schweigrohr" grows only in North America and during the war cannot be exported in adequate quantities. Dr. KOCH'S attempts to grow this plant from seed cultivated in hothouses have been successful, it is true;

221 Document No-046a, in Ibid.

but the process is very slow and the yield is not sufficient to permit carrying on experiments on a large scale.

Dr. Koch is hopeful that this will be remedied if it were possible for us to obtain permission for him to build a larger hothouse. I promised him this.

For the time being this is the first and only practical step to promote the project.

I shall continue reports periodically.

Heil Hitler!
(S) Pohl
SS Obergruppenführer and General of Waffen SS

Document No-046b[222]
Office of U.S. Chief of Counsel

The Reich Leader SS
Führer's H.Q., 11 June 1942
Personal Staff
Diary No. 1230/42
Bra/Bu
Re: Medical sterilization.

To SS Obergruppenführer Pohl
BERLIN.

Dear Obergruppenführer,

I have informed the Reich Leader SS of your letter of 3 June 1942. He asks you to see to it without fail that a large hot-house is set up as soon as possible for Dr. Koch. He considers the experiments extremely important.

The Reich Leader SS asks you to continue to send in further reports.

Heil Hitler!
signed (illegible)
SS Obergruppenführer
W 16.10

222 Document No-046b, in Ibid.

Document No-044[223]
Office of U.S. Chief of Counsel

Confidential Reich Matter
Document reference

During a consultation on the Wewelsburg on 19 June 1942 with SS Obergruppenführer POHL, I mentioned, among other things, the desire of the Reichsführer to investigate still more thoroughly what the ingredients are of the plant SCHWEIGROHR which may be considered for sterilization. The Reichsführer SS wished it to be determined if similar effective ingredients are contained in the plants which are to be found here or in any area accessible to us in Europe.

The present support of the work of Dr. KOCH of the Madaus-Institute shall be continued to the fullest extent.

The Reichsführer SS also requests that with the ingredients of this plant on hand sterilization experiments shall now in any case be carried out in the concentration camps.

SS Obergruppenführer POHL agreed to take the necessary steps at once.

22 June 1942
BRA/V
(S) BRANDT
SS Obergruppenführer

Document No-039[224]
Office of U.S. Chief of Counsel

Secret
The Deputy Gauleiter of the Lower Danube
To: The Reichsführer
Pg. Heinrich HIMMLER
Berlin SW 1
Prinz-Albrechtstrasse 8

It was established by an extensive series of experiments on rats, rabbits and dogs that in the administration or injection of caladium extract male animals became genitally unfit and females unreceptive.

223 Document No-044, in Ibid.
224 Document No-039, in Ibid.

It is clear that these observations could be of tremendous importance if alterations of genital power or fecundity could also be successfully brought about in human beings by the administration of Schweigrohr extract. Research on human beings themselves would, of course, be necessary for this. Accordingly, the director of my Racial-Political Office points out that the necessary research and human experiments could be undertaken by an appropriately selected medical staff basing their work on the Madaus animal experiments in cooperation with the pharmacological institute of the Faculty of Medicine of Vienna, on the persons of the inmates of the gipsy Camp of Lackenbach in the Lower Danube.

It is quite clear that such research must be handled as a nationally important secret matter of the most dangerous character, because enemy propaganda could work tremendous harm all over the world by the knowledge of such research, should it become known.

Heil Hitler!
Yours faithfully
(S) K. Gund
SS Oberführer

Document No-040[225]
Office of U.S. Chief of Counsel

The Reichsführer SS
Field-Command
Personal Staff
1336/42 Top secret Bra/V.
29 August 1942
Dort.Zch. Schd-310/42 g.
Top Secret !

To the Deputy Gauleiter in Lower Danube
SS Oberführer K. GERLAND
Vienna 9
Wasagasse 10

225 Document No-040, in Ibid.

Dear Sir:

I can inform you that the subject of your enquiry addressed to the Reichsführer has already been known since last March and dealt with. SS Obergruppenführer POHL and SS Gruppenführer Dr. GRAWITZ are attending to it.

There are difficulties insofar as the plant in question grows only in North America and on account of the war is not obtainable in sufficient quantities. The growing in hot houses is a very tedious process and the yield does not seem sufficient to carry out the planned experiments on a larger scale.

I would be very thankful if you could inform me, whether the plant in question is possibly at the disposal of Dr. FEHRINGER and what he considers the possibility of obtaining it.

On the return of the Reichsführer SS I shall submit your reply together with your letter, a copy of which I have already forwarded to the SS Obergruppenführer Dr. GRAWITZ.

Heil Hitler!
by order of
(Signed) BRANDT
SS Obersturmbannführer

Document No-043[226]
Office of U.S. Chief of Counsel

THE DEPUTY DISTRICT LEADER (Gauleiter) IN LOWER DANUBE (Niederdonau)
Vienna IX, 14 October 1942
Wasagasse 1A
310/42 Top Secret Ge/Go.

To: SS Obersturmbannführer R. BRANDT
o.V.i.A.
Personal Staff of the Reich Leader of
BERLIN SW 11
Prinz-Albrechtstrasse 8

226 Document No-043, in Ibid.

Dear Comrade Brandt:

...Unfortunately, I must give a negative reply to your question as to whether Dr. FEHRINGER has the plant in question available. He considers the procurement of *caladium seguinum* possible by chemical means.

It is also conceivable that one or another of the hot-houses which are located in our climatically preferable district (Gau) could be used for experimental purposes, in order to be able to cultivate the plants at least to a sufficient extent for experimental purposes.

I should be grateful if I could obtain the opinion of the Reich Leader in this matter and suggest, that Dr. FEHRINGER collaborate with SS Obersturmbannführer Dr. LOLLING.

Heil Hitler!
yours
(S[igned]) K. GERLAND

As indicated by the above documents, the *caladium seguinum* experiments could never really get off the ground because the plant needed for production of the "drug", even in experiments, could not be obtained.

The technique of injecting liquid substances into the uterus proved easier to test. The goal was to produce sterility by causing inflammation in the fallopian tubes that would prevent passage of the ova into the uterus.

Office of U.S. Chief of Counsel[227]
Subsequent Proceedings Division apo 124-A, U.S. Army

Staff Evidence Analysis
By: Henry Sachs
Date: 30 Aug 1946
Doc. No-211
Title and/or general nature: Letter from Clauberg to Himmler through Ogruf Schmauser
Re: sterilization of female prisoners
Date: 30 May 1942
Source (Location of original, etc.): Berlin Document Center
Language: German

227 Letter of Dr. C. Clauberg to Himmler, on sterilization of female prisoners 30 May 1942, Nuremberg Document 211, in Mendelsohn, ed., *The Holocaust: Selected Documents,* vol. 9, pp. 150–154.

Persons, firms or organizations involved:
Ogrf. Schmauser
Dr. Rudolf Brandt
Obstbf. Dr. Arlt
Prof. Dr. Clauberg

To be filed under these reference headings:
Same as above
Experiments on human beings
Concentration camps – Auschwitz
Concentration camps – General

Summary (Indicate page nos.): This is a five page letter containing a blueprint for the conducting of various experiments regarding the reproductive capability of women. One series of these planned experiments deals with the sterilization of female concentration camp inmates. Clauberg had written to Himmler before. He mentions a letter of 5 June 1941 in which he, apparently, suggested the establishment of a Forschungsinstitut für Fortpflanzungsbiologie (Research Institute of Propagation Biology) a pet project of his. Brandt had answered for Himmler on 19 June 1941 promising to contact him as soon as possible, but nothing had happened. He states that the main difficulties he had encountered in his research work on propagation problems had been connected with the supply of female concentration camp inmates needed for his experiments. In a conversation he had had with Dr. Arlt, the latter had advised him to approach Himmler in this matter. Apparently Clauberg had already seen Himmler.

He is now submitting a list of the material needed for the establishment of an experimental plant: personnel, animals, instruments, an X-ray apparatus, housing facilities, stables and cages, etc., and 5 to 10 female concentration camp inmates, the latter to be used for his experiments on sterilization without open operation (bloodless sterilization). As the place for his experimental plant he suggests the concentration camp Auschwitz.

Concluding his letter he stresses the fact that he is asking only for the barest necessities but hopes that some day his "Forschungsinstitut für Fortpflanzungsbiologie des RFSS" (Research Institute of Propagation Biology of the Reichsführer SS) will become reality. Pages 4 and 5 of the document contain a brief draft of the "Forschungsinstitut" including a chart.

■

One of the goals of the Propagation Biology Institute, Clauberg notes in an attached draft, would be "to evaluate the method of sterilization without operation (bloodless sterilization) on women unworthy of propagation and to use this method continually after it is finally proved efficient".[228] Himmler, favorably inclined towards the proposal, first refers Clauberg to the women's camp in Ravensbrück, then to Auschwitz. He also suggests that sterilizing males by X-ray be investigated.

Translation of Document No-213[229]
Office of U.S. Chief of Counsel

Reichsführer SS
Personal Staff
(handwritten remark:
Journal Number 1266/42, returned 31 October 1942 by
Bra/Dr., Pol. Administration K.)
Führer Headquarters 10. July 1942
Top secret
1.) Professor CLAUBERG (handwritten remark): W 1–10, 1–5–43,
10–7–43
Königshütte

Dear Professor:

Today the Reichsführer SS charged me with transmitting on his wish that you go to Ravensbrück after you have had another talk with SS Obergruppenführer POHL and the Camp Physician of the women's concentration camp Ravensbrück, in order to perform there the sterilization of the Jewesses according to your method.

Before you start your job, the Reichsführer SS would be interested to learn from you how long it would take to sterilize a thousand Jewesses. The Jewesses themselves should not know anything about it. As the Reichsführer SS understands it, you could give the appropriate injections during a general examination.

Thorough experiments should be conducted to investigate the effect of the sterilization largely in a way, that you find out after a certain time, which you would have to fix perhaps by X-rays, what kind of changes have taken place. In the one or the other case a practical

228 Ibid.
229 Document No-213, Office of the U.S. Chief of Counsel, in *Trials NMT.*

experiment might be arranged by locking up a Jewess and a Jew together for a certain period and to see then, what results are achieved thereby.

Translation of Document No-216[230]
Office of U.S. Chief of Counsel

Memorandum on Conference

Führer – Headquarters July 1942
Top Secret!
1 copy.

On 7 July 1942, a discussion took place between the Reichsführer SS, SS Brigadeführer Professor Dr. GEBHARDT, SS Brigadeführer GLUECKS and SS Brigadeführer CLAUBERG, *Königshütte.*

Topic of the discussion was the sterilization of Jewesses. The Reichsführer SS has promised SS-Brigadeführer Professor CLAUBERG that the Auschwitz concentration camp will be at his disposal for his experiments on human beings and animals. By means of some fundamental experiments a method should be found which would lead to sterilization of persons without their knowledge. The Reichsführer SS wanted to get another report as soon as the result of these experiments would become known, so that the sterilization of Jewesses could then be carried out in actuality.

It should also be examined, preferably in cooperation with Professor Dr. HOHLFELDER an X-ray specialist in Germany, in what way sterilization of men could be achieved by X-ray treatment.

The Reichsführer SS called the special attention of all gentlemen present to the fact that the matter involved was most secret and should be discussed only with the officers in charge and that the persons present at the experiments or discussions had to pledge secrecy.

(Signature) BRANDT
SS Obersturmbannführer

Clauberg reported to Himmler that his method was practically completed and that with ten assistants he would be able to sterilize 1,000 women a day.

230 Memorandum on Conference, Document No-216, in RG-30.00M.

Translation of Document No-212[231] Office of U.S. Chief of Counsel

Professor Dr. med C. CLAUBERG
Chief Physician of the Clinics for Women of the Knappschaft Hospital and the St. Hedwig Hospital
Telephone: 409-31
Königshütte O.S.
7 June 1943

To the Reichsführer SS Herr Heinrich Himmler
(Stamp)
Secret
Berlin
(Handwritten notations in shorthand – illegible)

Dear Reichsführer,

Today I am fulfilling my obligation to report to you from time to time about the state of my research work. In doing this I am – as before – adhering to the procedure to report only if the matter is essential. The fact that I after my most recent interview in July 1942 – [that] I could not do so before today, is due to temporary difficulties in detail against which I myself was powerless, and with which I could not bother you, Reichsführer. I mention as an example that only since February 1943 am I in possession of an X-ray installation, which is of great value to my special research. In spite of the short period of actually only 4 months, it is already today possible to report to you – Reichsführer – the following:

The method I contrived, to achieve the sterilization of the female organism without any operation is as good as perfected. It can be performed by a single injection inside from the entrance of the uterus in the course of the usual customary gynaecologic examination as known to every physician. If I say that the method is "as good as perfected", this means

1. Still to be worked out are only minor improvements of the method.
2. Already today it could be put to practical use in the course of our *regular* eugenic sterilizations and could thus replace the operation.

As to the question which you, Reichsführer, asked me almost one year ago, i.e. how much time would probably be required to sterilize 1000

231 Document No-212, in Ibid.

women by using this method: Today I can answer you with regard to the future as follows:

If my researches continue to give the same results as up to now and there is no reason to doubt that – then the moment is no longer far off when I can say: "by one adequately trained physician in one adequately equipped place with perhaps 10 assistants (the number of assistants in conformity with the desired acceleration) most likely several hundred – if not even 1000 per day".

In addition I should like to make a further request. It was SS Brigadeführer Dr. Blumenbuter, who finally managed to get me the one suitable X-ray installation. I am in urgent need of an other installation of the same kind and he informed me in February that he had such an other one stored in Berlin. He was ready to deliver it to me if I would secure your approval.

May I ask you, Reichsführer for this approval?

Heil Hitler!
(Signed) CLAUBERG
(handwritten)

The following depositions and testimonies are from former concentration camp prisoners who were victims of a sterilization procedure. Of special interest is the testimony of Dr. Dorotha Lorska from France, who, through the underground movement in the camp, was able to smuggle out descriptions of the experiments to inform the Free World.

Deposition of a Witness[232]

Extract

Interrogator: Dr. Barbas
Writer of the protocol: Stolarova
Experienced doctor: Dr. Jan Cespiva, certified expert
Witness: Margita Neumennova, born 16.9.1908 in Bytca, district Bytca
Interrogated in the process against Karl Clauberg

It was a dark room with a small X-ray machine, Dr. Clauberg gave the order for to me to lie on the gynecologic table and I could watch Sylvia

232 Deposition of Margita Neumennova for Interrogation of Klaus Clausberg, YVA, D. 33/4334.

Friedman who prepared an injection with a big needle. With this needle, Dr. Clauberg gave me an injection into the uterus. I had the feeling as if my abdomen would split from pains. I started to cry, so that people could hear it in the whole block. Dr. Clauberg shouted at me roughly, I should stop crying immediately or I would be brought back at once to the concentration camp of Birkenau.

I had unbearable pains. The substance of this injection was Jodipin. I know that another substance named Barium also was used for similar injections. After this experiment, I got a particular inflammation of my ovary. I had terrible pains, shivers and fever...

As a result of the experiments, Dr. Clauberg carried out on me, my life worthy of a human being as woman has become impossible to me. It is excluded to me, to live the normal life of a woman or to give birth to children.

Translation of Document No-875, RG-30.001M[233]

Deposition of Mudr. Zdenka, Nedvedova-Nejedla
September 6, 1945

I have seen Gypsy women prisoners enter and leave the X-ray room where they were sterilized by a method which according to my information had been tested in Oswiecim. This method was based on injecting an irritating solution into the uterus, most probably argentum nitricum together with contrasting solution to make possible an X-ray check of the performed operation. All sterilized women were immediately X-rayed after this operation. I examined these pictures with Mudr. Mlada-Taufrova, and I am, therefore, qualified to give evidence that in the majority of cases, said filling penetrated up to the end of the tubes (oviduct), in several cases even as far as into the abdominal cavity. This sterilization was performed even on Gypsy girls about 10 years of age. Only about the last 10 were given a Kelen narcosis on the intervention of SS-nurse Gerda. I nursed these children all night after the operation. All these girls were bleeding from the genitals and were suffering such pains, that I had to give them sedatives secretly. In the morning before the "appell", I transported these children, with the help of girls working in the revier, to their respective blocks.

233 Deposition of MuDr. Zdenka Nedvedova-Nejedla, 6 September 1945, Document No-875, Office of the U.S. Chief of Counsel, in RG-30.001M.

I have seen several German women before and after the operation who were detailed for sterilization on the ground of German racial laws. Also approximately 20 women on whom operational abortions were performed on order of the Gestapo (mostly women who returned from the brothels of various concentration camps for men "puffs"). These operations were performed by Dr. Treite.

Testimony of Dr. Dora Klein, Prisoner Physician from France[234]

...I nursed Clauberg's patients. I know that he carried out the experiments as follows: First, he injected some material into the woman's oviduct (fallopian tube). After the injection, he immediately took an X-ray of the uterus. In the case of certain women similar injections were administered repeatedly at intervals of a few weeks. As a result of the injections, the women sometimes had peritoneal irritation, pains, vomiting or high temperatures. From what I could determine, Clauberg's aim was to find a temporary or permanent method of sterilization simply by injecting a certain fluid into the oviduct (for obturation of the oviduct).

Testimony of Dorotha Lorska[235]

In June 1943, I was arrested in Paris for participation in the resistance movement and was handed over to the Gestapo after investigation by the collaborating French police. I arrived to Auschwitz in a transport from France on 2 August 1943. At the railway platform, I encountered for the first time an SS physician. This was Dr. Edward Wirths, who made on that day, or rather night, the "selection" for the camp. He ordered married women to line up and selected approximately 100; I was among them and that was how I got into Block 10. At that time, there were around 400 women there, Jewesses from 10 European countries. They all were guinea pigs for the SS doctors.

I was lucky to establish during the first days of my stay in Block 10, contact with the group of the resistance movement, with the help of a prisoner from the disinfection detail.

234 Deposition of Dr. Dora Klein (France), 0.33/4334, 0-2/507.

235 Testimony of Dorota Lorska, former inmate, Auschwitz–Birkenau, No. 52325 in IAC, *Inhuman Medicine*, vol. 1, pt. 2, pp. 81–98.

Following an instruction given by the resistance movement organization, I described at that time in a detailed and concise manner the experiments on the female prisoners in this Block, with special emphasis on the names of the SS men and other people, participating in these experiments.

This report, the first description of what was going on in the only female block in the Auschwitz camp, was at the end of 1943 smuggled out of camp by colleagues, Tadeusz Holuj and Stanislaw Klodinski. At that time, in 1943, I wrote:

> The following SS physicians are carrying out experiments on women prisoners in Block 10. Professor Karl Clauberg, Dr. Horst Schumann, Dr. Edward Wirths and Dr. Bruno Weber. Approximately 40 women are in two large rooms. From time to time the "used up material" is sent to the women camp in Birkenau and is being replaced with "new material" from the recently arrived transports. Clauberg's studio is on the ground floor, and is made up of a gynecological and a roentgenological room. The experiment consists of the injection with a syringe of approximately 10 ml of some turbid liquid into the cervix uteri of the selected married women. After the injection, an X-ray picture is taken of the reproductive organs. These injections are repeated at intervals of several weeks, always followed by a roentgenogram. The purpose is to cause an inflammation of the oviducts, leading to their occlusion and as a result to sterility. These injections are painful. Frequently symptoms of irritation of the peritoneum can be noticed, combined with fever, vomiting, pain in the hypogastrium.

In the light of documents, found after the liberation of the camp and of evidence, given by many SS men of the Auschwitz camp, it is possible to define even with greater precision and to analyze those pseudo-scientific experiments made with female prisoners in Block 10. It is a known fact that the sterilization of women was to serve the preparation of methods to sterilize entire nations of races, whom the Third Reich did not give the right to exist.

Here the SS physicians kept up with the ideologists and lawmakers; through such people as Clauberg and Schumann they industrially helped to find the possible methods of genocide.

A quote from Shelly Lore's book gives an insight into Clauberg's professionalism.

Block 10[236]

> Clauberg trained an SS man, SDG Buehning, a former hairdresser, in the method of sterilization through intrauterine injections, and the medical layman performed these sterilizations for about half a year. In addition, Clauberg relegated the execution of the procedure to a chemist of the Schering Factory, Dr. Goebel. Both of these men worked independently during Clauberg's absence, although a salpingography should never be performed by nonmedical personnel.
>
> The injections were extremely painful, caused high fever and inflammation. Some women even died as a result of them. When the experiments were completed, many of the guinea pigs were returned to Birkenau to be gassed, and fresh material for research arrived. A large number of the surviving guinea pigs were not only unable to conceive as a result of these experiments but were mentally and physically crippled by them.

This extract summarizing the sterilization experiment is from Colonel L. N. Smirnov, member of the Nuremberg Tribunal.

Opening Statement[237]

> Special hospitals, surgical blocks, histological laboratories and other departments were set up in the camp. But they were intended not for the treatment but for the extermination of people. Here the German professors and doctors carried out mass experiments on men, women, and children, who were in perfectly good health. They carried out sterilization experiments on women, castration of men, experiments on children, artificial infection of masses, on people with cancer, typhus and malaria, who were afterwards subjected to observation. They tested the action of poisonous substances on living persons.
>
> I would like to stress that experiments in the sterilization and castration of women and men were carried out on a particularly large scale. Whole blocks in the camp were especially designated for experiments using particularly effective methods of sterilization and castration.

236 Shelley, ed., *Criminal Experiments on Human Beings,* pp. 7–16.

237 *Trial of War Criminals, International Military Tribunal,* Part 8, February 27, 1946–March 1, 1946, Official Transcript published by his Majesty's Stationary Office, London 1947, pp. 7–11.

Experiments on women were carried out in the hospital blocks of the Oswiecim Camp. Up to four hundred women were detained simultaneously in Block 10 of the camp, and sterilization experiments were carried out on them by means of X-rays and subsequent removal of the ovaries, experiments in inoculation of cancer in the neck of the uterus and forced abortion, and in testing contrasting substances for X-raying the uterus.

...In Block 21 – that is another block, the women's block was No. 10 – mass experiments in castration of men were carried out for the purpose of studying the possibility of sterilization by X-ray. The castration itself was carried out some time after the X-raying process. These experiments in X-raying and castration were carried out by Professor Schumann and Dr. Dierring. It frequently happened that after the X-raying, one or both testicles of the subject were removed for examination.

I believe that it was not by accident that the experiments on people began with sterilization and castration. This was a quite natural result of the theories of German Fascism, interested in lowering the birth-rate of those people whom they considered to be vanquished. It was a part of Hitler's "depopulation technique" and in confirmation of this, I would now like to quote a very short excerpt from Rauschning's book, "The Voice of Destruction".

Hitler said to Rauschning: "And by 'destruction' I do not necessarily mean extermination of these people – I shall simply take systematic measures to prevent their procreation. There are many means by which a systematic and comparatively painless extinction of undesirable races can be attained, at any rate without blood being shed."

It is stated there that a statistical report by the commandant of the camp has been discovered in the archives of the camp. It has a column under the heading "Internees nominated for Experiments". This column reads as follows:

"Women subject to experiments: on 15th May, 1944 – 400
on 15th June – 413
on 19th June – 348",
and so on.

Finally documentation will be presented about sterilization experiments with the use of X-ray irradiation.

Translation of Document No-205[238]
Office of U.S. Chief of Counsel

Viktor BRACK
SS Oberführer
W 8, Voss-Str.4
Berlin
25 June 1942
Top Secret!
HH (sign)

To Reichsführer SS and Chief of German Police Heinrich HIMMLER
Berlin
Prinz-Albrechtstr. 8

Dear Reichsführer,

...Among the 10 millions of Jews in Europe are, I figure, at least 2–3 millions of men and women, who are fit enough for work. Considering the extraordinary difficulties, the labor problem presents us with, I hold the view that these 2–3 millions should be specially selected and preserved. This can however only be done, if at the same time they are rendered incapable to propagate. About a year ago I reported to you that agents of mine have completed the experiments necessary for this purpose. I would like to recall these facts once more. Sterilization, as normally performed on persons with hereditary diseases, is here out of the question, because it takes too long and is too expensive. Castration by X-rays however is not only relatively cheap, but can also be performed on many thousands in the shortest time. I think, that at this time it is already irrelevant whether the people in question become aware of having been castrated after some weeks or months once they feel the effects.

Heil Hitler!
Yours, (Signed) Viktor Brack

238 Document No-205, Office of the U.S. Chief of Counsel, in RG-30.001M.

Translation of Document No-206[239]
Office of U.S. Chief of Counsel

The Reichsführer SS
XIa/126 (handwritten)
1314/42 (handwritten)

11 August 1942
SS Senior Col.
(SS Oberführer) Brack (figure 11 – handwritten)
Berlin W 8
Field Headquarters (Feld Kommandostelle)
Voss-Strasse 4
Top secret
4 copies
4th copy

1. Dear BRACK!

It is only today that I have the opportunity to acknowledge the receipt of your letter of 23 June. I am positively interested in seeing that the sterilization by X-rays is tried out at least once in one camp in a series of experiments.

I will by very much obliged to the... Reichsleiter BOHLER if to begin with, he would place the expert physicians for the series of experiments at our disposal.

I will mail a copy of this letter to the Reich Physician SS (Reichsarzt SS) and to the competent Chief of the Main Office (Hauptamtschef) for Concentration Camps.

Heil Hitler!
Yours
(Signed) H. HIMMLER

2. SS Lieutenant General *(SS Obergruppenführer)* POHL
3. SS Major General (SS Gruppenführer) Dr. GRAWITZ
   for information

By order Br. (handwritten)
SS Lieutenant Colonel (SS Obersturmbannführer)
(stamps:) 11 August 1942

239 Document No-206, in Ibid.

In his essay "Inhuman Medicine", Dr. Stanislaw Klodzinski gives a complete and vivid description of the sterilization and castration procedures performed in Auschwitz. The main goal was to find the most effective and reliable method for the "mass production" of sterilized males.

"Sterilization" and Castration with the Help of X-Rays in the Auschwitz Concentration Camp[240]

Viktor Brack presented Himmler in 1941 with a proposal for the sterilization of Jews with X-rays, stating in a letter "...If certain people are to be permanently made incapable of reproducing, then this can be achieved with the help of heavy X-raying, which causes castration with all the consequences..."

He further wrote: "It would be advisable to order people, who are to receive such treatment, to stand behind a small window, whereby they would answer questions or fill out some form, which would keep them for 2–3 minutes there. A clerk, sitting at the window, could handle the built in apparatus, in such a way, that the opening of the window would put the machinery into operation, i.e. two X-ray tubes/radiation must affect both sides. An installation with such X-ray tubes could in such a way sterilize an average of 150–200 people a day, which means that if there were 20 such installations, approximately 3–4,000 people could be sterilized a day."

Summing up, one could say, that, taking into consideration the present-day state of roentgenological technique, it would be possible to carry out sterilization with the help of X-rays on a mass scale.

In the middle of 1942 the Auschwitz camp was turned into the place where "sterilization" experiments were carried out.

Himmler, who was possessed by the idea to make use of the prisoners as labour for the armament industry of the Reich, and simultaneously to make provisions that they would not reproduce, wanted an inexpensive and quick method, on a mass scale.

Dr. Horst Schumann, made his appearance in the Auschwitz-Birkenau camp in November 1942. It was at that time that an "X-ray sterilization" center was active in the women's camp in Birkenau, in Block 30.

A day in Block 30 was as follows (description of prisoner Sonia Fischmann, the scribe of this block):

240 Klodzinski, in IAC, *Inhuman Medicine,* vol. 1, pt. 2, pp. 46–79.

> On the eve of a work day Dr. Schumann notified the camp employment department, that he wanted next morning 100 young and healthy women or men to be sent to the block. In the morning the block senior reported with the prisoners the doctor had asked for.
>
> At the beginning neither the personnel of the experimental block, nor the prisoners brought there, were aware of the purpose of Schumann's "examinations". Rumours spread that these "examinations" were connected with the typhus fever raging at that time in camp. The entire work of this block was surrounded with absolute secrecy. That is why entry was forbidden to this block to SS soldiers as well as to prisoners, and the personnel, working in Block 30, slept there, too.

After the arrival of Dr. Schumann, Sonia Fischmann notified him about the arrival of the prisoners, their number and nationality. In the waiting room the prisoners had to disrobe completely. Next their prisoner number was entered on a joint list by one of the women prisoners, from which the prisoners' names were later called and then they were taken individually into the X-ray room.

In this room two types of mobile seats had been installed. These were connected with the X-ray machines. The prisoners were told to place themselves in the proper position between the machines, in such a way that they were standing sideways to the booth, in which Schumann was sitting. At that moment Dr. Schumann switched on the current. The "treatment" did not take more than several minutes. Due to this it was possible during the course of a few hours to sterilize quite a substantial number of prisoners. Later various after-effects of radiation were noted: burns and abscesses, mainly of the abdominal skin. I remember that women shortly after such radiation often suffered from nausea and also vomiting.

In the case of the male "guinea pigs" Dr. Schumann surgically removed some of the testicles, after having previously subjected them to X-ray radiation. Similarly, many ovaries were removed after the radiation for histological examination.

The preserved report, dated 16 December 1943, showed that during the period between 16 October 1943 and 15 December 1943 as many as 90 amputations of testicles were undertaken in the surgical department of the hospital of camp I in Auschwitz, 10 ovaries were removed and there was one case of surgical removal of the Fallopian tubes.

A witness, a prisoner-surgeon from Birkenau, Dr. Robert Levy, stated in his testimony that the testicles were removed in order to examine them under the microscope and find out about the results of the radia-

> tion. He also thought that these people were subjected to various doses of X-rays, to find out, which dose yields the expected result.
>
> Dr. Schumann subjected to radiation at one session an average of about 30 people. He carried out such a radiation 2–3 times a week.

Dr. Schumann worked not only in Birkenau but also in Auschwitz. Testimony of the following two witnesses, whose personal data and files are in the court in Frankfurt-am-Main, shows that among the female prisoners destined for gynecological experiments in Block 10 was a group of young Jewish girls from Saloniki.

These girls had served as experimental guinea pigs for Dr. Schumann. He had first X-rayed their ovaries, and then, several weeks later, performed laparotomies, during which one ovary was excised (ovariectomy). A few weeks afterwards, when the surgical wound had already healed up, the operation was repeated, and the excision of the second ovary took place. By means of the latter surgery the doctors were seeking data on the effects of the irradiation over time.

In October and November 1945, Dr. Matarasso of Salonika examined some fifteen former prisoners, men and women – who had been Schumann's guinea pigs and summarized the proceedings:

Proceedings Summaries[241]

> F. S., 20 years old, unmarried; Subjected to X-ray treatment, three months later operated. Present state: absence of menstruation, dizziness, attacks of perspiration, throbbing of the heart, frequent urinating, neuralgia.
>
> L. B., 20 years old, unmarried. Subjected to radiation, operated after four months. Since that time absence of menstruation. Present state: Disturbances connected with amenorrhoea, frequent dizziness, attacks of blushing, attacks of sweating profusely.
>
> D. V., 19 years old, married. Three times subjected to X-ray treatment, next operated on. Due to infection of the wound after surgery, bed-ridden for 3 months. Since that time absence of menstruation. Present state: amenorrhoea, dizziness, blushing, throbbing of the heart, frequent urination.

241 Dr. Matarasso's proceedings summaries.

> M. E., 30 years old. Subjected to X-rays, removal of one testicle. Examination on September 9, 1945 in Salonika revealed no spermatozoa.
>
> H. M., 20 years old. Bilateral removal of testicles; the first testicle in July 1943, the second in September 1943. Present state: breast slightly overdeveloped, sexual neurosis.

In his final remarks Dr. Matarasso mentions the fact that all subjects whom he examined suffered from slight psychic disturbances.

The ethical and legal side of these sterilization and castration experiments conducted by Horst Schumann and his colleagues in the Auschwitz-Birkenau concentration camp are a glaring violation of all the binding principles of medical experimentation. In effect, these were criminal acts, disguised as applications of "scientific method" to racial hygiene problems. In the context of the crazy fascist ideology, they were, in actuality, the first steps in the "Final Solution".

The testimony of victims follows.

Deposition of Gustava Winnowska, Taken in Stockholm, 18 September 1946[242]

> ...A doctor came from Auschwitz for a few days, possibly for a week, and worked all day. He was sterilizing Gypsy children by X-ray. The children used to come out crying after being sterilized, asking their mothers what had been done to them.
>
> Dr. Treite sterilised a young Gypsy child by abdominal operation on orders from Berlin. I saw her after the operation, she was about thirteen years old. Dr. Treite told me that Gypsy children had to be sterilised when they were young as they could have children when they were fourteen years old.
>
> (Signed) Gustava Winnowska

242 Deposition of Gustava Winnowska, taken in Stockholm, 18 September 1946, by Major Arthur Keith Mant, of the War Crimes Investigation Unit, detailed by Commander-in-Chief Baor, *Przeglad Lekarski,* No. 1: 1964/24, in RG-30.001M, p. 2.

Declaration of Aliza Barouch (nee Zarfati)[243]

> The first time they took a group of us Greek girls to Birkenau to irradiate our ovaries was in May/June 1943. They put us into a dark, locked and sealed room. We thought they were killing us. You could smell medicine in the air. We stood in the corner, holding each other, and then SS Dr. Horst Schumann arrived. He took one, Forforca (who now lives in Spain) and closed the door. The minutes were like eternity. What are they doing in there? Will she cry, will she scream? It was very frightening.
>
> I, at 15 the youngest of our group, looked through the key hole. I saw only legs. Fifteen to twenty minutes later she came out. Then Bella went in, then I. Schumann stood behind a glass divider. On my abdomen (front and back), he put a wooden board with many wires. Then I had to stand naked between two X-ray apparatuses. After 20 minutes, he let me go. It did not hurt.
>
> When Forforca came out she was snow-white and she felt like vomiting. The same with Bella. I thought, maybe they are poisoning us in there.
>
> It lasted a long time, until all 20 women had received their dosage of X-rays and were ready. We felt so miserable that it took us twice as long to walk back to Block 10 in Auschwitz since we had to vomit continuously. Afterward, we stayed in bed for 18 days.
>
> A little later, we lost all our hair and after the second irradiation experiment, our entire body was burnt and turned black and we had blood in the stool. All the other girls underwent radiation only twice, but Dora Gershon and I had to endure it three times. Dora does not want to talk about it, I am the only one who speaks out.

As the following letter to Himmler shows, for castration of men, the surgical method proved better than radiation. This, of course, meant that radiation of men for this purpose was discontinued.

243 Declaration of Aliza Barouch (nee Zarfati), in Shelley, ed., *Criminal Experiments on Human Beings*, pp. 81–83.

Translation of Document No-208[244]
Office of U.S. Chief of Counsel

Top Secret
Chancellery of the Führer of the NSDAP
Voss Strasse 4
Berlin W 8, 29 April 1944
Telephone No.: Local 120054
Long distance 126621
File No: IIa/Kt.

To the Reichsführer SS and Chief of the German Police Heinrich Himmler
Berlin SH II
Prinz-Albrechtstrasse

Dear Reichsführer!

By order of Reich Leader (Reichsleiter) Bouhler, I submit to you as an enclosure a work of Dr. Horst Schumann on the influence of X-rays on human genital glands.

Previously, you have asked Senior Colonel (Oberführer) Brack to perform this work, and you supported it by providing the adequate material in the Concentration Camp Auschwitz. I point especially to the 2nd part of this work, which shows that by those means a castration of males is almost impossible or requires an effort which does not pay. As I have convinced myself, the operative castration requires not more than 6 to 7 minutes, and therefore can be performed more reliably and quicker than the castration by X-rays.

Soon I shall be able to submit a continuation of this work to you.

Heil Hitler
(handwritten) Your much devoted
(Signature) Blankenburg

enclosure
(handwritten) 14/44/Top Secret

244 Document No-208, Office of the U.S. Chief of Counsel, in RG-30.001M.

Additional Bibliography on Sterilization Experiments

GLANVILLE WILLIAMS, *Sanctity of Life and Penal Law* (Warsaw: PZWL, 1960), pp. 71 ff; *SS im Einsatz* (Berlin: Kongress Verlag, 1957) p. 121; H. LANGBEIN, *Der Fall Dr. Horst Schumann;* D. CZECH, *Calendar of Events in the Auschwitz-Birkenau Concentration Camp* (Published by the State Museum in Auschwitz, 1958, 1960, 1962); SONIA FISCHMANN, *Block 30 – Roentgen Sterilization;* "Original records of the surgery room in Block 21", Archives of the State Museum in Auschwitz; J. SEHN, *Concentration Camp Auschwitz–Birkenau* (Warsaw, 1957), p. 98; "Evidence given by witness Dr. E. de Wind, former prisoner", Archives of the State Museum in Auschwitz; "Material of the camp resistance movement", Documents of the Main Commission for the Investigation of Nazi Crimes in Poland.

MISCELLANEOUS EXPERIMENTS

Experiments with Petrol and Benzene

Many German soldiers injected themselves with harmful preparations in order to get sick and thus avoid being sent to the front line. The Nazis, therefore, wished to identify the symptoms these preparations would cause.

The following experiments were described in an article by Dr. Philip Friedman, who, after World War II, was founder and director of the Central Jewish Historical Commission in Poland, and later became chairman of the European Coordination Committee of the Jewish Historical Commissions and Institute in Paris. His material is based on testimony of survivors of Auschwitz.[245]

Nazi doctors gave subcutaneous injections of petrol and benzene to test the reaction to these substances. The injections were made into the deep subcutaneous tissue of the legs of prisoners. After eight days, large phlegmones developed. These were incised, and the pus was sent in sealed containers to the Histological Institute of Breslau University.

245 Philip Friedman, "Nazi Crimes Against Humanity", *American OSE Review,* vol. 1, pp. 329. OSE was a Russian organization (Organization for the Protection of Health of Jews) founded in 1912. It sponsored a quarterly publication devoted to the problems of hygiene among Jews. The journal had an international editorial board, of which Albert Einstein was a member. The letters OSE are an acronym derived from the organization's Russian name.

The effects on the victims of these experiments were severe. The patients became very sick, the wounds did not heal, and they were sent to the gas chamber with the next transport.

Experiments with Various Pastes and Powders

Prisoners were subjected to the application of various chemicals which produced skin irritations and caused phlegmones and wounds. A variety of ointment pastes and powders were used for that purpose. The inflamed portion of the skin was excised together with the subcutaneous tissue and sent to the Breslau Histological Institute for analysis.

Experiment on Lead Poisoning

At the suggestion of Professor Werner Kollath of the Institute of Hygiene at the University of Rostock, Himmler's most senior hygienist, Mrugowsky, drafted a research proposal for a four-year study of the effects of long-term ingestion of minute quantities of lead. The following three physiological characteristics were evaluated independently: 1. problems of disturbances in sexual drive (libido); 2. problems/disturbances in the ability to engage in sexual intercourse (potency); and 3. problems of bringing forth healthy offspring (fertility).

Camp inmates were used for these experiments. Each male subject prisoner was introduced to a healthy female prisoner and the pair stayed partners for the duration of the experiment.

Anesthetics

Women were given a fatal dose of anaesthetic to measure the exact length of time required for death to occur.

Blood Volume

The arteries of victims were opened in order to find out whether five liters of blood would actually pour out.[246]

246 From Dr. Golse's evidence given before the Polish Investigation Commission, International Auschwitz Committee.

Electric Current

Dr. Koenig performed some experiments on Jews in Manowice, near Oswiecim (Auschwitz). He studied the effect of electric shock on the organism and killed many young men by directing high voltage electric current through their brains.

The most detailed evidence of these experiments is contained in an eyewitness report by Dr. Samuel Steinberg, a prisoner who was forced to work in the notorious Room 1 of Block 21.[247]

"Sleeping" Drugs

Studies of the actions of a certain sleeping drug were also made on the prisoners. There were two experiments, each on three prisoners who were ordered to drink coffee in which a powder had been dissolved. The first experiment ended with failure; the prisoners remained alive. The experiment was then repeated. The prisoners first had to drink alcohol, then coffee laced with a larger quantity of the poison. This time the experiment was successful; two patients died immediately, the other a day later.

Lipiodol Substitutes

Lipiodol was the contrast medium used in salpingography for visualization of the Fallopian tubes by X-rays. In the experiment to find a substitute contrast medium, Jewish women served as guinea pigs. The new contrast medium was injected via the uterus into the tubes. Some of the women had to undergo this procedure four or five times. Professor Dr. Karl Clauberg or his assistants usually made these studies themselves. The German physicians, of course, were totally indifferent to the sufferings of the women; they were interested only in their experiments.

247 See "Documents on World War II", Publication of the French Government, vol. 4.

Decontamination Experiments[248]

In 1943 Ludwig Werner Haase, Ph.D., claimed that he had developed a way of purifying drinking water that had been contaminated with chemical warfare agents. Haase's findings were tested out at the Munster camp at the end of summer in 1944.

On 20 December 1944, the SS Reich physician Helmut Poppendick informed Rudolf Brandt that the experiment would be conducted on 150 prisoners. Their water was to be poisoned with mustard gas. On 31 December 1944, Rudolf Brandt informed Poppendick that it was not necessary to continue with the experiments since the results could not be put into practice in a useful manner. Poppendick replied that chemical warfare agent experts Haase and Friese find it important to supplement the experiments with nitrogen mustard gas because the experiments conducted so far were confined to the usual "arsenic-chemical warfare agent" designation.

On 8 February 1945 Poppendick shared with Brandt that the research with nitrogen mustard gas had shown the same results as that with regular mustard gas. But he also noted that the harmful effects on the human body caused by the ingestion of mustard gas and related chemical warfare agents were still unknown. Thus Haase wanted to conduct further experiments, using at least 8 more prisoners who would be given the poison internally. This request was denied on the grounds of its irrelevance to the operations of the Third Reich.

Experiments to Convert Homosexuals to Heterosexuals[249]

Even though homosexuality was considered a crime in Germany (homosexuals would not reproduce the Aryan race!), homosexuality was quite common in the Waffen SS and also in the military camps.

Addressing this problem, hormone research was conducted by a Danish physician, Carl Peter Jensen, who called himself Carl Vaernet in Germany. He claimed to have developed a hormone capsule (crystallized male hormone) that needed to be implanted in the body of the subject, most of the time in the groin. His work impressed Himmler. It had two immediate uses: 1. as an aid to men

248 Klee, *Auschwitz,* pp. 177–179.

249 From a book by French scholar Jean Boisson, translated into Hungarian by Ágnes Pótfalusi as *A Rózsaszín Háromszög* [The Pink Triangle] (Budapest: Europa Kiadó, 1991), pp. 135–136. The title pink triangle refers to the fact that homosexuals in the camps were made to wear prison uniforms with a pink triangle sewn onto the shirt, positioned over the heart.

unimpaired, who exert themselves physically; and 2. as a means of artificially increasing birthrates by acting as an artificial male sexual gland. A female sexual gland was promised for September 1944.

Jensen-Vaernet claimed the greatest success with converts from homosexuality. In Copenhagen he had implanted two capsules into a homosexual, who, three months after the last transplant, had become engaged and started a normal life with a woman. Vaernet implanted the artificial hormone capsule in prisoners in Buchenwald. He wrote to Grawitz at the end of October 1944, that the capsule "3a" transformed homosexuals into heterosexuals and that "2a" had restored the sexual drive of an individual castrated seven years earlier. It is purported that the prisoners were clever enough to anticipate the expected outcome of the research and behaved accordingly. Of the fifteen prisoner subjects, two died as the result of Vaernet's experiments. After the war, Vaernet fled to Argentina.

CHAPTER 3

Nazi research and medical ethics

With the history of Nazi medical experimentation, as with other aspects of the Nazi record in Germany, judgment of the results requires our grappling with the moral dimensions of human existence and action. We cannot separate the Nazi experimental findings from their procedural context. And thus we cannot treat these results as we might treat others, obtained by ethical, professional means; indeed, if we think to use them at all, we must understand that we are making a moral philosophical statement about relationships between ends and means, that we are deciding that valuable results justify tortuous procedures.

We must also understand that the Nazi medical records disguise the truth of the procedures in sanitized, clinical description. Let me illustrate this by a quote from the New Scientist (20 February 1985), from a paper entitled "Citations of Shame".

> With the Nazi work, technique cannot be separated so easily from its moral dimension. Here the scientific results depended upon the protocols which were sown in iniquity. In many experiments, "control subjects" meant those denied treatment, who suffered most and died. "Sample size" meant truckloads of Jews. "Significance" was an indication of misery, and "response rate" a measure of torment. Behind the niceties of learned discourse were the horrors of torture.

In my evaluation of the Nazi research, I definitely do not claim to be value-neutral. The horror of the camps is part of my personal history. Would my reaction be different if the victims had not been my family members and friends? I think not. My personal feelings about the Nazi data are well expressed in a study by Baruch C. Cohen.

> After reviewing the graphic descriptions of how the Nazis conducted the experiments, it became increasingly difficult to remain objective regarding its subsequent use. The difficulty of objectively analyzing the use of

> Nazi data was further complicated by the use of the amorphous term, "data". "Data" is merely an impersonal recordation of words and numbers. It seems unattached to the tortured or their pain. Once [sic] cannot fully confront the dilemma of using the results of Nazi experiments without sensitizing one's self to the images of the frozen, the injected, the inseminated, and the sterilized. The issue of whether to use the Nazi data is a smokescreen from the reality of human suffering. Instead of the word "data", I suggest that we replace it with an Auschwitz bar of soap. This horrible bar of soap is the remains of murdered Jews. The image sensitizes and personalizes our dilemma. Imagine the extreme feeling of discomfort and the mortified look of horror upon discovering that one just showered with the remains of murdered Jews. The ghastly thought of the Nazis melting human beings (and perhaps even one's close relatives) together for a bar of soap precludes any consideration of its use. How could any civilized person divorce the horror from the carnage without numbing one's self to the screams of the tortured and ravaged faces of the Holocaust? Indeed, it is only with this enhanced sensitivity to the suffering that one can accurately deal with the Nazi "data".[1]

Despite my feelings on this matter, I wish to explore in these pages the complexity of the ethical questions brought forth in the camp experiments. The answers are still being disputed by specialists in the field of medical ethics, as well as philosophers and other writers. And so I offer this compilation of their opinions, along with commentary and a concluding statement of my own position, in order that readers may understand and judge the matter for themselves. My own position is constructed of the union of my personal history with both the convictions shaped in ethical debates and the knowledge gained through long years of research.

At this point in time, the year 2005, sixty years after the Holocaust was brought to an end by the Allied victory, a profound ethical question continues to confront us, indeed confronts us with renewed intensity: Is it morally acceptable, ever, to cite valuable medical data (if there are any?!) collected during the course of the Nazi medical experiments?

Before turning to the various answers that people offer to this question, let me mention that the Nazi concentration camp researches were not the very first unethical experiments. There are reports from Germany, and also France, pre-dating 1933, describing transplantations of cancerous breast tissue into

1 Baruch C. Cohen, "The Ethics of Using Medical Data from Nazi Experiments", on the website *Jewish Law Articles,* http://www.jlaw.com/Articles/NaziMedEx.html, April 28, 2004. Cohen's article appeared originally in *Midstream* (June/July 1989).

healthy breasts to see if the cancer will take root; inoculations of the female urethra with gonococcal bacteria to follow the course of the infection; inoculations of tuberculosis bacilli and gonococcal bacteria into the eyes of newborn infants to study these micro-organisms; to name only a few.

Even in the United States, unethical research occurred. Best known is the Tuskegee study, in which four hundred black prison inmates with syphilis were left untreated, in order that the natural history of the development of the disease might be observed. The inmates did not even know that they had syphilis! Another example comes from the Jewish Chronic Disease Hospital in New York, where twenty-two chronically ill patients were injected with live cancer cells to observe whether they were able to reject foreign cells. Even though their health was probably not affected at all by this procedure, again they were unaware that they were part of a research project wholly unrelated to their actual illnesses. Finally "The Beecher Exposé" that was published in 1966 should be mentioned. Henry K. Beecher, Professor of Research in Anesthesiology at Harvard Medical School, studied and evaluated one hundred published research papers and judged that twelve of them were not done ethically.

Unforgivable as all these instances are, neither in dimension nor in inhuman cruelty can they be compared to the experiments the Nazis performed in concentration camps. As Yale University law professor Jay Katz writes:

> The concentration camp experiments highlight the most appalling and gruesome forms of abuse that can be inflicted on human beings whenever the human rights of research subjects are utterly disregarded. When that happens... the immediate or soon-to-follow death of research subjects readily becomes a deliberate and integral part of the research design. This, to my knowledge, has never before or since been recorded in the annals of medical science... When science takes man as its subject, tensions arise between two values basic to Western society: freedom of scientific inquiry and protection of individual inviolability... When human beings become the subject of experiments, allegiance to one value invites neglect of the other. At the heart of this conflict lies an age-old question: When may a society, actively or by acquiescence, expose some of its members to harm in order to seek benefits for them, for others, or for society as a whole?[2]

2 Jay Katz, "Abuse of Human Beings for the Sake of Science", in Caplan, ed., *When Medicine Went Mad:* pp. 233–270, here 234–235. Katz's comment partially cites his earlier work *Experimentation with Human Beings*, p. 1.

Dr. Katz also writes in this paper: "If the data proved to be useless, the ethical dilemma of using the data and thus benefiting from evil is moot, but not the questions that the controversy over their use has raised: Can we benefit from evil without perpetuating evil? Are some deeds of history so barbarous that to feast by deliberate choice on their fruits makes cannibals of us all? Or is rejection of the fruit when humankind can benefit, a commensurate or even greater evil?"[3]

■

Benjamin Freedman's paper "Moral Analysis and the Use of Nazi Experimental Results" was published in the same volume as Katz's, a collection edited by Arthur L. Caplan titled *When Medicine Went Mad.* Freedman believes that the Nazi data can be used in certain circumstances. He begins his paper by noting that the question whether it is morally acceptable to use the Nazi experimental data can only arise, if it is accepted that these data, or some of these data, have valid scientific utility.

Freedman is an analytical philosopher and ethicist, and he attempts to construct a logical position shorn of subjective elements. Arguing from this strict analytical philosophical frame of reference, he concludes that the Nazi data, if it has been judged valid by medical specialists, may be used in strictly circumscribed conditions.

Along the way towards this conclusion, Freedman notes that many common arguments against using the data rely on unstated "symbolic" content. These arguments, which are listed below, may be valid given their premises, but they cannot answer the ethical philosophical question at hand.

> 1. The results could have been shown by "bench science", without recourse to human subjects.
> 2. Results are not to be trusted because the researchers were not trustworthy.
> 3. The results cannot be applied to people who were not subjected to the Nazi deprivations.
> 4. Editors of journals should refuse publication of data reached by unethical methods. This would deter researchers in the future from pursuing unethical means in their work.[4]

3 Katz, Ibid.
4 Ibid., pp. 144–145.

Dr. Freedman does not agree with those who argue that "by using Nazi data, we would prolong the Nazi project and perpetuate that evil". He believes instead that the terrible evil represented by the Holocaust cannot be changed by anything that happens now; that its terribleness is permanent. But this terribleness in itself does not constitute a valid analytical philosophical ethical argument against using the data. "The current scientific and medical use of these data is not an extension of the Nazi project. The use rather causally depends on that project; the project has perished, the remaining detritus has been co-opted for another purpose, one that is in fact quite antithetical to the intentions of the Nazis."[5]

As we see, Freedman's arguments are analytically disciplined and lead to a nuanced position based on a careful consideration of the logic of commonplace arguments. Yet he admits that the questions still honestly puzzle him.

■

The following quotations come from an article by Alan S. Rosenbaum, Professor of Philosophy at Cleveland State University, published in the *International Journal of Applied Philosophy* (1989, No. 4). The title of Professor Rosenbaum's paper is "The Use of Nazi Medical Experimentation Data: Memorial or Betrayal?"

> Some scientists have publicly [sic] declared their intention to make use of the data in order to advance current investigatory projects; others have expressed their unwillingness, on principles, to do so; some journal editors have decided not to publish articles which cite the Nazi protocols or other published references to the Nazi studies or to clinical studies based on this data; other editors will allow the publication of such articles if based on valid science and, further, they regard the unethical origin of the data as no absolute bar to publication.[6]
>
> The argument of "salvaging good from evil" uses quasi-religious language in support of the proposal to use Nazi data. It implies in some absolutist theological sense that a divinity could bless those who would find in evil something good which is worthy of preservation (i.e., using the data for some "good"). The assumptive moral reasoning in this argument is that there is both good *and* evil in the Holocaust and in the Nazi

5 Ibid., p. 146.

6 Alan S. Rosenbaum, "The Use of Nazi Medical Experimentation Data: Memorial or Betrayal?" *Journal of Applied Philosophy,* 4 (1989), pp. 59–67; here, p. 60.

medical experiments *per se,* an assumption which I categorically reject, especially in the light of the efforts of those who today seek to rewrite or revise history... inaccurately, often with the not-so-subtle intent of rehabilitating Nazism and Nazis.

Whether God would bless those who find and utilize good in evil I do not know. But, in my view, there is *no* good whatsoever in genocide and the experiments, nor in the Holocaust nor in the Nazi Reich. To presume otherwise is to diminish the singular immorality and criminality of the actions of the Nazi doctors. In other words, there is *no "good"* to be salvaged. Using the data is simply a matter of choosing to ignore its immoral beginnings.

The second argument for making current use of data may be framed in utilitarian language. It claims that since no further harm will befall the victims of the experiments, and since these sordid events are in the past, if the data can be used to save lives in the future, then despite their "unethical origins", they should be used today to promote a greater health or happiness for future generations of people, and also perhaps relieving their pain (unhappiness).

Unlike the first argument this one accepts the wholly immoral or evil nature of the experiments. But similar to the first one this argument falsifies both the continuous historical dimension of the scientific process of development and also the nature of the "ethical" consequences to ensue from using the data.[7]

The utility of saving the lives of persons, as important as this is, should include within its scope not only the "physical" but also the "moral" ("spiritual") aspect of human life, i.e., the quality of life is certainly at least as significant as physical longevity is. Accordingly, if using Nazi data violates a very basic moral principle (e.g., by respecting basic rights) even if future generations benefit in a limited way from their usefulness, then using the data may result in demoralizing our "moral" climate of opinion as to what is (not) permissible. In short, if immoral origins of "useful" data are of no consequence in deciding whether to use the data so obtained (which is precisely what this argument directs), not only is morality itself vitiated and its users degraded, but if future needs require it, there is no strengthened moral barrier against performing similar types of experiments in order to service those needs. In a related sense, the basic rights of some persons not to be used in this way would be bartered away for the arbitrary preservation of the rights of the beneficiaries. Therefore, in view of the unethical nature of the Nazi experimental data, the greater utility is not served by construing it as if ethical

7 Ibid., p. 63.

principles and respect for a proper moral climate are irrelevant. In brief, the argument that "a greater good" will be served if the data are used depends largely upon the concept and scope of goodness. That is, it would not include the victim's good nor the survivors' good, nor the "moral-spiritual" good of society's members.

Some researchers and writers have sought to excuse their intended use of the Nazi data by publicly disclaiming any approval of the unethical origins of the data. However, there is a basic principle of law which is analogous to a fundamental moral principle relevant in this case, namely, that is legally "wrong for someone to profit from one's own wrongdoing". Likewise, it is *prima facie* immoral for someone knowingly to profit from another's serious wrongdoing. The burden of exculpation lies with the researcher who seeks to excuse using the Nazi data; merely acknowledging their unethical origins does not seem to do the job, for the researcher, too, becomes tainted vicariously.[8]

Those who choose to use the Nazi data cannot be regarded as unethical in the same way, or to the degree that the original perpetrators are. But they certainly have an indefeasible burden of justifying or excusing their downgrading of the moral stigma which attaches to their intent in knowingly using such data to further their own research.[9]

Nazi medical science was not the result of mixing values and science, but of the wrong values influencing the practice of science (e.g., contempt for the idea of universal human rights). Among the lessons we are to learn from the medical-scientific experiments of the Nazis is not to rid science of values but rather to place science and technology in the service of those values which support all human life, consistent with the Hippocratic Oath.

Furthermore, using the data dishonors the memory of the victims because it is an important symbolic reenactment of the original acts and brings a retroactive veneer of legitimacy to them. It also trivializes medical killing and buries the unethical source of any positive contribution medical data may be presumed to make to contemporary science. Even if some dubious "good" somewhere down the line would accrue to using the data, this is hardly a fitting memorial. What would be a proper memorial in light of rememberance [sic] of the Holocaust is a commitment to respecting human rights found in explicitly rejecting the use of such data pressing the demand to find alternative sources of information. To justify using Nazi data by an appeal to scientific progress and eventu-

8 Ibid., p. 64.
9 Ibid., p. 65.

> al public benefit is simply wrong. We must choose to subordinate the practice of science to the (democratic and moral) values of civilization.[10]

Rosenbaum allows only two specific instances in which Nazi data may be used ethically:

> 1. If a direct and immediate link may be established between using *valid* Nazi data and saving a life, where no alternative data or techniques are acceptable, the data may be used provided that the recipient and the public generally are informed about the origin of the data so used, and that they approve…
>
> 2. The data may permissibly be used to illustrate in publications and discussions about the ethics of human experimentation the truly evil nature of certain types of experiments and what the implications are for those in medical science to take ethics seriously.[11]

An article published in the *Journal of Medical Ethics* by Steven G. Post of Case Western Reserve University in Cleveland, Ohio, "The Echo of Nuremberg: Nazi Data and Ethics", argues the following points:

> a) that as a prima facie duty unethically obtained data should never be used;
>
> b) that such data should be expunged from published works insofar as possible;
>
> c) that the editors of all journals that have in the past published Nazi data without a statement of moral condemnation should print such a statement now; and
>
> d) that science should at the moral minimum be sensitive to the emotions of the victims from whom it has pillaged data.[12]
>
> Researchers must come to an absolutely clear understanding that unethical human experimentation in the name of scientific progress is *never* justifiable and that the Nazi experience has partial roots in this doctrine of progress.[13]

10 Ibid., p. 66.

11 Ibid., p. 65.

12 Steven G. Post, "The Echo of Nuremberg: Nazi Data and Ethics", *Journal of Medical Ethics,* 17 (1991), pp. 42–44; here, p. 42.

13 Ibid.

> Ideally, all reference to Nazi data would be expunged from textbooks and future journal publications in order more forcefully to impress future researchers that unethically obtained data will never see the light of print. Yet the data is already a fixture in the research literature and cannot be "unlearned". At least the journals that have published the data should issue a clear condemnation of the means by which it was obtained and should avoid using such data in the future. Just as the state of Israel now calls on the German universities to apologize for using victims' body parts and tissues over the past four decades and return what parts remain for burial, so also should the Nazi data be as much as possible buried forever.
>
> Such condemnations serve the useful purpose of discouraging young researchers from engaging in unethical experimentation. They send the powerful message that the ends do not justify the means and that unethically obtained data must benefit absolutely no one, including the ambitious researcher...[14]
>
> Yet it is precisely in the aftermath of unethical experimentation that some opportunity to restore respect for the autonomy and dignity of the victims presents itself. To use the data without the consent of those who were violated is to violate the violated anew. Therefore, those who have been experimented on without consent have the ultimate right and authority to pass final judgement on the fate of data, whether it is useful or not.
>
> Many survivors of the Nazi experiments deeply resent the use of hypothermia and other data. Minimally, science should not proceed to use Nazi data without the consent of Holocaust victims, though even consent would not justify use insofar as any usage sends the wrong message to future scientists...[15]

In the *Journal of the American Medical Association* (9 February 1990), we find the article "What the Nazis Called 'Medical Research' Haunts the Scientific Community to This Day", by Terra Ziporyn. The writer is reporting on a conference called "Nazi Documents and the Nuremberg Code", which had been held at Boston University under the auspices of the Schools of Medicine and Public Health. Among the viewpoints discussed at the conference were the following:

> ...improvements in technology and discoveries since World War II are making the Nazi data less relevant...

14 Ibid., p. 43.
15 Ibid.

> ...concern for individual subjects takes precedence over a study's potential benefit to science or society, that informed consent is necessary but not sufficient in itself, and that studies are not ethical just because they are useful.[16]

We find in the journal *Science* (1988) the following:

> The literature is full of contradicting opinions and arguments. Frequently those who argue for publication say salvage some good from the ashes. Also that publications could be accompanied by references to the monstrous manner in which results were obtained.
>
> Others feel that under no circumstances should Nazi data be used. Their arguments are: None of these results are trustworthy given the heinous acts of the Nazis and studies conducted with malnourished, unwilling subjects are inapplicable to the population at large. Even if some of the results are scientifically valid, ethics is an equally important consideration.[17]

Arthur Caplan's book *When Medicine Went Mad* includes articles by survivors of the camp experiments. Among them is "Nazi Experiments as Viewed by a Survivor of Mengele's Experiments", written by Eva Mozes Kor. Kor writes:

> Regarding the Nazi data: I am appalled by anyone who seemingly is justifying the means by using the results of the Nazi experiments. In Auschwitz we were treated like a commodity; the hair was used for mattresses; the fat was used for soap; the skin for lampshades; the gold collected from the teeth of the dead went into the Nazi treasury, and many of us were used as guinea pigs. Today some doctors want to use the only thing left by these victims. They are like vultures waiting for the corpses to cool so they could devour every consumable part. To use the Nazi data is obscene and sick. One can always rationalize that it would save human lives, the question should be asked, at what cost?[18]

The followings remarks have been taken from an essay by Velvl W. Greene, "Can Scientists Use Information Derived from the Concentration Camps?" also printed in Arthur Caplan's *When Medicine Went Mad.* Greene is a member of

16 Terra Ziporyn, "What the Nazis called 'Medical Research' Haunts the Scientific Community to This Day", *Journal of the American Medical Association,* 263: 6 (9 February 1990), p. 791.

17 *Science* 240: 21(1988).

18 Eva Mozes Kor, "Nazi Experiments as Viewed by a Survivor of Mengele's Experiments", in Caplan, ed., *When Medicine Went Mad,* p. 7.

the faculty of Ben Gurion University Medical School in Beersheva, Israel. Part of his essay discusses the principles of Jewish medical ethics as they are relevant to the issue of using data from Nazi medical experiments.

> There is a growing body of [Rabbinic] responsa on questions of the Holocaust and there is a world of Halakhic literature on medicine. But the specific subject of Nazi data and whether we can use it in medicine and biomedical research today, has not been analyzed by any rabbinic authority...[19]

> The most important principle of Jewish medical ethics that pertains to the possible use of Nazi data is the principle of *Pikuach Nefesh* or saving a human life. This is a primary responsibility for every man but is particularly incumbent on physicians who have unique skills and knowledge. In the view of the Halakha, the physician acting as a healer is considered to be a special agent and partner of the Almighty... When involved in life-saving acts, his medical judgments carry more weight than most of the 613 commandments in the Torah...
>
> The Halakha, in innumerable instances, distinguishes between acts that are forbidden *a priori* and the consequences of acts that are already *ex poste facto.* If a forbidden act cannot be undone or reversed, the restrictions on deriving some benefit from the act, particularly if the benefits involve healing, are much less stringent...
>
> The rules about knowledge – in distinction to things – that may be acquired under questionable circumstances are even more liberal. The Halakha makes it very clear that if there is a choice between two physicians, one an observant Jew with no special competence, and the other completely unobservant, or even a heathen idolater, who might not have observed all the moral scruples while studying, but who is now an expert in diagnosis and therapy, you must choose the second!
>
> One more principle of Jewish Medical Ethics that bears relevance to the discussion: Judaism teaches that man is created in the image of God. Thus, the physical body... is considered inviolate... Jewish law does not sanction routine autopsies. They are permitted only in those cases where an immediate and urgent need exists for information essential to the treatment of other patients... But there is no absolute ban on autopsies. If, in the physician's opinion, the life of another human being can be saved or a deadly disease can be prevented, then permission for an

19 Vevl W. Greene, "Can Scientists Use Information Derived from the Concentration Camps? Ancient Answers to New Questions", in Caplan, ed., *When Medicine Went Mad,* pp. 155–170; here, p. 164.

autopsy should be granted. Similar Halakhic rulings have recently been issued with respect to authorizing donations of organs for transplantation.

It is quite evident, from the principles cited above, that rabbinic permission to use 45-year old data would probably be granted to any physician who can make a case that the information is pertinent to saving the life of his patient... If the use of Nazi data today does not involve committing murder, worshipping idols or illicit sex, its use for *Pikuach Nefesh* cannot be denied.

It should be emphasized, however, that this anticipated rabbinic ruling might not be directly applicable to [biomedical research]. There are parallels, to be sure, but there are also sufficient differences between *Pikuach Nefesh* and biomedical research to generate a reasonable atmosphere of doubt. The arguments cited above deal with direct benefit, with the here and now, with life and death, and with physicians' opinions. Under these circumstances, the rulings go beyond "permission" and sometimes become public "obligation". But the Halakha might say that since advancing biomedical knowledge provides only doubtful and delayed benefits for future patients who are as yet unknown, research is not, itself, a sufficient reason to risk the desecration of a martyr's memory or justification of a murderer. More important, since the data are old and of very questionable quality, considering the "scientific" standards that prevailed in the camps, an even greater shadow of doubt is cast on their potential benefit. Under these circumstances, the case for using the Nazi data becomes more and more ambiguous. Whether or not the potential benefit to life-saving practices of the future is of sufficient import, and whether denying a researcher access to data is equivalent to preventing a physician from exercising his professional judgment – these cannot be answered by speculation and must await an authoritative response from a recognized scholar.[20]

The bigger issue [bigger than the probability that the data's age and consequent out-of-dateness (sic) will soon mean that only those arguing against its use, will actually use it] is the double danger that the Nazi experiments and experimenters will become either over sensationalized or that they will become trivialized. In the first instance, the cruelty and bestiality and horror will place the Holocaust and the Nazi experiments beyond comprehension. They will stand so unique – a onetime historical aberration – so inhuman that no human can grasp it. It will become of legendary importance as a legend, but with little relevance to real life...

20 Ibid., pp. 165–167.

> At the other end of the spectrum is the possibility that Nazi experiments will simply be equated to unethical medical practices. Look what has happened to those other Holocaust memories: "Ghetto" today is almost a universal synonym for slum, with no shred of reference to either the misery or the heroism the word evokes; "genocide" is used by any politician in or out of the United Nations to refer to any military action his side is losing.[21]
>
> Instead of banning the Nazi data or assigning it to some archivist or custodial committee, I maintain that it be exhumed, printed, and disseminated to every medical school in the world along with the details of the methodology and the names of the doctors who did it, whether or not they were indicted, acquitted, or hanged. It should be taught in medical school classrooms, not during a special course in ethics or history, but as part of the anatomy, physiology, pathology, microbiology, and pharmacology portion of the curriculum. The data should be presented regularly during grand rounds and research symposia. Let the students, the residents and the young doctors know that this was not ancient history or an episode from a horror movie where the actors get up after filming and prepare for another role. It was real. It happened yesterday. It was "medical"; it was "scientific"; it was "contemporary" with the development of penicillin.[22]

Next I reprint sections of the previously cited article "The Ethics of Using Medical Data from Nazi Experiments", by Baruch C. Cohen. I have retrieved the article from the website *Jewish Law Articles* at http://www.jlaw.com/Articles/NaziMedEx.html. Cohen's article appeared originally in *Midstream* (June/July 1989).

> Nazi Concentration Camp science is often branded as bad science. First, it is doubtful that physiological responses of the tortured and maimed victims represented the responses of the people for [sic] whom the experiments were meant to benefit. Second, additional doubts about the scientific integrity of the experiments surface when we consider the Nazi doctors' political aspirations and their enthusiasm for medical conclusions that proved the Nazi racial theory. Finally, the fact that the Nazi experiments were not officially published nor replicated raises doubts about the data's scientific accuracy.

21 Ibid., pp. 168–169.
22 Ibid., pp. 169–170.

Doctor Jay Katz of the Yale University School of Law… suggests… that the experiments be republished in full detail so that no one may deny that they occurred. He would then condemn the data to oblivion. Dr. Katz dismissed the Nazi experiments with one phrase: "They are of no scientific value."[23]

…Brigadier General Telford Taylor, Chief Counsel for the Prosecution at Nuremberg, [stated] that the Nazi experiments were insufficient and unscientific, "a ghostly failure as well as a hideous crime… Those experiments revealed nothing which civilized medicine can use."[24]

Arnold Relman, Editor of the *New England Journal of Medicine,* similarly stated that the Nazi experiments were such a "gross violation of human standards that they are not to be trusted at all".[25]

Doctor Leonard Hoenig, Assistant Professor of Medicine at the University of South Florida College of Medicine, categorized the Nazi experiments as "pseudo-science", since the Nazis blurred the distinction between science and sadism. The data was not recorded from scientific hypothesis and research, but rather, it was inspired and administered through racial ideologies of genocide…[26]

Allen Buchanan, Philosophy Professor at the University of Arizona, is also a member of the Human Subjects Review Committee at the University of Minnesota. He believes that bad ethics and bad science are inextricably linked together… [having found that ethically sound experiments are also scientifically sound] he concluded that since the Nazi experiments were unethical, they were, by equation, scientifically invalid.[27]

Doctor Leo Alexander, a Major in the United States Army Medical Corps, and the psychiatric consultant to the Secretary of War and to the Chief Counsel for War Crimes at the Nuremberg Doctors' Trial, wrote a report evaluating the Nazi hypothermia experiments at Dachau… [He found] that parts of the Nazi data on hypothermia were not dependable because of inconsistencies found in Rascher's lab notes… [He concluded

23 Baruch C. Cohen, "The Ethics of Using Medical Data from Nazi Experiments".
24 Ibid., pp. 16–17.
25 Ibid., p. 17.
26 Ibid.
27 Ibid.

that] the experts agree that the Nazi experiments lacked scientific integrity."[28]

[Cohen writes additionally]: Ultimately the argument[s] as to whether the experiments were scientific or not, or whether the doctors were medically competent or not, leave one with the impression that had such experiments been "good" science and the doctors medical professionals, these facts would some how change our impression of the doctors and their experiments. This is not true. The sadistic evil of the Nazi butchery is in no way lessened by its scientific value. Conferring medical or scientific validity on the Nazi murders is not an option for consideration...

...Arguably, when the wickedness of the experiment has been very great, then only a colossally important objective can justify its use. Those that wish to use the data have to satisfy the burden of proof, which becomes greater in proportion to the wickedness of the experiment.

It is easy to see the futility of advocating the data's use when the intended benefit to society is trivial and moderate. Conversely, if the intended benefit is to save lives, most would agree that the data should be used.[29]

Dr. Howard Spiro, of the Department of Internal Medicine at Yale University, insists that no one honors the memory of the dead victims by learning from experiments carried out on them. Instead, we make the Nazis retroactive partners in the victims' torture and death.[30]

Lord Immanuel Jakobovitz, Chief Rabbi of the British Commonwealth of Nations and the pioneer of Jewish Medical Ethics, said that using the Nazi data offers not a shred of meaning to the 6,000,000 deaths. In fact, use of the data would serve to dishonor them even more so.[31]

Europe's collective memory is about to become history. Especially since most of the witnesses have died, and the Nazi saga becomes subject to greater distortions and reinterpretation. It is therefore incumbent on our society to confront the collective sets of conflicting memories *now* before the events of this era, and its implications fade.[32]

28 Ibid., pp. 11–18.

29 Ibid., pp. 21–22.

30 Ibid., p. 36, note 43, citing H. Spiro, "Let the Nazi Data Remind Us of Evil", Letter to the Editor, *The New York Times* (24 March 1988).

31 Ibid., note 44, citing Jakobivitz, "Some Modern Response on Medical-Moral Problems", *Jewish Medical Ethics,* 1 (May 1988).

32 Ibid., "Conclusion", p. 35.

Kristine Moe, a science fellow at the Massachusetts Institute of Technology, published an article in 1984, "Should the Nazi Research Data Be Cited", that tries to argue in favor of occasional use of Nazi data. She asserts:

> Despite the conventional wisdom, many of the scientists I spoke to regard the Nazi data as useful and necessary to their work. Typical was the comment by Dr. John S. Hayward of the University of Victoria in British Columbia, who uses the Nazi measurements of the rate of body cooling in cold water: "I don't want to have to use this data, but there is no other and will be no other in an ethical world. I rationalize it a little bit. But to not use it would be equally bad. I'm trying to make something constructive out of it. I use it with my guard up, but it's useful."[33]

In constructing her argument, Moe draws from fellow researchers, philosophers and medical ethicists, as follows:

> [On the hypothermia researcher Robert Harnett of Louisiana Technical University, who has cited the Nazi data]: He [Harnett] admits that they are weak. He uses them only to corroborate more reliable experimental results and case reports of accidental hypothermia.[34]

> [From Allen Buchanan of the University of Arizona]: I found that in the vast majority of cases [reviewed in five years of work on a human subjects review committee at the University of Minnesota] the experiments that are ethically unsound are also scientifically unsound. Very rarely have I seen an experiment that is very good and valuable that has serious ethical problems. Most of the time, if there was an ethical consideration, it could be eliminated without destroying the scientific value.
>
> [Buchanan, Moe reports, feels that the citation of unethical research in medical texts and articles is widespread and very difficult to eliminate. He suggests that the solution may be] some kind of concession… to the fact that we are evolving standards of acceptability.
>
> [Buchanan continues]: How unethical would research have to be where a person should avoid any reference to it? Is there some kind of "line of horribleness" over which you don't cross? I don't think there's any kind of formula you can give. Even with the Nazi work, if you came across some experimental data that you thought would save lives right

33 Kristine Moe, "Should the Nazi Research Data Be Cited", *The Hastings Center Report,* December 1984, pp. 5–7, here, p. 5.

34 Ibid., p. 6.

now, then you could say: As a general rule, we shouldn't use it, but in this particular case, the benefit would be so great, and after all, we're not in any danger at this point of becoming Nazis. You have to look at the data in the political context. In some countries, using that kind of data might be more dangerous than in others.[35]

The late Henry K. Beecher argued in a classic article ["Ethics and Clinical Research"] that information obtained in an unethical manner should not be published lest there be "an odor of hypocrisy" in medicine. He drew an analogy between the publication of unethically obtained data and the inadmissibility in court of unconstitutionally obtained evidence... "Even though suppression of such data (by not publishing it) would constitute a loss to medicine in a specific and localized sense", Beecher wrote, "this loss, it seems, would be far less important than the far-reaching moral loss to medicine if the data thus obtained were to be published".[36]

The specific standards of the *New England Journal of Medicine* would prevent citation of the Nazi hypothermia experiments according to [the editor, Dr. Arnold] Relman. References must come from peer-reviewed journals; the hypothermia information comes from Alexander's military report. [Some of the modern references to the Nazi data could, however, escape detection under that rule.] Some scientists published information collected second-hand from Alexander's report, by citing other journals that had cited Alexander directly. For example, Nazi data are included in several citations in the *Journal of the American Medical Association* and the *Annual Review of Physiology*.[37]

Relman's guidelines are further complicated by the fact that some of the Nazi experiments were published in German wartime medical journals. These reports were about Nazi experiments with typhus and malaria vaccines in which prisoners were deliberately infected and left untreated to serve as a control group.

[Relman maintains]: "I would allow references to it only if it were an article about ethical research."[38]

35 Ibid.

36 Ibid., see Henry K. Beecher, "Ethics and Clinical Research", *New England Journal of Medicine*, 274 (1966), pp. 1354–1360.

37 Ibid., p. 6.

38 Ibid., no other source indicated by Moe.

Robert J. Levine, Chairman of the Human Investigation Committee at Yale University School of Medicine, takes a somewhat different view. He declares: "If in the judgment of an editor an article is scientifically sound but ethically questionable, the decision should be to publish the article along with an editorial in which the ethical questions are raised. The author should be notified that this is what is to be done and invited to prepare a rebuttal to be published simultaneously."[39]

[Ronald Banner, member of the Jewish Ethical Medical Study Group in Philadelphia told Moe]: "I'm not against someone citing (the experiments), but I'm chagrined that someone would refer to those experiments without mentioning something about the way the information was gained. It shows a lack of conscience. There are times that something, morally, stinks so bad that you have to hold your nose even while you refer to it."[40]

[Moe closes her article with the following observations]: Uncritical censorship is not the answer, though. That would raise a regrettable parallel with the tactic of the Nazis themselves. According to the Berlin correspondent for the *Journal of the American Association* in 1939, medical students in Germany were forbidden from citing Jewish sources in their doctoral dissertations unless the citations were "indispensable".

Scientists have learned from other ugly moments in history. Jewish doctors imprisoned within the walls of the Warsaw ghetto in World War II kept extensive clinical notes on how the residents, many of them children, died of starvation. The notes were smuggled out of the ghetto and now are published as a landmark study on hunger disease [Hunger Disease, ed. Myron Winick (New York: Wiley, 1979)]. The survivors of Hiroshima and Nagasaki provided a tragic opportunity to understand more about radiation sickness.

To justify the use of Nazi data in a research article, I would expect scientists to use the findings only in circumstances where the scientific validity is clear and where there is no alternative source of information. To the volumes of data involved, a layman cannot know what can be considered scientifically valid among all the Nazi experiments. However, the experts in each field should critically evaluate the data before using it.[41]

39 Ibid., citing Robert J. Levine, *Ethics and Regulation of Clinical Research* (Baltimore, MD: Urban & Schwarzenberg, 1981), p. 20.

40 Ibid., p. 7.

41 Ibid.

Moe's article elicited several responses from other professionals, whose letters appeared in the *Hastings Center Report* of August 1985.

> [From Monroe H. Freedman, Professor of Law at Hofstrau University, director of the United States Holocaust Memorial Council from 1980 to 1982, and subsequently a senior advisor to the chairman of the Council, criticizing Moe's assertion that "uncritical" censorship is not the answer. "That would raise a regrettable parallel with the tactics of the Nazis themselves by forbidding the citation of Jewish sources unless the citations were indispensable"]: There is no such parallel.
>
> As Ms. Moe recognizes, the Nazi experiments on human beings were horrifyingly, cruel, unethical, and of questionable reliability. Jewish medical authorities were not censored by the Nazis for any of those reasons, or for any other rational reasons, but solely because of anti-Semitism. The suggested parallel, therefore, is illogical and insensitive. Indeed, the salient parallel is that Jews were the victims in both instances.[42]

> [From Leonard J. Hoenig, M.D., Assistant Professor of Medicine at the University of South Florida]: I do not believe that we can, in good conscience, cite data that were acquired through the brutal killing and torture of innocent persons. To do so would, in my opinion, lend a measure of undeserved dignity to these wicked studies and at the same time insult the memory of the victims by seeming to justify their murder. Further, it would suggest that our respect for human life and dignity can be disregarded once the crimes have already been committed.
>
> I sincerely hope that medical students and physicians alike will join me in rejecting Moe's very mistaken conclusions. Let us recognize the Nazi data for what they really represent: crimes against humanity. These atrocities deserve no worthy mention in our medical literature.[43]

> [And from Dr. Howard M. Spiro of the Yale University School of Medicine]: To the suggestion by Kristine Moe that data from the experiments on humans in the Nazi concentration camps should be scrutinized for the "possibility that some good may be salvaged from the ashes", let me express a different opinion. We need to express our revulsion at some activities even if that revulsion means losing something irreplaceable. I cannot agree that we honor the memory of the dead by "learning" from experiments carried out on their bodies. We make them retrospective guinea pigs by a strained utilitarian argument. Studies of

42 Letter from Monroe H. Freedman, *The Hastings Center Report,* August 1985, p. 31.
43 Ibid.

> starvation carried out by the physicians in the Warsaw Ghetto offer an entirely different example. Those observers did not create the conditions under which they themselves were suffering yet studying. Their work deserves honor...
>
> The best argument that I have heard in favor of preserving the Nazi data is to preserve evidence that those experiments were in fact carried out. "Revisionists" suggest that there were no concentration camps and no millions of deaths. Preserving the data from the experiments provides evidence against these intolerable claims. As long as the data are available, evidence that at least some people did some bad things in Nazi Germany cannot be denied.[44]

Opinions today still diverge sharply whenever the question of using Nazi data plays a role in decisions about research or publishing. I turn now to three recent examples and provide relevant citations to illustrate the ethical complexities of the question.

The Environmental Protection Agency Study on Phosgene Gas Air Pollution

The E.P.A. (Environmental Protection Agency) reported in 1988, on its findings in a study of phosgene gas as an air pollutant. Phosgene, of course, is one of the poisons tested by the Nazis in the concentration camps. It has been used in chemical warfare twice, during World War I and more recently, in the Iran-Iraq War. Its use was anticipated in any subsequent wars in the Persian Gulf. Phosgene also has peaceful uses, in the manufacture of pesticides and plastics; the U.S. alone annually produces a billion pounds of the substance.

The E.P.A. study sought to identify dangers associated with phosgene-created air pollution. The Nazi data provided examples of recorded dose-response in humans, and thus were inserted into the original report, even though, as John Vandenberg, the E.P.A. officer in charge of the project, admitted, it was not clear that the dose-response results of tests on animals would have differed from human test results.[45]

44 Ibid., pp. 31–32.

45 On the statement by John Vandenberg, see Marjorie Sun, "EPA Bars Use of Nazi Data", *Science* 240: 4848 (1 April 1988), p. 21.

When the study was presented, twenty-two agency scientists signed a letter of protest, specifically objecting to the study's reliance on the Nazi data. In response, the E.P.A. administrator, Lee M. Thomas, ordered the deletion of the data from the study. But news of the conflict reached the mainstream press and gave contemporary meaning to the ethical dilemmas posed by the Nazi data. Excerpts from critical press statements follow:

> [From *The New York Times,* 23 March 1988, quoting Hugh Kaufman, an official in the E.P.A.'s toxic waste program]: "My understanding is that they threw people in a room and broke open a vial of phosgene gas and counted how long it took for them to die. That is pseudo-science, and the people working on these things for the agency are making basic scientific calls we use to make standards and regulations."[46]
>
> [From Michael Weisskopf, writing in *The Washington Post,* 24 March 1988]: "The source of that information is so morally repugnant that I can't think of a situation where we want to use it."[47]
>
> [From Judith Bellin, one of the toxicologists who drafted the protest letter, the following, as reported by Marjorie Sun in *Science* (1 April 1988): These Nazi data] were flawed on several counts... The reports themselves note that the prisoners were "almost all in a weak and underfed condition." They did not say how pulmonary edema was measured. Different kinds of controls should have been used. The weight and sex of the subjects were not recorded...[48]

Some scientists defended the initial decision to use the data.

> [John Vandenberg, the E.P.A. project officer for phosgene explained]: We won't argue that the experiments were well reported or well designed, but compared to what we had, they offered a measure of improvement. They obviously had a lot of flaws, but we felt compelled to use it because it provided dose-response data.[49]

46 Philip Shabecoff, "Head of E.P.A. Bars Nazi Data in Study on Gas", *The New York Times* (23 March 1988).

47 Michael Weisskopf, "EPA Bars Use of Nazi's Human Test Data After Scientists Object", *The Washington Post* (24 March 1988), First Section, p. A17.

48 Ibid.

49 Ibid.

[Todd Thorslund, vice president of I.C.F. Clement Associates, Inc., the Washington environmental sciences consulting firm that reviewed the data, stated] that the poor health of the prisoners was not necessarily a negative because it only meant that the Nazis used a conservative model. The lack of information about sex and weight of the subjects was not important in this case because phosgene is so toxic that "it's the dose in the air that makes the difference".[50]

[*The New York Times* (23 March 1988) reported that Ila Cote, another E.P.A. toxicologist who worked on the study, said that] there were some indications of a serious health threat from phosgene, particularly to people living around plants that make or use it. She said that "ethical issues are real", and that she was sympathetic to those who expressed their ethical concerns. "But my personal opinion is that when data is collected in an unethical fashion, it is important in protecting public health and is not available in any other way, I would use it."[51]

[Judith Bellin is reported in *The Washington Post* as having said that the protest letter had noted that] "some" believe that such data, if scientifically sound and verifiable data should be used if some good can result. But it went on to say that others feel that to use such data debases us all as a society, gives such experiments legitimacy, and implicitly encourages others, perhaps in less exacting societies, to perform unethical human experiments... The Nazi data on phosgene should have been rejected on scientific grounds.[52]

[Sharply different views are expressed by Alan C. Nixon in the 14 November 1988 issue of *The Scientist.* He quotes himself from an article in *The Vortex,* a publication of the California Section of the American Chemical Society]: "In view of the fact that there is practically no human dose-response data on the toxicity of phosgene available, the action of Thomas to exclude the data seems mindless. If even one human being loses his/her life because this data is not available, I think Thomas et al. could reasonably be charged with, at least, manslaughter... [Nixon concludes with] I think it is wiser to separate our consideration of the value of data from the morals of the gatherers or their supporters. In the case of the phosgene results, let us accept the data as a memorial to the unfortunate victims and use it to save other human lives. Thus, the suffering

50 Ibid.
51 *The New York Times* (23 March 1988).
52 *The Washington Post* (24 March 1988).

> of the wretched prisoners would not be in vain. To reject the information on the grounds that the source is unsavory smacks of intellectual dishonesty and muddied thinking."[53]

The Pernkopf Anatomy Atlas Controversy

The dilemma that arises when the principle of freedom of information is brought into conflict with ethical considerations about medical experimentation is well exemplified in the worldwide dispute over a Viennese anatomy atlas, the *Topographische Anatomie des Menschen* (Topographical Anatomy of Man), authored by Professor Eduard Pernkopf. Dr. Pernkopf, professor and director of the Anatomy Institute of Vienna, joined the Nazi Party in 1933 and the Storm Troopers (Brown Shirts) in 1934. One month after Hitler invaded Austria in 1938, Pernkopf was appointed dean of the faculty of the University of Vienna, where he helped to guide the *Gleichschaltung* of the Viennese medical profession. His inaugural lecture (4 April 1938) as dean of that prestigious faculty was printed in the first edition of the *Wiener Klinische Wochenschrift* to appear after the reorganization.[54]

In his lecture, entitled "National Socialism and Science", Pernkopf declared that the principles of National Socialism must permeate education and science and that freedom, in the liberal sense, leads to chaos, which cannot be permitted in science. National Socialism, he maintained, was devoted to the practical solution of problems, among them two that the disciplines of anatomy and embryology were well equipped to address: the specific criteria of physical constitution and race. The curriculum at the medical school in the future would change to include race physiology, race psychology and race pathology. The role of medicine henceforth would consist of "furthering the propagation of the fit", while "eliminating the unfit and the defective". Pernkopf's atlas, which is acknowledged to be an excellent textbook, even a classic, contains several paintings by Nazi professionals, among them Erich Lepier, who signed his paintings with a swastika; and Karl Endtresser and Franz Batke, who signed their names with the SS symbol.

53 Alan C. Nixon, "Opinion: If the Data's Good, Use It – Regardless of the Source", *The Scientist*, 2: 21 (14 November 1988), p. 9.

54 All material for this section is derived from an excellent article "Ethics and Access to Teaching Materials in the Medical Library: The Case of the Pernkopf Atlas", by Michel C. Atlas of the Kornhauser Health Sciences Library at the University of Louisville in Louisville, Kentucky, published in the *Bulletin of the Medical Librarians' Association*, 89: 1 (January 2001), pp. 51–58.

At the end of World War II Pernkopf was not charged with war crimes. He was, however, held in an Allied prison camp near Salzburg for three years. Upon being released, he returned to Vienna where his anatomy institute had been largely destroyed by Allied bombing. He was stripped of all titles and appointments but was allowed to continue work on his atlas at the Neurological Institute of the Medical School of the University of Vienna. He died of a stroke in 1955.

In March 1955, Yad Vashem (The Israel Holocaust and Martyrs' Remembrance Authority) asked Austria and the University of Vienna to investigate the possibility that the cadavers that served as models for the atlas illustrations might have come from concentration camps. The Yad Vashem representative asked that the investigation be conducted by outside authorities. Yad Vashem also asked for both a public commemoration of the victims in the event that the investigation confirmed the camps as a source of "specimens", and a published acknowledgment in every future edition of the atlas, commemorating the victims and outlining Pernkopf's personal history.

The public outcry about the atlas started a bit later, with a letter to the editor of the *Journal of the American Medical Association* in November 1996. Its two authors, Howard A. Israel, a dental surgeon at Columbia University, and William E. Seidelman, a physician at the University of Toronto, alerted readers to the Yad Vashem request, and noted that atlas illustrations "contained expressions of Nazi sympathies" and that the specimen cadavers may have been victims of Nazi terror.[55]

A wide range of opinion, some of it heated, was elicited by the *JAMA* letter. It is documented in the *Bulletin of the Medical Librarians' Association,* in the article by Michel C. Atlas already cited. Selections from his documentation follow:

> Abraham Foxman, national director of the Anti-Defamation League, said that the research findings of heinous crimes or atrocities should not be used even if it would do good, because it would retrospectively cleanse the atrocity and possibly justify similar acts in the future.[56]

55 For the complete letter text, see "Letters", *Journal of the American Medical Association,* 276: 20 (27 November 1996), p. 1633.

56 Atlas, "Ethics and Access", p. 54, citing Vedantam S. (29 July 1997) Panel examining issue of science using knowledge gained by unethical means. [Knight-Ridder/Tribune News Service]. Retrieved January 13, 2000, from NewsBank online database (NewsFile Collection. Record No. 008430D1D26761664CC75), on the Internet at http://infoweb.newsbank.com.

The current author [Atlas], [Garrett] Riggs, [Vevl W.] Greene, and others believe that the active use of the atlas itself is the most fitting tribute to those who died for it... Using this atlas allows these cadavers to speak to us from [more than a] half a century ago. They make us reexamine and again repudiate the Nazi beliefs that created a society that killed them.[57]

Howard Spiro at the Program for Humanities in Medicine at Yale University says [that] to him the Pernkopf pictures serve a double role: they teach anatomy and they remind us of the horror that any "objective" science can impose. The brilliant depictions of Pernkopf atlas are transfiguring; in each, I heard the scream of a person...[58]

Edward B. Hutton, Jr., president of Waverly, Inc., the American publisher of the atlas, recognizes that Pernkopf was a Nazi and emphasizes that his company rejects Pernkopf's views. But they "separate Pernkopf, the man, from the work because of the lack of evidence as to the true origin of the cadavers used in the atlas".[59]

Malcolm Hast, of Northwestern University Medical School, who reviewed the book for *JAMA,* said that as it was one of the most beautiful anatomy books published, the book should continue to be used. He believed that if something was good, it could not be thrown away anymore than the knowledge already gained from it could be expurgated from readers' minds.[60]

Ernest April, an anatomist at Columbia University's College of Physicians and Surgeons, believed that one could not detract from the fact that the book was phenomenal, complete, thorough, and authoritative, despite the knowledge that Pernkopf was not a good person and belonged to the wrong party.[61]

57 Atlas, "Ethics and Access", p. 54, citing G. Riggs, "What Should We Do About Eduard Pernkopf's Atlas?" *Academic Medicine,* 73: 4 (April 1998), pp. 380–386; and V. W. Greene "Can Scientists Use Information Derived from the Concentration Camps", Caplan, ed. *When Medicine Went Mad,* pp. 155–179.

58 Atlas, "Ethics and Access", p. 54, citing H. M. Spiro, "The Silence of Words – Some Thoughts on the Pernkopf Atlas", *Wiener Klinische Wochenschrift,* 110: 4–5 (27 February 1998), pp. 183–184.

59 Atlas, "Ethics and Access", p. 54.

60 Ibid., citing N. Wade, "Doctors Question use of Nazi's Medical Atlas", *The New York Times,* (26 November 1996), Section C.

61 Ibid.

> [Michel Atlas, began the conclusion to this article saying that] a core tenet of medical librarianship is freedom of access to information. It is considered unethical for libraries and librarians to act as censors, even when the material is controversial. The sentiment is captured by The American Library Association's Library Bill of Rights, which states that "[m]aterials should not be excluded because of the origin, background or views of those contributing to their creation" and "[m]aterials should not be proscribed or removed because of partisan or doctrinal disapproval". There is no prohibition, however, to librarians adding statements that alert the reader to controversial or erroneous material. Adding such statements directly to material in public library holdings is ethical and especially important when works may contain material that may have violated the ethical standards of the medical community.[62]

Since August 1997, the Rector's Office of the University of Vienna has provided all libraries with an insert entitled, "Information for Uses of Pernkopf's Atlas". After describing Pernkopf's political history, the insert states that "currently, it cannot be excluded that certain preparations used for the illustrations in this atlas were obtained from victims of the National Socialist regime. Furthermore, it is unclear whether cadavers were at that time supplied to the Institute of Anatomy at the University of Vienna not only from the Vienna district court but also from concentration camps. Pending the results of the investigation, it is therefore within the individual user's ethical responsibility to decide whether and in which way he wishes to use this book."[63]

■

Certain Nazi experiments arguably were rigorously enough designed to contain valid and valuable data. But this opinion is by no means shared by everyone. Thus the vexing question still taunts: Can these data be used by ethical researchers and publishers, and, if so, in what circumstances? The following documents illustrate this issue in the context of a modern controversy over Sigmund Rascher's hypothermia experiments at Dachau concentration camp.

62 Ibid., p. 56, citing American Library Association, "Library Bill of Rights" (Chicago, Illinois: The Association), at http://www.ala.org/work/freedom/lbr.html.

63 Ibid., p. 53, here citing P. Malina, "Eduard Pernkopf's Atlas of Anatomy or: The Fiction of 'Pure science' " [English translation], *Wiener Klinische Wochenschrift,* 110: 4 (27 February 1988), p. 196.

Controversy Over the Data from the Nazi Hypothermia Experiments

"Can Evil Beget Good? Nazi Data: A Dilemma for Science" is the title of an article by Barry Siegel, published in the *Los Angeles Times* on 30 October 1988. Siegel reported on a newly erupted controversy over the use of Nazi medical experiments, this time in the form of the question whether the hypothermia data could justifiably be cited.

The Nazi data for the Dachau experiments had first surfaced for public consumption in the 1945 report prepared by U.S. Army Major Dr. Leo Alexander who was charged with uncovering evidence of Nazi medical atrocities. Dr. Alexander had reviewed the documents on the hypothermia experiments at Dachau contained in Heinrich Himmler's personal files. His report on the matter, "The Treatment of Shock from Prolonged Exposure to Cold, Especially in Water", summarized the procedures and the findings of the experiments and provided essential materials for the Nuremberg War Crimes Trials. Alexander detailed the horrors of the experiments, but he also noted that the hypothermia data seemed to have authentic value, unlike some of the other Nazi data. The horns of an ethical dilemma were succinctly present in his assessments.

At first classified, Alexander's report eventually entered the public domain, the original in the Library of Congress archives and copies in various university libraries. Its contents thus became available to anyone who might wish to use them.

In 1987 the report reached the desk of Robert Pozos, a physiologist at the University of Minnesota who was researching hypothermia. Pozos was impressed, alarmed, conflicted after having read the report. He could not escape the fact that the Nazi data offered the only directly measured evidence of the effects on human subjects of exposure to cold. Yet he knew that the data had been obtained in an unethical manner.

Faced with a disturbing moral dilemma, Pozos consulted a colleague at Minnesota, the biomedical ethicist Arthur L. Caplan. After talking with Pozos, Caplan published an article in the local *St. Paul Pioneer Press Dispatch,* outlining his own position on the matter. Siegel's *Los Angeles Times* article summarizes Caplan's argument as follows: "Make it hard to locate the data. Do not give identifying credit to Nazi scientists. Make those who use the data explain where it came from. Apply a moral judgment, but let the data be used." Siegel then directly quotes Caplan: "The prevention of the death outweighs the protection of the memory... The victim's dignity was irrevocably lost in vats of freezing liquid forty years ago. Nothing can change that."[64]

Caplan's article created a furor, which acquired almost apocalyptic dimensions in some hands. Proponents of using the data were talking of redemption. Siegel records the following reactions:

> [From Efraim Zuroff, the Israeli representative to the Simon Wiesenthal Center]: "If Pozos dedicated his study to the memory of those victims of the Nazis, it would serve as a nice way of reminding people about the horrible experiments."
>
> [From a concentration camp survivor]: "I wore a number in Dachau... I have two Belgian friends, who went through the procedures of Dr. Rascher... I see no reason why the results obtained should not be used for further research."
>
> [From Edwin S. Fletcher]: "A research physiologist with the U.S. Air Force saw those Dachau papers... We debated the same questions that Dr. Pozos confronted and we came to the same conclusion, but with few qualms and no guilt. We were doing the best we knew to make amends for the sacrifices of those wretched victims."
>
> [From an unnamed medical doctor]: "As a child of survivors of the Holocaust, I've strong empathy for those opposed to the data's use... Nevertheless, as a physician who deals with children and has seen them comatose, brain-damaged and dead from hypothermia, my sense is that to save one child through the use of this information is worthwhile."

Opponents of the data's use spoke with equal fervor.

> [From Dennis Klein, director of the International center for Holocaust Studies for the Anti-Defamation League of B'nai Brith]: "There's just no two ways about it... No way should they be used... I cannot accept the results as legitimate... One has to draw the line."
>
> [From Abraham Foxman, national director of the Anti-Defamation League]: "It goes to legitimizing the evil done."

64 Barry Siegel, "Can Evil Beget Good? Nazi Data: A Dilemma for Science", The *Los Angeles Times* (30 October 1988), Front Section. Recovered through the *ProQuest Newspapers* website at http://proquest.umi.com.

> [From Dr. Arnold S. Relman, editor of the *New England Journal of Medicine*]: "I don't see how any credence can be given to the work of unethical investigators... Given the source of the information and the way in which it was obtained, how can anyone believe it? How can anyone want to believe it?"
>
> [From Rod Martel, whose grandmother died in a concentration camp]: "I offer this challenge to the hypothermia researchers... As you page through the research, have next to it actual photos of Jews being tortured in the name of research and see how long you are able to analyze data. Better yet, think of your mother or father floating in that tank and see if your beliefs about this subject hold up."

The intensity of the furor provoked by Caplan's column might suggest that the data have never before been used. In fact, that is not the case; at least forty-five citations appeared between 1945 and 1988, when the Hastings Center published a search on the subject. Siegel's article notes two outstanding examples, in which prestigious institutions overlooked the source of the data: a July 1946 article in the *Journal of the American Medical Association,* authored by G. W. Molnár, a University of Rochester physiologist who expressed no sense of moral dilemma while writing about hypothermia survival rates; and a 1955 report by a team of physicians at the Children's Hospital in Washington, which cited the data and noted their potential value for the development of body-cooling techniques in connection with pioneering open heart research. Pozos, it seems, was simply the first scientist to pose the ethical question in a public manner.

Pozos, himself, always remained seriously conflicted by the findings in Alexander's report and troubled by the moral dilemma they posed. Siegel reports his words: "Ethicists never answer a question," he said. "They raise one question, which raises another question and another. I want guidelines. I want to know if the data is good. Should we use it? Or the data forever be banned?"[65]

■

Since 1988, several scientists have reviewed the Nazi data with the intent of determining their reliability and validity. Their answers may eventually lay the question about using them to rest, at least for conscientious scientists. A letter to the editor of the *Journal of Medical Ethics* (1991), by Dr. Gershon B. Grunfeld of the Department of Medical Humanities, Southern Illinois University School of Medicine, in Springfield, Illinois, succinctly points out this fact.

65 Ibid.

> Steven G. Post argued recently for a duty not to use data of Nazi experiments; his argument is made even stronger considering the fact that the data from these experiments are scientifically worthless.
>
> Examinations of the results of Nazi experiments revealed critical deficiencies in scientific method even by the standards of the 1940s. For example, during the infamous hypothermia experiments at Dachau, data were faked by the prisoners responsible for recording the measurement. Similar evidence was revealed in Joseph Mengele's study of heterochromia. Sigmund Rascher's work on high altitude and hypothermia, done at Dachau, was rejected by three different German universities when he tried to submit it to fulfill the requirement for a higher doctorate degree. Given the fact that the work was rejected by at least one German expert, who was later sentenced to death by the Nuremberg Tribunal for his own medical crimes, it is doubtful that ethical considerations were the reasons for these decisions.
>
> In light of the above, any use or presentation of "data" from the Nazi experiments as scientific fact is unethical.[66]

The print media have ensured that the reading public learns of the new negative assessments of the validity of Nazi data. In an article published in the *New York Times,* dated 27 May 1990, Nicholas Wade wrote:

> Probably some degree of taint has to be accepted in medical experiments from the past. But even that tolerance applies only to valid science. The Nazi hypothermia study does not even attain this status, a reminder that any experiment grossly deficient in ethics is likely to be defective in other ways as well.[67]

Dr. Robert L. Berger, a Harvard Medical School surgeon, is reported by the *Wall Street Journal* (17 May 1990) as saying that the Nazi hypothermia data are useless, that the results of the Dachau experiments were

66 Gerson B. Grunfeld, "Letter to the Editor", *Journal of Medical Ethics,* 17 (1991), p. 162. Gershon cites the following: Stephen G. Post, "The Echo of Nuremberg: Nazi Data and Ethics", *Journal of Medical Ethics,* 17 (1991), pp. 42–44; R. L. Berger, Nazi Science – The Dachau Hypothermia Experiments", *New England Journal of Medicine,* 322 (1990), pp. 1435–1440; W. Neff, "Report on his Experiences", *Nuremberg Tribunal,* ND 908, Sheet 60; Lifton, *The Nazi Doctors,* p. 362; and O. Reinhardt, "The 'Nazi Doctors' Debate", *Medical Journal of Australia,* 153 (1990), pp. 645–647.

67 Nicholas Wade, "The Editorial Notebook: The Errors of Nazi Science", *The New York Times* (27 May 1990), Section 4, p. 12; courtesy of the website *LexisNexis,* http://web.lexis-nexis.com.

> "riddled with inconsistencies" and contained evidence of data falsification and fabrication. "On analysis, the Dachau hypothermia study has all the ingredients of a scientific fraud, and rejection of the data on purely scientific grounds is inevitable. They cannot advance science or save human lives."[68]

Lawrence K. Altman, in "Nazi Data on Hypothermia Termed Unscientific", an article in the *New York Times* (17 May 1990), stated:

> A continuing debate over using Nazi data on hypothermia is moot, a new analysis suggests, because the concentration camp experiments in which the data were obtained were scientifically unsound.
>
> The report concludes that data from the experiments, in which prisoners were thrown into tanks of ice water, are worthless because the research relied on scientifically unsound methods, was carried out erratically and was largely fraudulent.
>
> The analysis said the hypothermia experiments conducted at the Dachau concentration camp in Germany in 1942 and 1943 have [as noted by Dr. Robert Berger, heart surgeon at the New England Deaconess Hospital and Harvard Medical School in Boston] "again all the ingredients of a scientific fraud and rejection of the data on a purely scientific grounds is inevitable".[69]

■

It is clear from the material that I have quoted that the ethical dilemma – is it morally permissible to use or cite the data of immoral, unethical Nazi medical experiments – is far from being settled. And until it is settled, no universal consensus on the proper way to proceed can be reached.

The most important arguments against the use of these data can be summarized as follows.

> 1. The experiments were unscientific, improperly designed and conducted. They were conducted on people starved and overworked, in the camps – their data cannot be applied to healthy people.
>
> 2. The results were often "modified", even fabricated, to satisfy the expectations of superiors.

68 "'Nazi Hypothermia Data is Useless,' Surgeon Says – A Wall Street Journal news Roundup", *Wall Street Journal* (17 May 1990), p. A-1; courtesy of the website *ProQuest Historical Newspapers*, http://proquest.umi.com/pqdweb?index.

69 Lawrence K. Altman, "Nazi Data on Hypothermia termed Unscientifc", *The New York Times* (17 May 1990), p. B-11; recovered through the website *ProQuest Historical Newspapers.*

3. The experiments were grossly unethical, e.g., subjects were not informed of the procedures or purposes or dangers; they were forced to participate, denied the opportunity or right to refuse; suffering was knowingly, willfully inflicted; the result in many instances was death.

4. If the Nazi data are allowed, this use might suggest implicit acceptance of Nazi methods; future scientists, less sensitive to the atrocities accompanying the experiments, might feel encouraged to cross the line

5. Use of the data would provide a form of defense of the perpetrators.

6. Users of the data become perpetrators themselves.

The arguments in favor of using the data can be summarized in this manner:

1. Good may come out of evil. Thus the victims did not suffer or die in vain.

2. The victims would have wanted the experiments to be publicized, and the data, whenever possible, utilized.

3. Citation of the data would glorify the memory of the victims.

4. To the still existing and active Holocaust deniers, published experiments would serve as proof of what really had happened.

5. The data are in the public domain, available to everybody. It would take governmental action to prohibit their use. We should never agree to any kind of censorship.

6. In some cases, the data might help to save lives today. In such instances, not using them would be morally wrong.

The Reverend Richard John Neuhaus, author of the widely known book, *The Naked Public Square: Religion and Democracy in America,* wrote: "For those of us in the West, the Holocaust is probably the only culturally available icon of absolute evil."[70]

My question is: Can we simultaneously repudiate and benefit from such an evil? If decided to benefit from such an evil, will we perpetuate evil?

My answer to these questions is best expressed in the words of Edmund Cahn: "To possess the end and yet not be responsible for the means, to grasp the fruit by disavowing the tree, that has, throughout the ages, been mankind's chief hypocrisy."[71] Therefore, my personal belief is that whatever the benefit to mankind might possibly be, the results of the Nazi experiments should be con-

70 "The Use of Metaphors and Analogies Concerning the Holocaust in Contemporary Bioethical Debates", Typescript of a Lecture by The Reverend Richard John Neuhaus, given at the conference "The Meaning of the Holocaust for Bioethics", in 1993, in Minnesota, p. 6.

71 Edmund Cahn, quoted by Jay Katz in "Abuse of Human Beings for the Sake of Science", in Caplan, ed., *When Medicine Went Mad,* pp. 269–270.

demned to oblivion. We should not be using them because their use may dehumanize us as conducting the experiments dehumanized the Nazi doctors.

I oppose censorship, yet I would approve editorial policies that refuse permission to publish articles making use of such data. I would also approve of scientific organizations and institutions suggesting on ethical grounds that researchers avoid using the data. I most certainly would applaud investigators whose individual conscience prohibited use of the data.

If, in any paper or lecture, the data are used, I would urge journals and scientific organizations to require the inclusion of a detailed description of the data's provenance. (A short footnote would not be sufficient!) I would also urge editors to insist that authors describe in detail why they have decided in favor of using the Nazi data.

Rabbi Emil Fachenheim has written that "we must grant Hitler no posthumous victories".[72] I most emphatically feel that acting in any manner other than what I have just described will mean exactly that!

72 Quoted in Richard John Neuhaus, "The Way They Were, The Way We Are", in Caplan, ed., Ibid. p. 217.

CHAPTER 4

Ethical Codes

In 1947 the judges of the military "Doctor's Trial" charged with trying Nazi war criminals issued a document born of the horrors and grief suffered by victims of World War II. The document in question is known as the Nuremberg Code, and it codifies the moral lessons drawn from the tribunal's trials of Nazi physicians.

This document is justly famous, but it is neither the first nor the last word in the history of ethical codes. I offer a brief summary of earlier codes and of developments since Nuremberg.

The codes of ethics of concern here began developing shortly after the revolutions in eighteenth-century America and France ushered in the so-called modern era. Experimental science, which had developed in the pre-revolutionary era, assumed central significance in this new human world. But, as this approach to science became codified and institutionalized, it became clear that the ethos of the enterprise, with its commitment to objectivity and controlled test design, did not, in itself, guarantee that scientists would restrain themselves out of concern for the interests and well-being of their human research subjects.[1]

The earliest known statement of ethical principles relating to this subject appeared just after the turn of the nineteenth century in Thomas Percival's 1803 book *Medical Ethics*.[2] Percival asserted that new remedies or other treatments should be given only after consultation, "according to the nature of the case", with physicians or surgeons. In the United States, William Beaumont's 1833 code is the earliest known example. Beaumont asserted that the subject's voluntary consent is necessary; also, that if the experiment causes distress or if "the subject becomes dissatisfied", the project must be abandoned.

1 I am partially indebted for this historical material to Jay Katz, "Development of Codes of Ethics", Chap. 2 in *A History of Experimentation,* pp. 37–39.

2 Thomas Percival, *Medical Ethics* (1803; reprinted 1975, 1976). See also C. D. Leake, ed., *Percival's* Medical Ethics (Baltimore, 1927).

The Frenchman Claude Bernard is credited with the first formulation of a code specifically designed for medical research. He stated that doctors should never perform on a "man an experiment which might be harmful to him in any extent, even though the result might be advantageous to science". In other words, Bernard recognized that the rights of the subject should take priority over the interests of science.[3]

In an intriguing twist, given subsequent history, the first country to issue a formal, legal directive on medical research ethics was Imperial Germany. In 1900, the Prussian Minister of Religious Educational and Medical Affairs prohibited experimentation on any but competent adults who had been properly advised of the possible adverse consequences.

The regulation failed to curtail abuses, especially in drug trials. Therefore, the German Ministry of the Interior published further *Richtlinien* (Guidelines) in 1931. These regulations included requirements for testing on animals before humans and for informed consent. They specifically prohibited experiments on children that "might endanger them in the slightest degree". Interestingly, these legally binding regulations were still on the books during the Nazi regime.

By far the most important document in the history of the development of the ethics of medical research is the "Nuremberg Code", which was formulated in August 1947 at the end of the Doctors' Trial in Nuremberg.

Evelyn E. Schuster, Ph.D., succinctly describes the proceedings at Nuremberg in the Doctors' Trial:

> The main trial at Nuremberg after World War II was conducted by the International Military Tribunal. The tribunal was made up of judges from the four allied powers (the United States, Britain, France, and the former Soviet Union) and was charged with trying Germany's major war criminals. After this first-of-its-kind international trial, the United States conducted twelve additional trials of representative Nazis from various sectors of the Third Reich, including law, finance, ministry, and manufacturing, before American Military Tribunals, also at Nuremberg. The first of these trials, the "Doctors' Trial", involved twenty-three defendants, all but three of whom were physicians accused of murder and torture in the conduct of medical experiments on concentration camp inmates.
>
> ...The Doctors' Trial began on December 9, 1946 and ended on July 19, 1947. The case was heard by three judges and one alternate. Thirty-two prosecution witnesses and fifty-three defense witnesses, including

3 Ibid.

> the twenty-three defendants, testified. A total of 1,471 documents were introduced into the record. Sixteen of the twenty-three defendants were found guilty; seven of them were sentenced to death by hanging, five to life imprisonment, two to imprisonment for twenty-five years, one to imprisonment for fifteen years, and one to imprisonment for ten years. Seven were acquitted. The sentences were confirmed by the military governor, and, after the U.S. Supreme Court declined to review the case, the executions were carried out at the Landsberg prison.[4]

The egregious excesses of the Nazi doctors clearly spawned the Nuremberg Code, but the actual author of the document is unknown. The chief prosecutor at the Doctors' Trial, General Telford Taylor, believed that Harold Sebring, who was one of the U.S. judges at Nuremberg, was the author. But the American physicians Leo Alexander and Andrew Ivy, both of whom helped prosecute the Nazi doctors at Nuremberg, have also been named as authors. Careful reading of the trial transcript, of all the background documents, and of the final judgment reveals that the authorship was most likely shared, for the famous Ten Principles of the Nuremberg Code actually grew out of the trial itself.

The judges at Nuremberg realized the importance of the famed Hippocratic Oath, with its vows to safeguard the life and welfare of patients, but they concluded that this oath was not sufficient to protect human subjects in medical research. For this a set of principles that focused on the subject's human rights was required. The judges accordingly articulated ten principles centered not on the physician but on the research subject, insisted on a more comprehensive and absolute informed consent requirement, and introduced the new right of the subject to end an experiment. These principles are known as "The Nuremberg Code".

> 1. The voluntary consent of the human subject is absolutely essential.
>
> This means that the person involved should have legal capacity to give consent; should be so situated as to be able to exercise free power of choice, without the intervention of any element of force/fraud, deceit, duress, overreaching, or other ulterior form of constraint or coercion; and should have sufficient knowledge and comprehension of the elements of the subject matter involved as to enable him to make an understanding and enlightened decision. This latter element requires that before the acceptance of an affirmative decision by the experimental subject there should be made known to him the nature, duration, and purpose of the experiment; the method and means by; which it is to be con-

4 Schuster, "Fifty Years Later", p. 1437.

ducted; all inconveniences and hazards reasonably to be expected; and the effects upon his health or person which may possibly come from his participation in the experiment.

The duty and responsibility for ascertaining the quality of the consent rests upon each individual who, initiates, directs or engages in the experiment. It is a personal duty and responsibility which may not be delegated to another with impunity.

2. The experiment should be such as to yield fruitful results for the good of society, unprocurable by other methods or means of study, and not random and unnecessary in nature.

3. The experiment should be so designed and based on the results of animal experimentation and a knowledge of the natural history of the disease or other problem under study that the anticipated results will justify the performance of the experiment.

4. The experiment should be so conducted as to avoid all unnecessary physical and mental suffering and injury.

5. No experiment should be conducted where there is an a priori reason to believe that death or disabling injury will occur; except, perhaps, in those experiments where the experimental physicians also serve as subjects.

6. The degree of risk to be taken should never exceed that determined by the humanitarian importance of the problem to be solved by the experiment.

7. Proper preparations should be made and adequate facilities provided to protect the experimental subject against even remote possibilities of injury, disability, or death.

8. The experiment should be conducted only by scientifically qualified persons. The highest degree of skill and care should be required through all stages of the experiment of those who conduct or engage in the experiment.

9. During the course of the experiment the human subject should be at liberty to bring the experiment to an end if he has reached the physical or mental state where continuation of the experiment seems to him to be impossible.

10. During the course of the experiment the scientist in charge must be prepared to terminate the experiment at any stage if he has probable cause to believe, in the exercise of good faith, superior skill, and careful judgment required of him, that a continuation of the experiment is likely to result in injury, disability or death to the experimental subject.[5]

5 Ibid., p. 1436.

By insisting that medical investigators alone cannot set the rules for the ethical conduct of research, even when guided by beneficence and Hippocratic ethics, and by adopting a human rights perspective that acknowledges the centrality of informed consent and the right of the subject to withdraw, the Nuremberg Code has changed forever the way both physicians and the public view the proper conduct of medical research on human subjects.

■

Since the formulation at Nuremberg, medical ethical principles have continued to develop. One significant revision was generated within the World Medical Association, which had been established in 1947. Its founding members were physicians from Europe, the British Empire, and the United States, who had first gathered in London, during the Second World War, for a meeting of the British Medical Association. The Eighteenth Assembly of this group, held in 1964, in Helsinki, produced a revision of the Nuremberg principles. Known as the "Helsinki Declaration", this new ethical code was viewed by the medical profession, not as a legal document, but rather as a guide. On the matter of consent, it loosened the restrictions of the Nuremberg Code: the Nuremberg Code makes informed consent an absolute cornerstone of ethical research, thereby excluding the mentally ill, the unconscious, and the very young from participation in medical experiments, but the Helsinki Declaration allows proxy consent on such subjects. The latter also makes a clear distinction between therapeutic and non-therapeutic research; therapeutic research always must be justified by its potential benefit for the patient. Perhaps most importantly, the Helsinki Declaration recommends that "research projects be considered by a specially appointed independent committee".

The 1980s witnessed additional developments in medical ethics. In 1982 two groups, the World Health Organization and the Council for International Organizations of Medical Sciences, put out the *Proposed International Guidelines for Biomedical Research Involving Human Subjects.* This statement, published because of concern that research might be moved to developing countries by firms and individuals seeking to avoid restrictions and to minimize expenses, aimed at preventing such abuses. These new guidelines recommended the formation of review committees by national or local health administrations or national councils. This point, "a nation should not allow or support in a country, research which does not conform to ethic review standards at least equivalent to those in force within the nation", was reinforced at the International Summit Conference on Bioethics in Ottawa, in 1987 and subsequently adopted by the Economic Summit nations.[6]

6 Ibid.

The Belmont Report, a document formulated in 1989 in deliberations of the National Commission for the Protection of Human Rights, went further.[7] This report, "Ethical Principles and Guidelines for the Protection of Human Subjects of Research", was accepted by the U.S. Department of Health, Education and Welfare. It outlines three basic ethical principles:

> 1. respect of persons; a principle which mandates the acknowledgment of the autonomy of the individual and the protection of individuals with diminished autonomy;
> 2. beneficence (the imperative to do no harm); a principle which demands the maximization of possible benefits and minimization of possible harms;
> 3. justice (fairness in distribution).

Application of these principles translates into:

> 1. informed consent (information, comprehension and voluntarism);
> 2. assessment of risks and benefits;
> 3. selection of subjects on two levels, the social and the individual. The last point speaks to the fact that experiments using subjects from a single special ethnic, racial, or social group, etc., are not always valid, because the principle of random selection has been violated. Random selection helps also to ensure that the potential benefits of any experiment will be spread across socio-economic classes; similarly that potentially harmful research will not be limited to underprivileged or otherwise impaired individuals.

■

All these codes represent significant progress in our consciousness that ethical principles must guide medical research. Codes alone, however, cannot protect the research subject or ensure ethical experimentations, for codes simply formulate principles. In determined hands not really guided by moral concerns, such codes may do nothing more than hide ongoing, unethical conduct. To put the ethical principles into practice, we must have effective enforcement mechanisms. And finally we must also always remember that the Hippocratic Oath has lost none of its relevance: "I will use my power to help the sick, to the best of my ability and judgment; I will abstain from harming or wronging any man by it."

7 Belmont Report: "Ethical Principles and Guidelines for the Protection of Human Subjects of Research", Department of Health, Education, and Welfare, Publication No. (05) 78-0012 (Washington, D.C.: U.S. Government Printing Office, 18 April 1979), vol. 1, Appendix, p. 3.

Appendix

THE DOCTORS*

ACKERMANN, DR. JOSEPH: research assistant to Dr. Waldemar Hoven; participated in the carbon monoxide experiments conducted at Buchenwald.[1]

ADAM, DR. OTTO: camp doctor at Sachsenhausen and Flossenbürg; tested poison-laced ammunition on humans. He was acquitted in 1962, and thereafter practiced medicine in Hammelburg/Unterfranken.[2]

BABOR, DR. KARL: camp doctor, first at Dachau, then at Groß-Rosen and Natzweiler; participated in experiments with phlegmones and sepsis, which caused the deaths of 600–800 involuntary prisoner-subjects. At the war's end, he went underground and was eventually traced to Addis Ababa, Ethiopia.[3]

BAERENDT, DR.: conducted experiments in Dachau with T-stoff, an explosive that was being tested as a substitute for powder.[4]

BAUMKÖTTER, DR. HEINZ: Erster Lagerarzt (senior physician) at Sachsenhausen; also served in Mauthausen and Natzweiler; conducted hepatitis and *Zyankali* (potassium cyanide) capsule experiments on camp inmates; tried by a Russian court in 1947 and sentenced to life imprisonment with compulsory labor.[5]

BECKER-FREYSENG, DR. HERMANN (Stabsarzt): 1933, joined the NSDAP; 1934, intern at the Robert Koch Institute in Berlin; 1940, drafted into the Luftwaffe; 1943, promoted to Stabsarzt [captain in the medical corps]; 1941–44, in the central offices of the Air Force

* In some cases first names could not be found.

1 Aziz, *Doctors of Death*, vol. 3, p. 104.

2 Klee, *Auschwitz*, pp. 49, 176.

3 Ibid., pp. 49, 149; Affidavit of Dr. Franz Blaha, Document No-3249-PS, Exhibit No. USA-663, in *Trial IMT*, vol. 5, p. 171.

4 Interrogation Summary No. 40 of Wolfram Sievers, 17 August 1946, YVA, JM/6027, p. 3.

5 Klee, *Auschwitz*, pp. 43 and 43 n. 117, 49, 176 and 176 n. 116; *Documented Report of the Sachsenhausen Trial*, SWA Verlag, Berlin, 1948, cited in Mitscherlich and Mielke, eds., *The Death Doctors* (London, 1962), p. 167; UNWCC, p. 534.

Medical Services, first served as a consultant on aviation medicine in the Luftwaffe's Bureau of Medical Inspectors (Amt des Sanitätsinspekteurs der Luftwaffe), and later as Chief of Aviation Medicine. He was charged at the Nuremberg Doctors' Trial with war crimes in the high altitude, seawater and freezing (hypothermia) experiments carried out at Dachau on behalf of the Luftwaffe; also for participation in the sulfanilamide, hepatitis and typhus experiments conducted at other camps; sentenced on 20 January 1947, to twenty years imprisonment. He served only ten years.[6]

Beiglboeck (Beiglböck), Dr. Wilhelm (Stabsarzt): an Austrian-trained physician who worked at the University of Vienna Medical Clinic as an assistant to Professor Eppinger. Beiglböck was considered a talented and revolutionary medic. He was appointed Stabsarzt [captain] in the Luftwaffe's medical corps in May 1941; 1944, appointed professor at the University of Vienna; also served as chief physician of the University Medical Clinic; was stationed in June 1944, at the Paratroopers Hospital in Tarvis, Italy. On behalf of the Luftwaffe, Beiglböck supervised the seawater experiments at Dachau. The Nuremberg tribunal sentenced him in 1947 to fifteen years imprisonment, but he was released in 1951. Beginning in 1952 he worked as the head physician at a clinic in Buxtehude; died in 1963 at the age of fifty-eight.[7]

Berger, Dr. Arno or Bruno (also Beger, Bruno): The names Berger and Beger appear in sources in a confusing manner, in the permutations Arno Berger, Bruno Berger and Bruno Beger. A Dr. Arno Berger appears in sources as a camp doctor at Ravensbrück. The names Arno Berger, Bruno Berger and Bruno Beger have all been used to indicate an anthropologist who assisted with the selection of individuals for Hirt's skelton collection at the Strasbourg Institute. Ernst Klee reports that Bruno *Beger* was born in 1911, the son of an officer; 1934, entered the SS (highest rank, SS Hauptsturmführer); 1937, joined the NSDAP; trained as an anthropologist under race biologist Prof. Hans Günther and 1940, obtained his doctorate (Dr. rer. nat) in 1940; employed in the Ahnenerbe; 1941/42, participated in the selection of individuals for Hirt's Jewish-Bolshevik skull collection and in 1943 assisted with the selections at Auschwitz of individuals who were sent to Natzweiler, gassed, and their bodies transported to Hirt, as specimens for the skeleton collection. Beger worked in the "Ahnenerbe's Abteilung der Forschungsstätte für Innerasien", which from July 1943 to the end of the war, was headquartered at Schloss Mittersill in Salzburger Land. It is likely that Bruno Beger is identical to Arno Berger/Bruno Berger.[8]

6 Interrogation of Dr. Hermann Becker-Freyseng, 12 November 1946, YVA, JM/5964, p. 1; UNWCC, p. 533; Burman, ed., *The First German War Crimes Trial*, p. 247; Klee, *Auschwitz*, p.254.
7 Interrogation of Professor Dr. Oskar Schroeder, 2 October 1946, YVA, JM/6025, p. 12; Interrogation Summary No. 240 of Dr. Konrad Wilhelm Philipp Schaefer, 4 October 1946, YVA, JM/6021, pp. 1–2; Hoedeman, *Hitler or Hippocrates*, p. 176; Klee, *Auschwitz*, p. 252.
8 Interrogation Summary No. 48 of Wolfram Sievers, 20 August 1946, YVA, JM/6027, p. 3; Klee, *Auschwitz*, pp. 49, 257, 359–360, 360 n. 47, 371–374.

BERNING, DR. HEINRICH: associate professor at Hamburg University with expertise in edema, especially in cases of starvation. Berning led "famine experiments", in which Soviet prisoners were starved so that the physiological effects of malnutrition could be studied; published his results in 1949, in an article entitled "Dystrophy". He was appointed medical director of the Hamburg General Hospital in 1963, and continued in that position until 1974.[9]

BICKENBACH, DR. OTTO: professor on the medical faculty of the University of Strasbourg, particularly renowned in the Third Reich as an expert on gasses. Bickenbach helped to oversee experiments in the concentration camps exploring the effects of phosgene gas on human subjects. At his first trial for war crimes, he was sentenced to twenty years imprisonment. Because several witnesses had failed to appear for this trial, his case was reopened and the sentence commuted to twenty years hard labor. In 1956, he left Germany for an unknown destination, having been granted early release.[10]

BLEIBECK, DR.: physician from Vienna who helped to conduct the seawater experiments at Dachau.[11]

BLOME (BLOHME), PROF. DR. KURT (Generalarzt): cancer researcher, in 1939 appointed deputy to Leonardo Conti, the Reich Chief of Public Health and NSDAP's Reich Health Leader. Blome assisted Conti with his NSDAP duties; thus acted as chief of the Reich Medical Association and as nominal chief of both the Main Office of Public Health of the Nazi Party and the National Socialist Medical Association. In 1943 he was appointed Commissioner for Cancer Research under Hermann Goering, but here, "cancer research" was simply a code name for a top-secret program of research on biological warfare agents; Blome testified before the International Military Tribunal at Nuremberg that, with this appointment, he was given full authority over the covert research ("in dieser Eigenschaft, als Bevollmächtigter für die Krebsforschung, wurde ich im Jahre 1943 Bevollmächtigter für die gesamte biologische Kriegsforschung"). His Institut für Krebsforschung (Institute for Cancer Research), on the grounds of the former Nesselstedt Monastery outside Posen, was engaged in developing biological weapons.

After the war an American military tribunal acquitted Blome; the CIA recruited him and assigned him to the "Paperclip" program at Camp King, but shortly thereafter, French authorities arrested him, convicted him of war crimes and sentenced him to twenty years imprisonment.[12]

9 G. J. Annas and M. A. Grodin, eds., *The Nazi Doctors and the Nuremberg Code*, pp. 32–52; Klee, *Auschwitz*, pp. 258–259, 360.

10 Paul Hoedeman, *Hitler or Hippocrates*, pp. 148–149; Mitscherlich and Mielke, eds., *Doctors of Infamy*, p. 80.

11 Testimony of Dr. Franz Blaha, in *Trial IMT*, vol. 5, p. 186.

12 Excerpt of Affidavit of Kurt Blome, Document No-471, in *Trial IMT*, vol. I, RG-30.001M, p. 1; Interrogation Summary No. 40 of Wolfram Sievers, 17 August 1946, YVA, JM/6027, p. 2; Klee, *Auschwitz*, pp. 87–91, on pp 87–88, citing "Aussage Kurt Blome, 1 March 1950, Verfahren 2 Js 389/49 OstA Hannover; Nuremberg Document No-538; Bericht ZSt über

BLUMENREUTHER, DR. (probably CARL BLUMENREUTHER); a "Dr. Blumenreuther" worked on the sulfonamide experiments. Dr. Carl Blumenreuther (SS Brigadeführer), born 16 November 1881 in Berlin, graduated in 1916 from the Kaiser-Wilhelm-Institute with a specialty in gas warfare; joined the NSDAP in 1937, and served as Chief Pharmacist of the SS Totenkopfverbande; worked at Oranienburg, 1936–40; became head of the Department of Chemical and Pharmaceutical Services in the Health Department of SS Headquarters (Sanitätsamt des SS Führungshauptamtes). Blumenreuther's department supplied pharmaceuticals for research to the concentration camps.[13]

BODMANN, DR. FRANZ VON: Standortarzt (chief physician) at Auschwitz; also worked 1941–42 at Neuengamme and Lublin, and 1943 at Natzweiler; gave phenol injections to subjects of the experiments; committed suicide 25 May 1945 in Markt Pongau.[14]

BOGAERTS, DR. CARL: physician from Brussels who was associated with the typhus experiments on Gypsy inmates at Natzweiler. Bogaerts carried out autopsies on the bodies of those Gypsy subjects who died during the experiments.[15]

BRACHTEL (BRACHTL), DR. MED. RUDOLF ADALBERT (SS Hauptsturmführer): born 1909 in Gaya/Sudetenland; listed as a member of the NSDAP, SA and SS, and as a member of the National Socialists Doctors Association; SS camp doctor at Dachau (15 April 1941–1 December 1942). In the Dachau trials, witness Michalowski spoke of a Dr. Brachtel (Brachtl) who was an assistant to Karl Klaus Schilling. Dr. Brachtel was involved in the experiments on freezing (hypothermia), liver biopsy, and the malaria drug Atabrine (R 1610).[16]

BRACK, VIKTOR (SS Oberführer): Born 1904 in Haazen; studied economics in Munich; one of Hitler's earliest disciples; 1929, joined the NSDAP; 1932, appointed to the NSDAP office in Munich, working under Philipp Bouhler; 1933, moved to Berlin after

---

den RFR. 413 AR-Z 501/67 vom 9.7.1970, Bl. 20.). For more on the nature of the Posen facility, including the likelihood that Russian prisoners were used as experimental subject, see Klee, op. cit., p. 89, citing Nuremberg Doc. No-3061 and p. 90, citing Nuremberg Document USSR-510; see also "The CIA-Nazi Connection" Quote is from "The CIA-Nazi Connection". See also the United States Holocaust Memorial Museum website.

13 Interrogation of Joachim Mrugowsky, 27 August 1946, YVA, JM/6006, p. 2; Klee, *Auschwitz*, pp. 30, 140, 203; Scharsach, *Die Ärzte der Nazis*, p. 212; MacLean, *The Camp Men*, p. 44; and Dörner, ed., *The Nuremberg Medical Trial*, p. 77.

14 Klee, *Auschwitz*, pp. 49, 410, and 410 ns 60–61.

15 Henri Chretien, "'Scientific' Experimentation", *Le Médecin Français*, 41 (25 May 1945), p. 8.

16 Testimony of Leo Michalowski, Dachau, 13 May 1945, Translation of Document No-2428-PS, in RG-30.001M, p. 2; Extracts from the Review of the Proceedings of the General Military Court in the Case of the United States vs. Weiss, Ruppert, et al., held at Dachau, Germany, Translation of Document No-836 [856], in RG-30.001M, p. 6. See also MacLean, *The Camp Men*, p. 47; BDC SS Officer Files A3343 SSO-096; and BDC A3340-RAK-005. Dr. Brachtel is likely the Dr. Bracht mentioned in Hoedeman, *Hitler or Hippocrates*, p. 23.

Bouhler was named Chief of Hitler's Chancellery (Chef des Kanzlei des Führers); 1936, appointed Chief of Bureau II (Chef des Amtes II) in the chancellery; December 1939–August 1941, assigned to T4 (his codename was "Jennerwein") and given responsibility for the administrative details of the euthanasia program (Aktion T4); 1942, joined the Waffen SS; charged at Nuremberg with "special responsibility for, and participation in, sterilization experiments and the euthanasia program". Brack was sentenced to death on 20 August 1947 by the Nuremberg tribunal and hanged on 2 June 1948.[17]

Brandt, Dr. Karl (SS Gruppenführer and Waffen SS Generalleutnant): Born 1904, in Mühlhausen, Alsace (then part of Germany); 1928, became a medical doctor; joined the Nazi party in January 1932 and the SA in 1933; July 1934, commissioned as an SS Untersturmführer; by June 1943, had risen to the rank of SS Brigadenführer; transferred in 1943 from the Allgemeine SS to the Waffen SS with an equivalent commission, Generalmajor (Major General); April 1944, promoted to Generalleutnant, Waffen SS.

Brandt, who served as Hitler's personal physician, 1934–1944, eventually rose to become the most powerful physician in the Reich. In 1939, working conjointly with Philipp Bouhler, he organized and instigated Aktion T4, the euthanasia program through which the Nazis killed sick and handicapped patients. On 28 July 1942, he was made Plenipotentiary for Health and Medical Services. His task was to coordinate certain activities of the civilian medical service (under the direction of Dr. Leonardo Conti), with the activities of the military medical services (under Dr. Siegfried Handloser). In September 1942, Hitler gave Brandt more formal powers by naming him Generalkommissar für Sanitäts- und Gesundheitswesen. Brandt was also a member of the Reichsforschungsrat, the board responsible for research. His power in this arena increased on 5 December 1943, when Hitler gave him the authority to see that the activities and programs of the medical and public health services addressed the goals of Nazi scientific research. In this capacity, Brandt founded the Bureau for Medical Science and Research (directed by Paul Rostock) and the Bureau for Planning and Industry (headed by Admiral Major [medical] Alfred Fikentscher). In August 1944, Brandt was elevated for the final time, when Hitler made him Reichskommissar für das Sanitäts- und Gesundheitswesen. He was now responsible for health services throughout the Reich.

In this high office Brandt was authorized to issue instructions on health matters to the medical organizations of the government, party and armed services. Brandt ordered the research on the effects of gas warfare. Trial evidence revealed that he was involved

17 Interrogation of Dr. Viktor Brack, 14 October 1946, Translation of Document No-426, in RG-30.001M, p. 3; Burman, ed., *The First German War Crimes Trial,* pp. 216–217, 243–244. See also Document No-205, Office of U.S. Chief of Counsel, Letter from Brack to Himmler. On Brack's codename at T4, see Lifton, *Nazi Doctors,* p. 141, posted on the Mazal Library website at www.mazal.org/Lifton.

with top-level planning for the euthanasia program and medical experiments on humans. Brandt was actually arrested by the Gestapo on 16 April 1945, and condemned to death by a court in Thuringia, but he was released on 2 May 1945, only to be arrested again, this time by the British, on 23 May 1945. He was brought before the U.S tribunal at Nuremberg in the so-called Doctors' Trial (United States of America vs. Karl Brandt et al.). Brandt was found guilty of war crimes in connection with the experiments on freezing (hypothermia), malaria, *Lost* (mustard gas), sulfa drugs, bone, muscle and nerve transplantation and bone regeneration, seawater, infectious hepatitis, sterilization and typhus, and with war crimes and crimes against humanity for his participation in the euthanasia program. He was executed on 2 June 1948 at Landsberg Prison in Bavaria.[18]

BRANDT, RUDOLF (SS Standartenführer): not a physician. Born 1909, in Frankfurt; studied law in Berlin and Jena; 1932, joined the NSDAP; 1935, SS Untersturmführer; Persönlicher Referent (Personal Advisor) to Himmler; Ministerial Counsellor and Chief of the Ministerial Office of the Reich Ministry of the Interior. As Himmler's personal assistant, Brandt maintained close relations with Wolfram Sievers, head of the Ahnenerbe, and consequently was involved in coordinating many of the experiments with involuntary human subjects in the concentration camps. At the Doctors' Trial in Nuremberg, Brandt was charged with and found guilty of war crimes connected with the experiments on high altitude, freezing (hypothermia), malaria, mustard gas (*Lost*), sulfanilamides, jaundice, sterilization, typhus, and seawater. He was also found guilty of exterminating both Jews and Poles, the former as subjects for August Hirt's skeleton collection and the latter as allegedly incurable victims of tuberculosis. A charge of war crimes in the bone, nerve, and muscle experiments was dismissed. He was sentenced to death by hanging; sentence carried out 2 June 1948.[19]

BREUER, DR. SERGIUS: worked at the Deutsche Versuchsanstalt für Luftfahrt (German Experimental Institute for Aviation). He was responsible for distributing Sigmund Rascher's final report on the high altitude experiments to departmental experts and also served as Dr. Kurt Blome's deputy for cancer research.[20]

18 Interrogation Summary No. 322 of Karl Gebhardt, 17 October, 1946, YVA, JM/5979, p. 2; Declaration of Wolfram Sievers, Evaluation Report No. 98, Combined Intelligence Objectives Subcommittee, 13 June 1945, YVA, JM/10046, p. 2; Interrogation of Dr. Hermann Brack, 14 October 1946, Translation of Document No-426, in RG-30.001M, p. 2; Klee, *Auschwitz*, pp. 141–143; Burman, ed., *The First German War Crimes Trial*, pp. 124, 129–138, 141–142, 365; "Jewish Virtual Library"; "Wikipedia"; and "Bioprofiles".

19 Burman, ed., *The First German War Crimes Trial*, pp. 129–138, 156, 191–197, and 365; *Jewish Virtual Library;* General Telford Taylor's Opening Statement at the Nuremberg Doctors' Trial, posted on the United States Holocaust Memorial Museum website.

20 Interrogation of Wolfram Sievers, 28 October 1946, YVA, JM/6027, p. 9; Handwritten note, "Cancer Research", Translation of Document No-690, in RG-30.001M, p. 1.

BRUNNER, DR. KARL: doctor at Hohenlychen; participated in Karl Gebhardt's research experiments.[21]

BUTENANDT, PROF. ADOLF (also JOHANN): born 1903; died 1995; 1939, awarded the Nobel Prize in chemistry for research on sex hormone but was not allowed by the Nazis to accept the award; received the award finally in 1949; during the war headed the Kaiser-Wilhelm Society's Biochemical Institute in Berlin; collaborated on Robert Ritter's anthropological studies of gypsies; Müller-Hill reports that Joseph Mengele regularly sent blood samples taken from his experimental subjects at Auschwitz to this institute for analysis; Butenandt denied the report but did nothing when Müller-Hill elected to publish it anyway. After the war Butenandt served as president of the Max-Planck Gesellschaft.[22]

CAPESIUS, VICTOR: born 1907, in Reussmarkt, Romania; chief SS pharmacist; served in Auschwitz during the war; worked with Bruno Weber on chemicals for "brain-washing"; sentenced to nine years imprisonment after the war.[23]

CLAUBERG, DR. KARL: born 1898, in Wuppertal into a family of craftsmen; served in the infantry in World War I; studied medicine after the war and advanced to become physician-in-chief at the University of Kiel Gynecology Clinic; 1933, joined the NSDAP and was appointed professor of gynecology at Königsberg University; 1942, asked Himmler for permission to perform experimental human sterilizations; December 1942, was sent to Auschwitz with permission to do the experiments. Clauberg was given Block 10 in the main camp as an experimental site. There he worked on a "cheap and efficient" method of sterilizing women: injecting acid liquids, without anaesthetics, into the uterus of thousands of Jewish and Gypsy women. He also sterilized women by radiation and surgery; bragged that, with his methods, one doctor and ten assistants could sterilize one thousand women in a day. As the Allies approached Auschwitz, he fled to Ravensbrück. It is estimated that he subjected seven hundred Ravensbrück prisoners to his procedures.

In 1948 the Soviet Union brought Clauberg to trial and sentenced him to twenty-five years imprisonment. Seven years later he was pardoned and returned to the Federal Republic of Germany. Shortly thereafter he gave a press conference at which he boasted of his scientific work in Auschwitz. Then he proceeded to set up a new medical practice. The Bundesärztekammer (West German Federal Physicians' Chamber) eventually decertified him but only after the application of severe outside pressure. In 1955, after survivor groups protested, Clauberg was arrested. He died in 1957, shortly before his trial was to begin.[24]

21 Interrogation Summary No. 54 of Joachim Mrugowsky, 27 August 1946, YVA, JM/6006, p. 5; Klee, *Auschwitz*, pp. 158, 202.

22 Müller-Hill, "Genetics After Auschwitz", *Holocaust Genocide Studies*, 2: 1 (1987), p. 8; anecdote related to Dr. Alfred Pasternak.

23 Dr. Alfred Pasternak Personal Notes.

24 "Jewish Virtual Library"; Kater, *Doctors Under Hitler*, p. 1; "Doctors of the Holocaust".

Conti, Dr. Leonardo: born 1900 in Switzerland; 1933, appointed Staatskommissar für das Gesundheitswesen (State Health Commissioner) in the Prussian Ministry of the Interior; 1939, replaced Dr. Gerhard Wagner as Reichsgesundheitsführer (Reich Health Leader) responsible for all civilian medical services in the Reich; also replaced Wagner as Reichärzteführer (NSDAP member charged as leader of the medical profession after *Gleichschaltung*). As Reichsgesundheitsführer, Conti was subordinate to Dr. Wilhelm Frick, Minister of the Interior, until 1943, when Himmler assumed Frick's duties. Within the NSDAP structure, Conti was subordinate to Martin Bormann, NSDAP Chancellor. After July 1942, when Hitler made significant changes to the structure of medical services, Dr. Siegfried Handloser was given a position in military health matters equal in rank to Conti's in civilian health. Both men had to work with Karl Brandt, as Hitler had charged Brandt, who reported directly to him, with coordinating key aspects of civilian and military health services. Conti was taken into custody and imprisoned by the American military; he hanged himself in October 1945, before he could be brought to trial. Among other things, his suicide note indicates that he had inspected Kurt Blome's so-called Cancer Institute at Posen, which was actually dedicated to developing biological warfare agents, and that Blome had informed him of his plan (*Absicht*) to do experiments on human subjects.[25]

Cremer (Craemer), Dr. Hans-Dietrich: Oberstabsarzt (Chief) of the research station in Sankt Johann in Tirol, which focused on the special medical problems of mountain troops; specialist in dietetics; professor and director of the Institut für Ernährungswissenschaften at the University of Giessen; involved with Sigmund Rascher in conducting the hypothermia experiments.[26]

Dachfinney, Prof.: conducted malaria experiments at Dachau.[27]

Delmotte, Dr. Hans: born 1917, in Alsace; camp physician at Auschwitz; worked at the Rajsko Hygiene Institute in Auschwitz under Dr. Bruno Weber, especially with spotted fever (typhus). According to Professor Geza Mansfield, "some regard Delmotte as one of the most decent and responsible doctors at Auschwitz (and not only in regard to the Hippocratic Oath). He was the only one who protested openly against the selections

25 See General Telford Taylor's Opening Statement at the Doctors' Trial, Nuremberg, for a description and organizational chart demonstrating the relationship between Hitler, the Reich administration including the armed forces, the NSDAP, and the place of military and civilian health services within these structures. Reproduced on the United States Holocaust Memorial Museum website. See also Klee, *Auschwitz*, p. 139. On Conti's suicide note, see Klee, op. cit., p. 89, citing Nuremberg Doc. No-3061.

26 Dr. Sigmund Rascher, "Memorandum Concerning Cooperation of SS Physicians of the Mountain Troops", 6 November 1942, Nuremberg Document No-319, in RG-30.001M, p. 1; Klee, *Auschwitz*, pp. 236, 239.

27 Extracts from the Testimony of Prosecution Witness August H. Vieweg, 13, 16 December 1946, in *Trials NMT*, vol. 1, p. 303.

and stated that he did not want to be in a slaughterhouse. He considered it was his duty as a physician to save lives and not to destroy them." In 1945 he committed suicide.[28]

DEUSCHL, DR. HANS: one of the supervisors of medical experiments at Dachau, a personal friend of Himmler's and head of the Doctors' Führer School at Alt-Rehse; member of the SS; served on the eastern front in Estonia, near Fellin; recommended "radical measures" to deal with sick Russian prisoners. Himmler asked Deuschl in summer 1943 if he would be willing to supervise medical experiments at Dachau; Deuschl accepted; benefited personally, receiving chocolate, cognac, flowers, china and fresh fruit from Himmler; was also able to acquire a house in Starnberg, at the foot of the Bavarian Alps, formerly the residence of a Jewish family.[29]

DIERRING: worked with Dr. Horst Schumann on sterilization experiments at Auschwitz.

DIETZSCH, DR. ARTHUR: a prisoner-doctor, who served as Kapo (captain) of the medical experiments ward at Buchenwald; had authority over the prisoners on the ward and was accused of mistreating them; worked with Dr. Ding-Schuler on the typhus experiments; was brought before the American Military tribunal at Dachau in the trial of Buchenwald camp staff (U.S. vs. Josias Erbprinz zu Waldeck-Pyrmont); sentenced to fifteen years imprisonment.[30]

DING (DING-SCHULER), DR. ERWIN (SS Sturmbannführer): born 1912 in Bitterfeld, the illegitimate son of Baron von Schuler and a girl by the name of Braun; the baron was a doctor in Grimma/Sachsen, notorious for his dissipated life. A rich shopkeeper of Leipzig adopted the infant and gave him the name Ding. In 1933, Ding joined the NSDAP and the SS; was chief of Buchenwald's Block 46, where all the camp prisoners chosen as experimental subjects were housed.

At Buchenwald, Ding supervised or observed experiments with poisoned ammunition; infected patients with typhus in order to experiment with potential cures (and accidentally infected himself with the disease); was chief at Buchenwald of the Department of Spotted Fever and Virus Research of the Waffen SS Hygiene Institute (Abteilung für Fleckfiebor- und Virusforschung am Hygiene-Institut der Waffen SS); wrote the report "On Treatment of Typhus with Acridine Derivates."[31]

28 Comments of Prof. Geza Mansfield in Shelley, ed., *Criminal Experiments on Human Beings*, pp. 306–307, 322.

29 Proctor, *Racial Hygiene*, pp. 218–219; Himmler to Deuschl, n.d. and Deuschl to Himmler, 24 January 1942, NS 19/3382, B (Archives of the Reichsführer SS, Himmler).

30 "Nazi Doctors and Other Perpetrators of Nazi Crimes"; and "Dachau Scrapbook: Buchenwald Trial".

31 Dr. Alfred Balachowsky, "Statement Concerning Experiments and Research about Exanthematous Typhus at Buchenwald Camp", 24 May 1946, Translation of Document No-484, in RG-30.001M, p. 1; Translation of Document No-582, in RG-30.001M; Klee, *Auschwitz*, pp. 50, 174; "Nazi Doctors and Other Perpetrators of Nazi Crimes".

DOHMEN, DR. ARNOLD (also Dohman): (Stabsarzt [captain] in the Forschungsstätte der Heeressanitätsinspektion [Research Laboratory of the Army Medical Inspectorate] and Führer, Allgemeine SS); a bacteriologist who assisted Kurt Gutzeit with hepatitis experiments at Auschwitz; also worked at Sachsenhausen. Dohmen reportedly felt uneasy about using human subjects and expressed his concerns to Gutzeit, who rebuked him.[32]

DOLLING, DR. [possibly Enno Lolling; see that entry] (SS Standartenführer): chief of Büro D III, Sanitätswesen und Lagerhygiene (Medical Services and Camp Hygiene); participated at Natzweiler in research to develop a new type of typhus serum.[33]

EGG, DR. MARTIN: a physician in the Waffen SS; did cancer research in the camps.[34]

EISELE, DR. HANS KURT: physician and Waffen SS officer who worked at Mauthausen, Buchenwald (1941–43), Natzweiler and Dachau. He has been judged one of the worst of his kind among the physicians who worked at Buchenwald. Eisele's experiments included vivisections, injections of apomorphine to observe vomiting; injections of Evipan (a dangerous new drug, also known as Evipal and Evipan-natrium); unnecessary amputations and operations, performed without anaesthetics and followed by the murder of the patients. He was reported to have arbitrarily selected able-bodied Jews for murder by means of Evipan injection. He is known to have murdered Dutch Jews on the sick ward by ordering "Reviersperre" [ward closing] and giving them lethal injections. He eliminated TB patients the same way. He spent the last two-and-a half months of the war at Dachau. At war's end Eisele was tried and condemned to death by hanging at two Dachau trials, United States vs. Weiss, Ruppert, et al. (staff from Dachau camp); and United States vs. Josias Erbprinz zu Waldeck-Pyrmont (staff from Buchenwald camp). In 1948, a War Crimes Board commuted his sentence to life imprisonment. He was pardoned in 1952. German authorities financed his purchase of a medical practice in München-Passing, but in 1958, after ex-prisoners discovered his whereabouts, he fled to Cairo and set up a new practice under his own name; he was a favorite physician among the local aristocracy. German attempts at extradition were unsuccessful. Eisele died in Cairo on 3 May 1967; his file disappeared from the German Ministry of Justice.[35]

32 Document No-01, in *Trials NMT,* vol. 1, p. 495; Mitscherlich and Mielke, eds., *The Death Doctors,* p. 165; Klee, *Auschwitz,* p. 259; Annas and Gronin, eds., *The Nazi Doctors and the Nuremberg Code,* pp. 32–52.

33 Letter from SS Sturmbannführer Brandt to SS Obersturmbannführer Sievers, 21 March 1945, in *Trials NMT,* vol. 1, p. 144; See also Letter, SS Standartenführer to SS Obergruppenführer Pohl, 19 May 1944, in *Nazi Conspiracy and Aggression,* Supp. A, pp. 1270–1271; "Inspektion der SS-Totenkopf-Standarten-Lexikon der Wehrmacht," at http://www.lexikon-der-wehrmacht.de/Gliederungen/SSTotenkopfStandarten-R.htm. Material re: Enno Lolling as possible correct name comes from Weindling, *Nazi Medicine and the Nuremberg Trials,* pp. 39, 54. See also Dörner, ed., *Nuremberg Medical Trial,* p. 115.

34 Interrogation Summary No. 48 of Wolfram Sievers, 20 August 1946, YVA, JM/6027, p. 4.

35 Hoedeman, *Hitler or Hippocrates,* pp. 120–138; Hackett, *The Buchenwald Report,* pp. 68–81, 228–230, 369–371; Klee, *Auschwitz,* p. 50.

ELLENBECK, DR. HANS-DIETER (SS Hauptsturmführer): employed by the SS Führungsamt, Amtsgruppe D, Amt XVI (Department for Blood Preservation) in Berlin-Lichterfelde; worked at Buchenwald; participated in typhus research; conducted nutrition experiments; studied the oxygen levels in blood samples that had been taken from patients doing various tasks and exercises; artificially produced starvation edema in patients.[36]

ENTRESS, DR. FRIEDRICH-KARL: Waffen SS doctor; born 1914 in Posen; 1939, passed state medical examinations; served as Lagerarzt at Gross-Rosen, Auschwitz and Mauthausen; euthanized patients with phenol injections; in March 1943, succeeded Dr. Hellmuth Vetter as principal SS doctor at Auschwitz/Monowitz, the sub-camp that supplied prison-laborers to the local I. G. Farben factory; Entress made "selections" of sick laborer-prisoners whenever the number of sick exceeded 5% of the total Monowitz camp population; condemned to death at the trial of Mauthausen staff (U.S. vs. Hans Altfuldisch et al.) in Dachau; executed 28 May, 1947, along with four other SS doctors.[37]

EPPINGER, PROF. HANS: associated with the University of Vienna Medical Clinic, where his students included Wilhelm Beiglboeck; sent to Dachau to work on the hepatitis and seawater experiments.[38]

ESSER: involved in hepatitis experiments.[39]

FEHRINGER, DR.: Gauhauptstellenleiter (district administrator) who was Director of the Office of Racial Policy in the Niederdonau District (Rassenpolitisches Amt, Niederdonau); conducted sterilization research: a letter from SS Oberführer Gund to Himmler (24 August 1942) reports that Fehringer favored conducting experiments on human subjects (Gypsies) to test Madaus's method of sterilization (by means of dumbcane extract); recommended seeking support from the pharmaceutical institute at the University of Vienna; *Gutachter* (evaluator) for T4, 6 September 1940–13 January 1941.[40]

36 *Trials NMT,* vol. 1; "Nazi Doctors and Other Perpetrators of Nazi Crimes"; Klee, *Auschwitz,* p. 50. See also www.mazal.org/archives/nmt/01/NMT517.

37 "Dachau Scrapbook: Mauthausen"; IAC, *Inhuman Medicine,* vol. 1, pt. 2, p. 116; Klee, *Auschwitz,* pp. 20, 20ff, 50, 400, 407, 419ff, 443; and Pasternak personal notes.

38 *Trials NMT,* vol. 1, p. 499; Klee, *Auschwitz,* p. 244.

39 *Trials NMT,* vol. 1, p. 499.

40 "Nazi Doctor Database"; also Letter, SS Oberführer Gund to Himmler, 24 August 1942, in *Trials NMT,* vol. 1, pp. 716–717; Yad Vashem-YIVO *The Holocaust, The Nuremberg Evidence,* 237; Klee, *Deutsche Medizin im Dritten Reich*; Scharsach, *Die Ärzte der Nazis,* p. 119. A Dr. med. Anton Fehringer was a member of the NSDAP, SA, NSD-Ärztebund, and Ärztekammer Niederdonau (Niederdonau Physicians Chamber), per BDC A3340-RAK-010.

FINKE, DR. ERICH (Stabsarzt, Luftwaffe): doctor, associated with Kiel University; worked on freezing (hypothermia) experiments with Sigmund Rascher at Dachau; authored a comprehensive research report, "Freezing Experiments with Human Beings," which he delivered in Nuremberg at conference on casualties at sea and in wintertime, held 26–27 October 1942.[41]

FISCHER, DR. FRITZ ERNST (Waffen SS Sturmbannführer): physician and surgeon; 1935, joined the SS; 1936, received his medical degree from the University of Hamburg; 1939, joined the NSDAP and moved over into the Waffen SS; served first as a medical officer with a combat division; transferred to the SS Hospital at Hohenlychen as an assistant surgeon; worked at Hohenlychen with Prof. Karl Gebhardt on the effectiveness of sulfanilamide in gangrene; also conducted bone transplantation experiments at Ravensbrück. He was convicted at the Nuremberg Doctors' Trial, 20 August 1947, for war crimes in connection with the sulfanilamide and bone, nerve and muscle experiments; sentenced to life imprisonment but served only fifteen years.[42]

FLOSSNER, OTTO: Director of the Nutrition Physiology Department of the Reich's Health Department; served as an adviser on nutrition experiments in concentration camps.

FREITAG, DR.: Stabsarzt and Oberarzt in the Institut für Flugmedizin (Institute for Flight Medicine) of the Deutschen Versuchsanstalt für Luftfahrt, Berlin-Adlershof; research assistant to Siegfried Ruff.[43]

FUGGER, FRANZ (or ANDREAS): born, 1920 in Mettnitz, Austria; an SS Unterscharführer working at Auschwitz's Institute of Hygiene under Dr. Hans Muench; participated in malaria testing. After the war he changed his name to Creigher and lived in Friesnach/Kärnten.[44]

FUSSGAENGER (FUSSGÄNGER), DR.: doctor of medicine and natural philosophy; pharmacologist with I. G. Farbenindustrie A.G. Höchst; a consultant in experiments with I. G. Farbenindustrie drugs Akridin Granulate and Rutenol, carried out under SS auspices at Buchenwald; no evidence of membership in any NSDAP organization.[45]

41 Interrogation Summary No. 374 of Wolfram Sievers, 28 October 1946, YVA, JM/6027, p. 1; Interrogation of Dr. Siegfried Ruff, 22 October 1946, YVA, JM/6020, p. 21; Memorandum of Dr. Sigmund Rascher, 17 May 1943, Translation of Document No-230, in RG-30.001M, p. 2; Fischer, *Nazi Germany*, pp. 479–497; Klee, *Auschwitz*, p. 50.

42 Affidavit of Fritz Ernst Fischer, in *Nazi Conspiracy and Aggression*, vol. 8, pp. 635–42; Interrogation Summary No. 322 of Karl Gebhardt, 17 October 1946, YVA, JM/5979, p. 1; Interrogation of Herta Oberhauser, 31 October 1946, YVA, JM/6009, p. 8; Klee, *Auschwitz*, p. 153; Burman, ed., *The First German War Crimes Trial*, p. 186.

43 Interrogation of Dr. Siegfried Ruff, 22 October 1946, YVA, JM/6020, p. 23; Klee, *Auschwitz*, pp. 215, 236, 515.

44 Shelley, ed., *Criminal Experiments on Human Beings*, pp. 305, 324.

45 Opening Statement of Prosecutor Brig. General Telford Taylor, 9 December 1946, in *Trials NMT*, vol. 1, pp. 50–52; see also BDC A3340-RAK-012; and Kogon, *Theory and Practice of Hell*, p. 156.

GABERLE, DR. ALOIS: 1943–45, camp doctor at Sachsenhausen; participated in experiments testing poisonous ammunition and *Zyankali* (potassium cyanide) capsules on inmates; sentenced to three years, three months imprisonment by the Landesgericht Münster (district court) in 1962.[46]

GALNZKEN, DR. (SS Gruppenführer): a member of the Superior Committee dealing with typhus experiments in Buchenwald.[47]

GEBHARDT, PROF. DR. KARL (SS Gruppenführer, Waffen SS Generalleutnant; president of the German Red Cross): a pupil of the famous Lexer; school friend and medical advisor to Himmler; 1923, participated in the unsuccessful Munich Putsch; 1933, joined the NSDAP; 1935, joined the SS; 1933, appointed Chefarzt (Chief Physician) at Hohenlychen Hospital; 1940, appointed as consulting surgeon of the Waffen SS; 1943, served as chief clinical officer of the Reichsarzt SS und Polizei (Oberster Kliniker, Reichsarzt und Polizei); commissioned to find a cure for gangrene at Hohenlychen; in charge of sulfonamide tests and bone transplantations at Ravensbrück; helped to develop methods of mass sterilization; carried out brain experiments at Hohenlychen. Charged at the Nuremberg Doctors' Trial with war crimes in connection with the high altitude, freezing, malaria, *Lost* (mustard gas), sulfanilamide, bone, muscle and nerve transplantation, seawater, hepatitis, sterilization, typhus and incendiary bomb experiments. Sentenced to death by hanging at the Nuremberg Doctors' Trial and executed on 2 June 1948 at Landsberg Prison.[48]

GENZKEN (GENTZKEN), DR. KARL (SS Gruppenführer and Waffen SS Generalleutnant): born 8 June 1895, Preezt/Holstein; studied medicine in Marburg/Lahn; 1912, doctor of medicine and commissioned in the Medical Service of the German Navy; served throughout World War I; 1919–34, private medical practice in Preetz; 1926, joined the NSDAP; 1934, re-commissioned as a reserve officer in the Navy Medical Service; 1936, was transferred to the Medical Department of the SS; 1940, assigned to the branch which became the Waffen SS; served as chief surgeon of the SS Hospital in Berlin and director of the department charged with supplying medical equipment to, and the supervision of medical personnel in, the concentration camps; May 1940–end of the war, Chef des Sanitätsamtes der Waffen SS (Chief of the Medical Office of the Waffen

46 Klee, *Auschwitz*, pp. 51, 176.

47 Dr. Alfred Balachowsky, Statement Concerning Experiments and Research about Exanthematous Typhus at Buchenwald Camp, 24 May 1946, Translation of Document No-484, in RG-30.001M, p. 3.

48 Interrogation Summary No. 54 of Joachim Mrugowsky, 27 August 1946, YVA, JM/6006, p. 4; Interrogation of Herta Oberhauser, 31 October 1946, YVA, JM/6009, p. 4; Statement of Dr. Herta Oberhauser, Translation of Document No-487, in RG-30.001M, p. 3; IAC, *Inhuman Medicine*, vol. 1, pt. 1, pp. 38–39; Affidavit of Fischer, *Nazi Conspiracy and Aggression*, vol. 8, pp. 635–642; Klee, *Auschwitz*, pp. 152, 158; Burman, ed., *The First German War Crimes Trial*, pp. 123–138, 151–152, 227–230; "Nazi Doctors and Other Perpetrators of Nazi Crimes".

SS); involved in the camp experiments on humans, especially as supervisor of Dr. Joachim Mrugowsky in the typhus and malaria experiments (1940–43). A defendant in the Nuremberg Doctors' Trial, Genzken was found guilty of war crimes in connection with the sulfanilamide and typhus experiments. He was sentenced to life imprisonment on 20 August 1947; sentence was reduced to twenty years. Genzken was released in 1954.[49]

GERL, PROF. KARL: worked on producing synthetic insulin, with which he experimented on diabetic camp inmates.[50]

GILDEMEISTER, DR. EUGENE: president of the Robert Koch Institute; regularly visited the experimental station at Buchenwald to supervise typhus experiments.[51]

GLÜCKS, RICHARD (SS Gruppenführer): chief of Department D (Concentration camps) of the SS Wirtschaftsverwaltungshauptamt (WVHA); responsible for the overall administration of the concentration camps; subordinate to Oswald Pohl, the chief of the WVHA; supervisor of Dr. Enno Lolling, head of Department D III in the WVHA; according to Wolfram Sievers, Glücks and Pohl selected the inmate-subjects for the camp experiments.[52]

GOEBEL (GÖBEL), JOHANNES: born 1891 in Berlin; pharmacologist for the Schering company; served as an assistant in Claus Clauberg's sterilization experiments at Auschwitz and Ravensbrück; helped Clauberg improve the X-ray tracing material used in the experiments; died 8 November 1952 in Bremen.[53]

GOHRBANDT, DR. ERWIN: surgeon; Director of Surgery at the University Clinic of Berlin; the chief medical advisor for aeronautical medicine at the Luftwaffe's Sanitary Services Division; participated in hypothermia experiments in Dachau and published a report on them in a leading surgical journal.[54]

49 Interrogation of Joachim Mrugowsky, 27 August 1946, YVA, JM/6006, p. 2; Affidavit of Joachim Mrugowsky, 17 October 1946, Translation of Document No-423, in RG-30.001M, p. 2; Klee, *Auschwitz*, p. 140. See also Dörner, ed., *The Nuremberg Medical Trial*, p. 92; and Burman, ed., *The First German War Crimes Trial*, pp. 124, 131, 133–134, 150, 193, 195, 366.

50 Burman, ed., *The First German War Crimes Trial*, p. 224; Klee, *Auschwitz*, p. 182.

51 "Diary of the Division for Research for Spotted Fever and Virus at the Institute of Hygiene of the Waffen SS", Translation of Document No-265, in RG-30.001M, p. 2.

52 Interrogation of Wolfram Sievers, 28 October 1946, YVA, JM/6027, p. 5; Document No-179, Letter from Himmler to Grawitz, 15 May 1944; and www.deathcamps.org/reinhard/wvha.html.

53 Shelley, ed., *Criminal Experiments on Human Beings*, p. 324; "Nazi Doctors and Other Perpetrators of Nazi Crimes".

54 Annas and Grodin, eds., *The Nazi Doctors and the Nuremberg Code*, pp. 32–52.

GRÄFE (GRAEFE; also GRAFE), DR. MED. HELLMUT: Dr. Haagen's assistant at Natzweiler in experiments with typhus (spotted fever); experimented on Polish inmates; justified working with human subjects with the words: "They are Poles. They are really not human beings"; last served as Obersturmführer and Stabsarzt in the RSHA (Reichsicherheitshauptamt); died 28 June 1952 in Hamburg.[55]

GRAWITZ, PROF. DR. ERNST-ROBERT VON (SS Obergruppenführer and SS Reichsarzt): born 1899; an internist whose father was a noted hematologist with the same name; 1935, became Himmler's chief Gestapo physician; vice-president of the German Red Cross; responsible for medical experiments conducted within the SS; supplied Zyklon B to Auschwitz gas chambers; directed Dr. Karl Gebhardt and Dr. Fritz Ernst Fischer in the sulfanilamide experiments at the SS hospital in Hohenlychen; 1945, committed suicide.[56]

GRESE, IRMA: a guard at Auschwitz; known as the "Blond Angel of Death"; reportedly beat female prisoners to death and assisted in medical experiments; especially fond of breast removal operations; condemned to death after the war.[57]

GROSS, DR. KARL JOSEPH: worked at the SS Hygiene Institute in Berlin; oversaw vaccine experiments in Mauthausen; experimented with vaccinations as cures for typhoid, paratyphoid and cholera; after the Mauthausen experiments went to Blome's "Institut für Krebsforschung" (on the grounds of the former Kloster Nesselstedt) in Posen; the institute was, in reality, a center for research into methods of biological warfare.[58]

GUDACKER, DR. HEINZ: head of pathology at Buchenwald in 1940.[59]

GUTZEIT, PROF. DR. KURT (SS Hauptsturmführer): born 2 June 1893 in Berlin; a gastroenterologist; 1934, professor of medicine at the University of Breslau; hospital consultant to the Heeressanitätsinspekteur (Army Medical Service); NSDAP member; at Auschwitz conducted hepatitis experiments on Jewish children, with Dr. Arnold Dohmen as an assistant; rebuked Dohmen for being concerned about the ethics of experimenting on human beings. In this respect he is reported to have noted that it is odd how difficult it is for people to take the step from experimentation on animals to experimentation on humans, when humans are in the end the most important thing: "Komisch, wie schwer [bei Versuch] der Schritt vom Tier zum Menschen ist, aber

55 Mitscherlich and Mielke, eds., *Doctors of Infamy;* Klee, Auschwitz, p. 368 and 368 n. 79.
56 Affidavit of Oswald Pohl, 23 June 1946, Translation of Document No-065, in RG-30.001M, p. 1; Affidavit of Fritz Ernst Fischer, in *Nazi Conspiracy and Aggression*, vol. 8, pp. 635–642; Kater, *Doctors under Hitler*, pp. 5, 24, 113, 116, 183; Klee, *Auschwitz*, p. 140.
57 Snyder, *Encyclopedia of the Third Reich*, McGraw-Hill Book Company, New York, 1976.
58 Klee, *Auschwitz*, pp. 88, 162, 310.
59 Ibid., p. 51.

schliesslich und endlich ist das letztern ja doch die Hauptsache." After 1945, Gutzeit did not return to Breslau University, but directed the Sanatorium Herzoghöhe at Bayreuth and the Klinik Fürsterhof in Bad Wildungen; died 28 October 1957.[60]

HAAGEN, DR. EUGEN (Oberstabsarzt): immunologist and viral specialist; 1933, produced the yellow fever vaccine; before the war worked briefly in the United States for the Rockefeller Institute; 1936, was appointed as professor of the Robert Koch Institute in Berlin; 1941, appointed Professor of Hygiene and Bacteriology at the Reichsuniversität Strassburg (German University in Strasbourg); later became the director of the SS Institute of Hygiene; 1943, chief doctor (Oberstabsarzt) and consultant for hygiene for the Luftwaffe; "requested through Wolfram Sievers of the 'Ahnenerbe' that one hundred concentration camp prisoners made available to him for experimentation on the effectiveness of spotted fever vaccines"; carried out the experiments in Naztweiler; conducted further spotted fever vaccine experiments on 200 additional prisoners in the summer of 1944; also used camp inmates for tests of vaccines for yellow fever, influenza, epidemic jaundice, and cholera; carried out additional hepatitis experiments at Sachsenhausen.

In November 1944, with the Nazis retreating, Haagen transferred his laboratory to Saalfeld-an-der-Saale in Thuringia; was captured there in April 1945 by American troops; interned in France in an American POW camp; November 1945, was transferred to Nuremberg Prison; June 1946, released and returned to Saalfeld, in the Soviet sector; appointed director of the newly founded Institute of Research on Tumors and Viruses in the Soviet sector of Berlin; 16 November 1946, left the Soviet sector of the city for a visit to the British sector; was arrested; January 1947, was handed over to the French and sent to Strasbourg; was indicted for criminal experiments on concentration camp prisoners at Natzweiler; sentenced to death and executed in Metz, France.[61]

HAAS, DR. RICHARD: headed the "Emil v. Behring" Spotted Fever research Institute in Lemberg; supplied spotted fever vaccine made from the intestines of lice to Buchenwald for the typhus experiments.[62]

HAFERKAMP, DR. HANS: Born 3 July 1906 in Duisburg; studied medicine in Göttingen, Bonn, Köln, and Düsseldorf; 1932, licensed as a physician; physical therapist and nat-

60 For the quotation and some biographical details, see *Die Zeit* 40/2003, "Von deutschen Ruhm" at A-DBE, citing the entry "Kurt Gutzeit" in *Biographische Enzyklopedie deutschsprachiger Mediziner,* 2 vols. (K. G. Saur, 2002). See also *Trials NMT,* vol. 1, p. 495; Mitscherlich and Mielke, *The Death Doctors,* p. 165; Annas and Grodin, eds., *The Nazi Doctors and the Nuremberg Code,* pp. 32–52; Klee, *Auschwitz,* pp. 259–260.

61 Statement of Rudolph Brandt, 14 October 1946, Translation of Document No-370, in RG-30.001M, pp. 1–2; Letters of Dr. Eugen Haagen to Dr. August Hirt, Translation of Document No-121 and No-123, in RG-30.001M; Interrogation of Professor Dr. Oskar Schroeder, 2 October 1946, YVA, JM/6025, p. 40; *Trials NMT,* vol. 1, p. 495. Quotes are from Brandt's statement.

62 "Diary of the Division for Research for Spotted Fever and Virus at the Institute of Hygiene of the Waffen SS", Translation of Document No-265, in RG-30.001M, p. 3.

ural cures specialist who collaborated with Rascher on the search for cure of cancer; at Dachau 1942–44; also participated in the polygal experiments and published a report of the results in the *Münchener Medizinischer Wochenschrift* (28 January 1944), indicating that it was research from the Ahnenerbe's Institut für Wehrwissenschaftliche Zweckforschung (Institute for Military Scientific Research).[63]

HAFERKORN: worked with Rascher in cancer research and conducted experiments on blood-coagulation.[64]

HANDLOSER, PROF. DR. SIEGFRIED (Generaloberstabsarzt): born 25 March 1885 in Konstanz; father a music director; attended the Kaiser-Wilhelm-Akademie für das militärärztliche Bildungswesen in Berlin, to train as a military medicine specialist; 1910, passed the medical state exams; fought in World War I; in the interwar period, trained as an internal medicine specialist at Giessen University Clinic, then directed a hospital department of internal medicine; 1928–32, served as Referent des Heeressanitätsinspektion des Reichswehrministeriums (Army Medical Services Advisor in the Reich Ministry of Armed Forces); 1935–38, worked as a military physician in Stuttgart and Dresden; 1938, appointed Chief Medical Officer of the German forces in Austria; 1940, appointed Heeressanitätsinspekteur (Chief of Army Medical Services); 28 July 1942, acquired additional duties and power when Hitler issued a decree commissioning him as Chef des Wehrmachtssanitätswesens (Chief of Armed Forces Medical Services), which charged him with coordinating and unifying the operations of the medical branches of the Army, Luftwaffe, Navy and Waffen SS. Like Conti, his counterpart in civilian medicine, Handloser had to work with Hitler's powerful confident Karl Brandt.

Handloser was convicted at the Nuremberg Doctors' Trial of war crimes in connection with experiments on freezing (hypothermia), malaria, *Lost* (mustard gas), sulfanilamides, bone, nerve and muscle, seawater, infectious hepatitis, and typhus. Evidence showed that he was particularly involved in the experiments at Dachau and Buchenwald. He was sentenced to life imprisonment at Landsberg Prison in Bavaria on 20 August 1947; died 3 July 1954.[65]

HARTMAN (HARTMANN), DR.: a doctor at Hohenlychen; assisted Karl Gebhardt in the performance of experimental surgeries at Ravensbrück.[66]

63 Weindling, *Nazi Medicine and the Nuremberg Trials,* pp. 198–199; Dörner, ed., *The Nuremberg Medical Trial,* p. 96; Klee, *Auschwitz,* pp. 51, 352.

64 Interrogation Summary No. 40 of Wolfram Sievers, 17 August 1946, YVA, JM/6027, p. 2.

65 "Diary of the Division for Research for Spotted Fever and Virus at the Institute of Hygiene of the Waffen SS", Translation of Document No-265, in RG-30.001M, p. 1; Klee, *Auschwitz,* pp. 193, 254; Burman, ed., *The First German War Crimes Trial,* pp. 124, 129–133, 143–144, 366; "Nazi Doctors and Other Perpetrators of Nazi Crimes"; "Wikipedia, the Free Encyclopedia [German]".

66 Testimony of Vladislava Korolewka, National Archives Record Group 238, M887, p. 828, posted on the National Holocaust Memorial Museum Internet website.

HEFELMAN[N] (or HEVELMANN), DR. HANS: a collaborator of Viktor Brack's on sterilization experiments. Dr. Hans Hefelman[n], born 4 October 1906, Dresden, son of a cloth manufacturer; 1931, NSDAP member; July 1932, doctorate in agriculture; worked under Rudolf Hess in the economic service department; 1936, moved to Department IIB of the Kanzlei des Führers der NSDAP (Nazi Party Leaders' Chancellery) under Viktor Brack's supervision; led the "Reich Committee for research on Hereditary and Constitutional Susceptibility to Severe Diseases", under the auspices of which the children's euthanasia program was carried out; in Aktion T4, the euthanasia program, served as Viktor Brack's deputy; 1941, drafted into military service. Hefelman went underground near the war's end; escaped to Argentina; 1955, returned to the Federal Republic of Germany (BRD) as business manager of a southern German textile firm; 1960, turned himself in to Munich authorities and was imprisoned; 22 May 1962, Hefelman and Heyde (arrested November 1959) both found guilty of the murders of thousands of adults and children; 1964, testified in the abortive euthanasia trial at Limburg. Brack testified at Nuremberg that he and Dr. Hefelman had proposed resettling Jews as an alternative to mass extermination. Hefelman reportedly had suggested Madagascar as a suitable location.[67]

HEIM, ARIBERT (HERBERT) F.: conducted private experiments in Mauthausen; specialized in the production of preparations of human heads, some of which were exhibited at the Pathology Museum (Block 27) of KZ Mauthausen-Gusen. This museum contained human organs prepared in conjunction with the SS Medical Academy at the University of Graz. Heim reportedly sent some heads to friends as special gifts and used some specimens as paperweights in his office.

Ernst Klee reports under the name "Aribert Heim" the following: SS Hauptsturmführer; born 28 June 1914 in Radkersburg/Steier, Austria; studied medicine at the University of Graz; 1935, entered both the NSDAP and the SA; 1938, moved into the SS and April 1940, to the Waffen SS; April 1941, sent to Buchenwald; 1941/42 also at Mauthausen; gave intravenous injections of benzene, phenol, and harmful chemicals, and observed the speed at which these substances killed the patients; was called "The Death Doctor" because he performed operations without anaesthesia. After the war, Heim was fined 510,00 DM ("wird verurteilt zu einer Sühnemassnahme von 510,000 DM"), by a de-Nazification court (*Spruchkammer)* in Berlin because he had promoted Nazi rule through [the] murders at Mauthausen. In 1962, having been indicted for the killing of many hundreds of concentration camp inmates, he went into hiding; is believed to have lived in Germany, Denmark, Argentina, and Brazil. In October 2005 the international press reported that he has been traced to Spain.[68]

67 Interrogation Summary No. 40 of Viktor Brack, 13 September 1946, YVA, JM/5967, p. 2; Dörner, ed., *The Nuremberg Medical Trial,* p. 98; Klee, *Euthanasie,* pp. 77–78; Yad Vashem-YIVO The Holocaust, *The Nuremberg Evidence,* p. 252; Proctor, *Racial Hygiene,* pp. 186–187, 193, 206; Scharsach, *Die ärzte der Nazis,* p. 74; Weindling, *Health, Race, and German Politics,* p. 622; Declaration of Viktor Hermann Brack, 14 October 1946, Translation of Document No-426, in RG 30.001M, p. 3.

68 *Doctors of the Holocaust,* website; Klee, *Auschwitz,* pp. 37–39, including footnotes; *Los Angeles Times,* Section A, 16 October 2005.

HEISSMEYER (HEISMEYER), DR. KURT (Oberarzt): doctor from Sanderhausen/Thuringia; educated at Marburg, where he joined the anti-Semitic fraternity Arminia; 1933, licensed to practice medicine; trained in Freiburg, also at the Davos-Clavadel [TB] Clinic and at Berlin's Auguste-Victoria Hospital; an uncle, August Heissmeyer, was a general in the Waffen SS und Polizei. Dr. Heissmeyer served as head physician at Hohenlychen; also as assistant to Karl Gebhardt on the surgery wards; authored a 1943 paper "Principles of Present and Future Problems of TB Sanatoriums", which argued that racial factors determine TB resistance and should be used to tailor specific treatments; spring 1944, proposed a series of TB experiments, to be conducted at Hohenlychen using patients as subjects. The Nazi leadership approved the proposal but moved the experiments to the Neuengamme concentration camp near Hamburg. Heissmeyer traveled to Neuengamme for the experiments, whose first subjects were inmate adults and final subjects, the children murdered at the SS's satellite camp Bullenhuser Damm. In April 1945, he fled to his parents' home; then moved to Magdeburg, opened a practice for lung diseases and practiced until his arrest in 1963.

A 1959 article in *Stern* magazine, which admonished Germans to teach their children about the Nazi atrocities and mentioned Bullenhuser Damm as an example of what should not be forgotten, spurred the discovery and arrest of Heissmeyer by East German authorities on charges of crimes against humanity. Although he originally denied charges, Heissmeyer eventually led interrogators to a cache of documents buried on the grounds of his former Hohenlychen home. His trial was 21–30 June 1966; sentence, life in prison; death, fourteen months later, of a heart attack.[69]

HILLMANN, DR. GÜNTHER: affiliated with the Kaiser-Wilhelm-Institut für Biochemie; Adolf Butenandt was his superior during the time of the Auschwitz experiments. Hillmann participated in comparative studies of proteins (Eiweiss) in racial groups, which used blood samples taken from inmates at Auschwitz. The experiments were sponsored by the Deutschen Forschungsgemeinschaft (DFG), directed by Verschuer, and carried out at Auschwitz by Mengele. After the war, Hillmann became an Associate Professor in Tübingen and later President of the German Society for Clinical Chemistry.[70]

HINTERMAYER, DR. FRITZ: the Erster Lagerarzt (chief doctor) at Dachau, in charge of carrying out the seawater experiments; sentenced to death by the General Military Court at Dachau on 12 December 1945.[71]

69 Declaration of Oswald Pohl, undated, YVA, JM/6013, p. 3; Affidavit of Oswald Pohl, 23 June 1946, Translation of Document No-065, in RG-30.001M, p. 2; Schwarzberg, *Murders at Bullenhuser Damm,* p. 3; Steven G. Friedman, "Terrorists in Hamburg in Redux", *Midstream: A Monthly Jewish Journal,* April 2002, at www.midstreamhf.com/200204/feature.html.

70 Müller-Hill, *Murderous Science,* pp. 72–73, and "Genetics After Auschwitz", *Holocaust Genocide Studies,* 2: 1 (1987), p. 8; Klee, *Auschwitz,* pp. 458–459.

71 Direct Examination of Dr. Franz Blaha, Military Government Court, Dachau, Germany, November 2, 1945, YVA, JM/10047, p. 9; UNWCC, p. 535; Klee, *Auschwitz,* p. 52.

HIPPKE, DR. ERICH: Generaloberstabsarzt and Inspekteur des Sanitätswesen der Luftwaffe (Chief of Medical Affairs of the Luftwaffe and Inspector of Medical Affairs); in charge of all aviation-related medical research; served as a troop medic in World War I; was associated before the Nazi era with the Hygiene Institute in Berlin and worked at various posts in Germany as a military hygienist; 1935, transferred to the Luftwaffe and began his rise to the top; left his posts on 31 December 1943; replaced by Oskar Schroeder; went into the Hitler Reserve; retired before war's end; provided testimony for the American Military Tribunal in the Milch case, as a witness for the defendant; was mentioned in the case as having ordered Rascher to undertake the Dachau research; went underground after the trial; died 1969 in Bonn.[72]

HIRT, PROF. DR. AUGUST (SS Hauptsturmführer): associated with the University of Tübingen (Allgem): affiliated with the factory Knoll AG, at Ludwigshafen, where he reportedly worked on penicillin; 1941–44, appointed chairman of the anatomy department at the University of Strasbourg; expert on cancer research and treatments for *Lost* (mustard gas) poisoning; 1942, began collecting skeletons of Jewish prisoners for the Ahnenerbe with assistance from Dr. Arno (Bruno) Berger [also known as Bruno Beger]. The collection was intended to demonstrate the superiority of the Nordic races. Before the arrival of French troops in Strasbourg, part of the collection was moved, according to some sources, to Schloss Mittersill in Salzburger Land, where Hirt's assistant Bruno Beger was stationed. Hirt was arrested at Strasbourg at the end of 1944 by French forces; 2 June 1945, committed suicide at Schonenbach/Neustadt.[73]

HOFFMAN, DR. HELMUT: a research assistant at Sachsenhausen, where Dr. Albert Widmann conducted mass killing experiments on Russian POWs; employed by Bayer-Leverkusen after the war.[74]

HOHLFELDER, PROF. DR. HANS (SS Standartenführer and Colonel in the Waffen SS Reserve): born 22 April 1891 in Wernigerode/Harz; 1915, received his medical license and appointed director of the Radiology Institute of the University of Frankfurt-am-Main; 1933, NSDAP membership; 1934, joined the SS; 1937, elected honorary member of the Royal Society; 1943, *Ordinarius* (professor) for radiology at the Reich University

72 Interrogation of Dr. Siegfried Ruff, 28 September 1946, YVA, JM/6020, pp. 2–3; Klee, *Auschwitz*, p. 253. See the article on the internet at http://www.geocities.com/ /~onion47/WEHRMACHT/LUFTWAFFE/Sanitäts Offizier/HIPPKE_Erich.html, for more details on Hippke's career and the report of his death date. For his testimony in the Milch case, see the transcripts of the American Military Tribunals at Nuremberg posted by the Mazal Library as the Green Series on the web at www.mazal.org/archive/nmt/02/ NMT02-t0875.html.

73 Interrogation Summary No. 39 of Wolfram Sievers, 16 August 1946, YVA, J/M6027, p. 3; Interrogation Summary No. 48 of Wolfram Sievers, 20 August 1946, YVA, J/M6027, p. 3; Declaration of Wolfram Sievers, Evaluation Report No. 98, Combined Intelligence Objectives Subcommittee, 13 June 1945, YVA J/M10046, p. 2; Mitscherlich and Mielke, eds., *Doctors of Infamy*, p. 214; Klee, *Auschwitz*, p. 360 n. 47; "Jewish Virtual Library".

74 "Nazi Doctor Database".

of Posen; chief of the SS-Röntgensturmbann (SS X-ray battalion) at Waffen SS Operational Headquarters Northeast; participated in experiments with X-ray examination of Polish TB patients in the Warthegau; also assisted with X-ray-sterilization experiments carried out on Jewish males; killed in battle, December 1944, on the German-Russian front.[75]

HOLLER, DR.: April-May 1943, tested Rutenol and Nitroacridin 3582 as typhus treatments at the Department for Spotted Fever and Virus Research of the Hygienic Institute of the Waffen SS, the SS experimental station in Buchenwald.[76]

HOLZ (HOLTZ), PROF. PETER: worked on cancer research with Rascher and Blohme.[77]

HOLZLÖHNER, PROF. DR. ERNST (Oberstabsarzt): professor of physiology in the medical school at the University of Kiel; Oberstabsarzt in the Luftwaffe Medical Corps, subordinate to the Luftwaffe Sanitary Inspectorate; worked with Sigmund Rascher on the high altitude and hypothermia experiments at Dachau; co-authored (with Dr. Finke) a research report called "Freezing Experiments on Human Beings", which he delivered at a Nuremberg conference on 26–27 October 1942; committed suicide after the war.[78]

HOOS, DR.: head of the Criminal Technical Institute (Kriminaltechnisches Institut or KTI) in Department V (RKPA) of the Reich Security Police Headquarters (Reichsicherheitspolizeihauptamt or RSHA); the KTI was an SS institute especially devoted to providing scientific aid (Hilfsmittel) in the fight against crime. Hoos recommended a drug derived from the plant *Plauderdoge* tried on camp inmates.[79]

HOVEN, DR. WALDEMAR (Waffen SS Hauptsturmführer): born 1903, Freiburg-im-Breisgau, into a wealthy family and hence able to travel in the Scandinavian countries and the U.S.; tried his hand at journalism in Paris; nicknamed "Babyface"; 1933, assumed his father's post as director of a sanatorium and began medical studies; 1934,

75 Dörner, ed., *The Nuremberg Medical Trial,* p. 103; *Trials NMT,* vol. 1, pp. 728, 775–776, 782–783, 794; Kater, *Doctors Under Hitler,* p. 130; Klee, *Deutsche Medizin im Dritten Reich,* pp. 135–137; IAC, *Inhuman Medicine,* vol. 1, pt. 1, p. 39; Memo from SS Obersturmbannführer Brandt, July 1942, in *Trials NMT,* vol. 1, p. 728; Affidavit of Rudolf Brandt, 24 October 1946, in Ibid, p. 775; Letter from Greiser to Himmler, 1 May 1942, in Ibid, p. 776; also Ibid, pp. 782–783, 794.

76 Dr. Erwin Ding [-Schuler], "On Treatment of Typhus with Acridin Derivatives", Translation of Document No-582, in RG-30.001M, pp. 2, 8–11.

77 Interrogation Summary No. 40 of Wolfram Sievers, 17 August, 1946, YVA, JM/6027, p. 2.

78 Cross Examination of Wolfram Sievers, 9 August 1946, in *Trial IMT,* vol. 20, p. 537; Interrogation of Dr. Hermann Becker-Freyseng, 12 November 1946, YVA, JM/5964, pp. 8–9; Klee, *Auschwitz,* pp. 236, 252; "Nazi Doctors and Other Perpetrators of Nazi Crimes", website.

79 For general background on the biological and natural scientific theories that supported Nazi approaches to crime, and on the application of these ideas in Nazi organizational structures, see Karsten Eule and Marco Siegert, *Kriminalistik im System der Kriminalwissenschaften,* on the web at www.marco-siegert.de/projektarbeit/KAP-03.htm.

joined the SS; 1937, joined the NSDAP; 1939, first appointment at Buchenwald as an assistant medical officer in the SS Hospital; 1941–43, served at Buchenwald as chief doctor of the hospital and worked with Dr. Erwin Ding on the typhus experiments. Carried out tuberculosis experiments for his dissertation (doctorate/University of Freiburg); also experimented with carbon monoxide, engaged in torture and gave patients lethal injections.

In 1943, he was removed from his position for a "finance swindle" and then arrested (September 1943) after he killed the man (Obersharführer Kohler) who had reported the financial wrongdoing; tried and sentenced to twenty months in prison for that crime. Hoven was one of the twenty-three defendants at the Doctors' Trial in Nuremberg. He was charged with war crimes in connection with the typhus experiments and euthanasia program and found guilty; sentenced 20 August 1947 to death by hanging and executed 2 June 1948 at Landsberg Prison in Bavaria.[80]

HUEBNER, PROF. WOLFGANG: participated in experiments at Dachau.[81]

JENSEN, DR. CARL PETER (CARL VAERNET): a Danish physician who called himself Carl Vaernet in Germany; conducted hormone research at Mauthausen; experimented with the implantation of artificial hormone-producing glands; was especially interested in trying to "cure" homosexuality; fled to Argentina after the war; may have worked in health administration in Buenos Aires.[82]

JUETTNER, DR. HANS: worked on the development of *Endstoff* (poison gas); also conducted diet experiments under the supervision of Prof. Dr. Ernst-Günther Schenk.[83]

KAHR, DR. KARL (SS Obersturmführer): graduate *(Absolvent)* of the SS Ärztliche Akademie in Graz, a training center for SS doctors; graduates of this institution were sent to Dachau concentration camp for further training. Kahr conducted polygal and surgical experiments at Dachau.[84]

KALK, PROF. HEINZ (Oberstabsarzt): worked with Dr. Eugen Haagen on hepatitis experiments at Sachsenhausen.[85]

80 Affidavit of Ferdinand Roemhild, Translation of Document No-434, in RG-30.001M, p. 1; Declaration of Gerhard Schiedlausky, 7 August 1945, Translation of Document No-508, in RG-30.001 M, p. 29; Hoedeman, *Hitler or Hippocrates; Trials NMT,* vol. 1, p. 685; "Nazi Doctors and Other Perpetrators of Nazi Crimes"; and Burman, ed., *The First German War Crimes Trial,* pp. 127, 133, 135, 177–178, 365.

81 Klee, *Auschwitz,* p. 246.

82 Klee, *Auschwitz,* pp. 163, 166; Hackett, *The Buchenwald Report,* pp. 369–371.

83 Interrogation Summary No. 39 of Wolfram Sievers, 16 August 1946, YVA, JM/6027, p. 4.

84 Klee, *Auschwitz,* pp. 34, 53; see also Translation of Document No-656, Memo from Kahr to Rascher, 10 December 1943.

85 *Trials NMT,* vol. 1, p. 496.

KASCHUB, DR. HEINZ: conducted experiments at Auschwitz with toxic substances applied to the skin; studied symptoms of liver disease.[86]

KATZENELLENBOGEN, DR. EDWIN: a former American found working at Buchenwald; originally one of the prosecution witnesses at the trial of Buchenwald staff (U.S. vs. Josias Erbprinz zu Waldeck-Pyrmont); eventually became one of the accused and was sentenced to life imprisonment for participation in the Buchenwald experiments; in America, had been a Harvard lecturer on abnormal psychology and a fellow for research in logic.[87]

KIESELBACH (KIESSELBACH), PROF. DR. ANTON (Unterarzt der Reserve): born 13 June 1907 in Kempenich/Rheinland; SA member; 1937, listed in the NSDAP membership; 1937–41, student of Dr. August Hirt at the Anatomical Institute/Greifswald; 1941, received medical license and drafted; stationed in the reserve military hospital at Oberhof/Thuringen. Although Kiesselbach was implicated in Hirt's crimes (especially the experiments with *Lost,* i.e., mustard gas, at Natzweiler), having been named as Hirt's assistant at Natzweiler and at Abteilung H in the "Ahnenerbe's Institut für Wehrwissenschaftliche Zweckforschung", he was never brought to trial; 1955, appointed professor of anatomy at the Anatomical Institute of the Medical University of Düsseldorf; 1960s, director of the University Medical School. Kieselbach was investigated in 1963–64, but charges were not filed against him.[88]

KIESEWETTER, DR. HERMANN: a physician from Magdeburg, experienced in bio-chemical research who was transferred by Grawitz from Magdeburg to Dachau; an SS member until 1938, requested reinstatement in May 1941; conducted phlegmone experiments, resulting in the deaths of hundreds of prisoners; conducted vivisections on prisoners to observe the human brain in action; worked at Dachau and Mauthausen; disappeared after the war, possibly to East Berlin.[89]

86 Klee, *Auschwitz,* p. 53.

87 Proctor, *Racial Hygiene,* pp. 298–299; "Dachau Scrapbook: Buchenwald".

88 Dörner, ed., *The Nuremberg Medical Trial,* p. 108; Kater, *Doctors Under Hitler,* p. 237, 360, n. 8 and *Das Ahnenerbe der SS 1935–1945,* pp. 248 and 426 n. 242.

89 Affidavit of Dr. Franz Blaha, Document 3249-PS, Exhibit No. USA-663, in *Trial IMT,* vol. 5, p. 171; Letter of Theodor Laue, SS Standartenführer, undated, Translation of Document No-408, in RG-30.001M, p. 2; Klee, *Auschwitz,* pp. 35 and 35 n. 83, 53, 146 and 146 n.19, 149. Klee, op. cit., p. 35 n. 83, reveals that Kiesewetter is supposed to have settled in East Berlin after 1945 ("Er soll nach 1945 in Qstberlin leben"). Kiesewetter was a member of the SS until March 1939, when he resigned; in 1941 he sought reinstatement, but Klee does not indicate whether or not his request was granted. There is confusion in sources about Hermann Kiesewetter and Rudolf Kiesswetter.

Theodor Laue, in the source cited above, says that a Hermann Kiesewetter, physician from Magdeburg, experienced in biochemical medicine and research, was transferred by Grawitz from Magdeburg to Dachau to partake in the experiments; Klee (op. cit., p. 146 and 146 n.19), notes that the Landesgericht (district court) in Munich could not judge whether

KIESEWETTER, DR. RUDOLF: experimented at Dachau with mineral salts as a therapy for sepsis; disappeared after the war. See the notes for comments about problems identifying and distinguishing Hermann Kiesewetter from Rudolf Kiesswetter.[90]

KITT, DR. BRUNO: born 1906; SS camp physician at Auschwitz, June 1942 until the evacuation; January 1945, moved to Neuengamme. Kitt is one of the men reported to have used human flesh in preparing the medium for bacterial cultures at the Rajsko Hygiene Institute. In May 1946 Kitt was sentenced to death by a British tribunal for crimes committed in Neuengamme; he was executed on 10 August 1946.[91]

KLEIN, DR. FRITZ: born 1888; served as a camp physician in Auschwitz from December 1943 to December 1944; then went to Neuengamme and Bergen-Belsen; at Auschwitz, Klein was initially Mengele's superior; with Mengele, he conducted experiments on dwarfs; did some experiments with petrol, benzene, pastes and powders; was sentenced 17 November 1945 by a British tribunal to death by hanging; sentence executed at Hamelin, on 13 December 1945.[92]

KLEIN, DR. HANS: chief pathologist at Hohenlychen; collaborator of Dr. Kurt Heissmeyer; analyzed glands removed from under the arms of children used in TB experiments, sent by Heissmeyer from Neuengamme, where children were being used as subjects for experiments; autopsied deceased subjects; not pursued after the war; became an instructor in forensic medicine at the Institut für gerichtliche Medizin (Institute for Forensic Medicine), Universität Heidelberg.[93]

KOLLER, DR.: worked with Dr. Kurt Heissmeyer on experiments at Hohenlychen.[94]

---

the man in question was a Dr. Kiesewetter or Kiesswetter. He also notes, without providing a date, that the Reichmedizinalkalendar officially lists a Rudolf Kiesswetter in Magdeburg. Given the lack of clarity in sources and the similarities in careers (both are listed as disappearing after the war; both worked at Dachau), it must be asked whether Hermann Kiesewetter and Rudolf Kiesswetter are perhaps the same individual, or in some way related. Perhaps Kiesewetter's request for reinstatement into the SS might have resulted in a transformation of names; perhaps the problem is one of simple transcription error.

Kiesewetter originally resigned from the SS in 1938 because his fiancée had a congenital hip problem on the list of conditions not acceptable in SS men or their families. He notes this in his 1941 request for reinstatement (Klee, op. cit., p. 35, citing "Antrag Kiesewetter [20 May 1941] an SS-Führungshauptamt. DC Unterlagen Kiesewetter").

90 Klee, op. cit., pp. 53, 146–147.

91 Shelley, ed., *Criminal Experiments on Human Beings*, pp. 315, 328; Klodzinski, in IAC, *Inhuman Medicine*, vol. 1, pt. 2, p. 165; Klee, op. cit., p. 53.

92 Declaration of Elisabeth Ovitz-Moskovitz, undated, YVA, 0.33/4334, p. 2; Shelley, ed., *Criminal Experiments on Human Beings*, p. 328; Klee, op. cit., p. 53; Aziz, *Doctors of Death*, vol. 2, p. 82; UNWCC, p. 535.

93 See Friedman, "Terrorists in Hamburg Redux", *Midstream: A Monthly Jewish Journal*, April 2002, posted at www.midstreamhf.com/200204/feature.html; also Schwarzberg, *The Murders at Bullenhuser Damm*, p. 28.

94 Affidavit of Fritz Ernst Fischer, 19 November 1945, Document No-228, in RG-30.001M, p. 13.

KÖNIG, DR. HANS WILHELM: SS physician; born 1912 in Stuttgart; served as a camp physician in Auschwitz; conducted experiments on dwarfs with Josef Mengele, used phenol to kill sick and healthy political prisoners, experimented with electric shock, and castrated young Jewish boys; supervised "selections" at Auschwitz. "His last known residence was in Holt-Colnrade. On May 4, 1945, his wife, Mrs. Dagmar Kalling-König, reported him dead. Dagmar is Swedish and lives in Uppsala. All inquiries as to whether Dr. König is living in Sweden have been unsuccessful, although the likelihood of his living there is very great."[95]

KÖNIG, DR. KARL: cooperated with Prof. Gerhard Rose in testing the efficacy of new synthetic remedies against malaria.[96]

KREBSBACH, DR. EDUARD: SS doctor, Chefarzt des SS und Polizei at Linz, Steyr, Wels, and KZ Mauthausen-Gusen; used injections to the heart to execute ill and unfit prisoners; nicknamed Dr. Spritzbach (Dr. Injection); transferred to Warwara after he shot a German soldier who had annoyed him; carried out selections and the liquidation of that camp in August 1944.[97]

KREIBICH, DR. EDUARD: sent in 1942 to Oranienburg/Sachsenhausen; was present for the tests in 1944/45, in which camp prisoners were killed with *Zyankali* capsules, then cremated.[98]

KREIENBERG, PROF. WALTER: a physiologist; conducted pressure-chamber (high altitude) research for the Luftwaffe. After the war, he became a professor of physiology at the newly established University of Mainz in 1948; received his first West German national award (Bundesverdienstkreuz) in 1971 and an upgraded one in 1977; was awarded the highest possible citation of that order in 1984; and was the recipient of the Paracelsus-Medaille (presented to him, as it had been to Albert Schweitzer earlier, by the German medical establishment) in 1987.[99]

KREMER, PROF. DR. MED. ET PHIL. JOHANN PAUL (SS Obersturmführer): born in 1883 in Etelberg; received both an M.D. and a Ph.D.; physician of the Waffen SS; assistant pro-

95 Declaration of Elisabeth Ovitz-Moskovitz, undated, YVA, 0.33/4334, p. 2; Declaration of Jakov Freimark, undated, YVA, 0.33/4334, p. 1; Declaration of Dr. Naum Wortman, undated, YVA, 0.33/4334, p. 2; Eva Mozes Kor, "Nazi Experiments as Viewed by a Survivor of Mengele's Experiments," in Arthur L. Caplan, ed., *When Medicine Went Bad,* p. 4; IAC, *Inhuman Medicine,* vol. 1, pt. 1, p. 116; Shelley, ed., *Criminal Experiments on Human Beings,* p. 329.

96 Extracts from Report of Professor Dr. E. Gildemeister Concerning the Activities of the Robert Koch Institute – Reich Institute for the Fight Against Infectious Diseases, Partial Translation of Rose Document II, Rose Defense Exhibit 27, in *Trial IMT,* vol. 1, p. 298.

97 "Jewish Virtual Library".

98 Klee, *Auschwitz,* pp. 54, 176 and 176 n.117.

99 Kater, *Doctors Under Hitler,* p. 2.

fessor at the University of Münster; 30 August 1942 to 18 November 1942, worked at Auschwitz; at the Block 28 clinic, main camp, was responsible for assessing prisoners seeking admission to the camp hospital and empowered to order euthanization; the killings were disguised as experiments; factors considered in selecting "subjects" included criminal history, medical history, and presence of the "Musselman state" (near death from starvation); some subjects were photographed; most were killed by phenol injection; Kremer ordered sections from the liver, pancreas and spleen so that he could study the effects of starvation on these organs.

Kremer was tried at the Auschwitz Trial in November–December 1947, with his diary and depositions as part of the evidence against him. The diary revealed that Kremer was involved in several so-called *Sonderaktionen* (special actions), in addition to the selections, in which prisoners were killed. In the matter of the mass exterminations, Kremer argued that he had not been directly involved, but the camp commandant, Rudolf Höss, maintained that there was no reason to assume that Kremer's duties had differed from those of any other SS doctor (supervision of the gassings and determination of the moment at which gas-chamber doors could be opened). The number of his victims could not be determined. Kremer was found guilty of war crimes and sentenced to death; sentence was commuted to life imprisonment. On 29 November 1960, a German Federal Republic court further reduced the sentence to ten years, with loss of civil rights for five years; the prisoner died in 1965.[100]

KUHN, PROF. DR. RICHARD: born 1900, in Vienna; educated at the Universities of Vienna and Munich; 1922, D. Phil. for work on enzymes; 1926–29, taught general and analytic chemistry in Zürich at the Eidgenössische Technische Hochschule; 1929, assumed responsibilities in Heidelberg in the chemistry institute that eventually was linked with other institutes to form the Kaiser-Wilhelm Institut für Medizinische Forschung (after 1950, the Max Planck Institut für Medizinische Forschung); was awarded the 1938 Nobel prize in chemistry for his research with enzymes, especially vitamins B2 and B6; could not accept the prize until after the war due to Nazi regime restrictions; recommended the addition of the food supplements Biosyn and Mycel to concentration camp diets; participated in a conference in which the results of the camp research were presented; experimented with the "sulfa" drugs Eugasin, Eleudron and Prontonsil; after the war, director of the Max Planck Institute for Medical Research; 1948–1966, sat as senator of the institute's governing organization, the Max Planck Gesellschaft; honorary senator thereafter.[101]

LAUCK, DR.: assistant to Klaus Schilling in Dachau (1944–45).[102]

100 "Jewish Virtual Library"; IAC, *Inhuman Medicine*, vol. 1, pt. 2, p. 116.
101 Declaration of Wolfram Sievers, Evaluation Report No. 98, Combined Intelligence Objectives Subcommittee, June 13, 1945, YVA, JM/10046, p. 2. On the nutrition conference, see Klee, *Auschwitz*, pp. 179–189.
102 Klee, op. cit., p. 54.

LAUER, PROF. DR. THEODOR (also LAUE): SS Standartenführer; was one of the participants in the Dachau sepsis/phlegmone experiments that caused 600–800 deaths; he was also instrumental in initiating the experiment to compare allopathic and homeopathic approaches in the treatment of phlegmone.[103]

LAUTENSCHLÄGER, PROF. EUGENE: employed at I. G. Farbenindustrie A.G. in Frankfurt; worked on typhus vaccines and therapeutic drugs; requested tests of vaccine and of the compounds Acridine Granulate and Rutenol on prisoners at Buchenwald; met with Drs. Ding, Weber, and Fussgänger about the experiments.[104]

LEMBEL: carried out hepatitis experiments.[105]

LESSER, DR. THEODOR: chemist and physician who collaborated with Dr. Wilhelm Beigelboeck on the Dachau seawater experiments.[106]

LETZ, DR. FRIEDRICH: took part in Dr. Otto Bickenbach's phosgene research with prisoners as subjects.[107]

LEWE, DR. VIKTOR: chief pathologist for research at Buchenwald and (1941–42) Sachsenhausen.[108]

LOCKEMANN, PROF. DR. GEORG: chemist affiliated with the Robert Koch Institute; role in testing on human subjects a drug called Orthromin.[109]

LOLLING, DR. ENNO (DOLLING): born 1888 in Cologne; chief of Department D III in the Wirtschaftsverwaltungshauptamt (WVHA, Office of Economic Policy) of the SS. The WVHA, headed by Oswald Pohl was responsible for administration, economic and construction affairs of the SS. It was divided into five departments, A–E. Department D, which was headed by Richard Glücks, was responsible for the administration of the

103 Affidavit of Dr. Franz Blaha, Document 3249-PS, Exhibit No. USA-663, in *Trial IMT,* vol. 5, p. 171; Klee, *Auschwitz,* pp. 146–147, text and notes. Two names appear in documents, Laue and Lauer. It is likely that these are variant spellings of the same name, though the documentary evidence is confusing.

104 Dr. Alfred Balachowsky, "Statement Concerning Experiments and Research about Exanthematous Typhus at Buchenwald Camp", 24 May 1946, Translation of Document No-484, in RG-30.001M, p. 14; "Diary of the Division for Research for Spotted Fever and Virus at the Institute of Hygiene of the Waffen SS", Translation of Document No-265, in RG-30.001M, p. 5. See also "The Mazal Archives". www.mazal.org/archives/nmt/01/nmt052.

105 *Trial IMT,* vol. 1, p. 499.

106 Interrogation Summary No. 240 of Dr. Konrad Wilhelm Philipp Schaefer, 4 October 1946, YVA, JM/6021, p. 2.

107 Hoedeman, *Hitler or Hippocrates,* p. 149.

108 Klee, *Auschwitz,* p. 54.

109 Testimony of W. Hoven, 24 October 1946, in *Trial IMT,* vol. 1, pp. 555–631, especially p. 567.

concentration camps. Of the four subdivisions in Department D, the third (III), called Sanitätswesen und Lagerhygiene (Camp Medical Services and Hygiene), directed by Dr. Lolling, was responsible for administering all medical and dental services in the camps.

As director of D III, Lolling provided an important link between the camps and the central administration of the SS. He was involved in Rascher's high altitude experiments at Dachau; the Zyankali (potassium cyanide) capsule and typhus vaccine experiments at Ravensbrück; collected human skin from all of the concentration camps for his own personal study; committed suicide on 27 May 1945, in the military hospital in Flensburg.[110]

LUCAS, DR. FRANZ BERNHARD: graduate of the SS Akademie in Graz, which was a training center for SS doctors; served at Auschwitz, Mauthausen, Struthof, Ravensbrück and Sachsenhausen; participated in sterilizations at Ravensbrück; assisted with the liquidation of the Gypsy camp at Auschwitz; after the war served as director of gynecology at Elmshorn Hospital; 1965, sentenced to three years, three months imprisonment in the Auschwitz Trials.[111]

MAGNUSSEN, DR. KARIN: assistant to Prof. Otmar Freiherr von Verschuer (director of the Kaiser Wilhelm Institute of Human Genetics and Eugenics in Berlin-Dahlem); assigned to study the anomaly of heterochromia in twins, using eyes from twins murdered by Mengele at Auschwitz.[112]

MADAUS, DR. GERHARD: an advocate of folk medicine, including homeopathy and "natural" means of healing; founder of the Biological Institute of Dr. Madaus in Dresden-Radebeul, directed by E. Koch, Ph.D. and M.D.; the institute published works on folk medicine and natural healing; the Madaus Annual Report of 1940 reported on the efficacy of the North American plant *caladium seguinium* (dumbcane) in sterilizing animals; report came to the attention of Dr. Fehringer, whose District Office for Racial Policy was investigating ways to reduce the unwanted minority populations in the Reich; Madaus was tapped for the human sterilization experiments at Auschwitz, using both medicinal and x-ray approaches. As examples of the Madaus publications, see G. Madaus, *Heilkunst: Monatszeitschrift für Psychotherapie, Medizin- und Naturheilkraft,* Jahrgang 4/5 (1920–24); Madaus, ed., *Abgekürzte homöopathische Pharmakopöe... nach Prof. W. Ostwald* (Radebeul: Selbstverl., 1931); *Aufwärts zur biologischen*

110 Interrogation of Wolfram Sievers, 28 October 1946, YVA, JM/6027, pp. 1, 6; Translation of Document No-008, in RG-30.001M, p. 1; Shelley, ed., *Criminal Experiments on Human Beings,* p. 330; "Nazi Doctors and Other Perpetrators of Nazi Crimes"; Weindling, *Nazi Medicine and the Nuremberg Trials,* pp. 39, 54; Dörner, ed., *The Nuremberg Medical Trial,* p. 115; for the WVHA and Lolling, see www.deathcamps.org/reinhard/wvha.html.

111 Klee, op. cit., pp. 34, 54 and 54 n.180, 467.

112 Astor, *The Last Nazi,* p. 98.

Therapie... (Radebeul: Madaus, 1934); *Taschenbuch für die biologische Praxis* (Radebeul-Dresden: Madaus, 1933).[113]

MAY, PROF. DR. EDUARD: assistant professor at the University of Munich; head of the Ahnenerbe's Institute of Entomology, which was located in Dachau; conducted malaria experiments; Wolfram Sievers testified that Himmler ordered the results of Schilling's malaria experiments passed on to Dr. May, but that Schilling refused to cooperate. The testimony also indicates that Himmler ordered two rooms at Dr. May's institute set aside for chemical and physiological experiments to be conducted by the Luftwaffe.[114]

MENGELE, DR. JOSEF: physician and member of the Waffen SS; performed medical experiments at Auschwitz, Gross-Rosen and Mauthausen; born 16 March 1911 in the southern German village of Günzberg; father a wealthy factory owner. In his twenties, Mengele studied anthropology in Munich at Ludwig Maximilian University, earning his doctorate in physical anthropology in 1935, then entered medical school (M.D., 1938, from Leipzig's Wolfgang Goethe University Hospital). His theses, "Racial Morphological Examinations of the Lower Frontal Jaw in Four Racial Groups" and "Examinations in Cases of Cleft Lips, Jawbones and Palates", were both published.

During his university years, Mengele served as a local leader of the national organization Stahlhelm (Steel Helmets), which was dedicated to the preservation of "Old Mother Germany". In 1939, he was drafted into the Wehrmacht and transferred quickly to the Waffen SS; served four years on the eastern front, then was sent to Auschwitz, where he stood on the ramp selecting twins and others for his medical experiments. He left Auschwitz as the Red Army was approaching, and finished out the war at Gross-Rosen and Mauthausen.

After the war, a long list of pseudonyms allowed Mengele to conceal his identity, among them: Helmut Gregor; G. Helmut; Fritz Ulmann; Fritz Hollmann; Jose Mengele; Peter Hochbeider; Ernst Sebastian Alvez; Jose Astiazi; Lars Ballstrem; Friedrich Edler von Breitenbach; Fritz Fischer; Karl Geuske; Ludwig Gregor; Stanislas Brosky; Fausto

113 "Nazi Doctors and Other Perpetrators of Nazi Crimes"; Dörner, ed., *Nuremberg Medical Trial*, p. 117; letters from Brandt to Pohl, Pohl to Himmler, and Gund to Himmler, in *Trials NMT*, vol. 1, pp. 715–718; Annas and Grodin, eds., *The Nazi Doctors and the Nuremberg Code*, p. 79; Carsten Timmermann, "Rationalizing 'Folk Medicine' in Interwar Germany: Faith, Business and Science at Dr. Madaus & Co.", *Social History of Medicine*, 14 (2001), pp. 459–482.

114 Interrogation of Wolfram Sievers, Evaluation Report No. 98, Combined Intelligence Objectives Subcommittee, 13 June 1945, YVA, JM/10046, p. 1; Cross Examination of Wolfram Sievers, 8 August 1946, in *Trial IMT*, vol. 20, p. 531; Klee, *Auschwitz*, p. 350. The Sievers testimony and cross examination can also be found at www.nizkor.org/hweb/imp/tgmwc-20/tgmwc-20-198-05.shtml, a website which reproduces documents from *Trial IMT*.

Rindon; Fausto Rondon; Gregor Schklastro; Heinz Stobert; Dr. Henrique Wollman; and "Beppo", his nickname within his family.[115]

Despite the false names, Mengele remained a fugitive until his death, forced to move repeatedly to evade authorities from Germany, Israel and the U.S. who were seeking to bring him to justice. He first lived in southern Germany, in the village of Mangoldig outside Munich, then in Argentina (Buenos Aires), Paraguay and finally Brazil. All attempts at extradition failed. Towards the end of his life, he slipped into poverty and paranoia, and died by drowning. The positive identity of his remains was made by a dental forensics expert and reported in the *New York Times,* 28 March 1986.

Mengele is notorious for his experiments at Auschwitz with twins, among them blood transfusions, psychological tests of endurance, removal of organs and limbs, sterilizations, sex changes, exposure to X-rays, lethal injections, studies of possibly race-specific proteins, experimental suturing of twins back to back, and various tests to study the transmission of twinning. Deaths among subjects, due to the experimental procedures, were frequent and welcomed as an opportunity for autopsies and other post-mortem studies. Organs and tissues from killed subjects were sent for further analysis to Mengele's mentor in Berlin-Dahlem, Professor Verschuer.

Mengele was also fascinated with the "freaks of nature" – dwarves, hunchbacks, imbeciles, hermaphrodites, giants, twins with heterochromatic eyes – and with rare diseases such as noma.

Lifton says of Mengele's scientific work: "It consisted of a combination of relatively ordinary scientific procedures with literally murderous scientific fanaticism."[116]

MERTENS, DR. ANTON: worked with Prof. Gerhard Rose in testing the efficacy of new synthetic remedies against malaria.[117]

MEYER, GEORG (FRANZ): used phenol injections on prisoners, both sick and healthy, at Auschwitz; see the next entry also; the two may signify the same individual.[118]

115 Useful references include: Gerald L. Posner. *Mengele: The Complete Story* (New York: McGraw-Hill, 1986); Lucette Matalon Lagnado and Sheila Cohn Dekel, *Children of the Flames: Dr. Josef Mengele and the Untold Story of the Twins of Auschwitz* (New York: William Morrow & Company, Inc., 1991); Christian Bernadac, *Devil's Doctors: Medical Experiments on Human Subjects in the Concentration Camps* (Geneva: Ferni Publishing House, 1978); Ben Abraham, *The Angel of Death: The Mengele Dossier* (Paris: France-Empire, 1967); Eva Morris Kor, "Nazi Experiments as Viewed by Survivor of Mengele's Experiments", in Caplan, ed., *When Medicine Went Mad;* Benno Müller-Hill, *Murderous Science* (Oxford: Oxford University Press, 1998); Nancy Siegel, *Twin Research at Auschwitz and Birkenau;* Gerald Astor, *The Last Nazi: The Life and Times of Dr. Joseph Mengele* (New York: Donald Fine Publications, 1985); *The International Commission on Inquiry into Josef Mengele's Crimes Resolution* (Jerusalem: Yad Vashem, 1985).

116 Lifton, *The Nazi Doctors,* p. 351.

117 Extracts from Report of Professor Dr. E. Gildemeister Concerning the Activities of the Robert Koch Institute – Reich Institute for the Fight Against Infectious Diseases, Partial Translation of Rose Document II, Rose Defense Exhibit 27, published in *Trial IMT,* vol. 1, p. 298.

118 IAC, *Inhuman Medicine,* vol. 1, pp. 2, 116; Klee, *Auschwitz,* p. 55.

MEYER, DR. GEORG: conducted research on tuberculosis at Sachsenhausen in 1937–1938.[119]

MEYTHALER, MAJOR DR. FRIEDRICH: an internist; consultant to the army; used English POWs for hepatitis research.[120]

MRUGOWSKY, PROF. DR. JOACHIM (Oberführer, Waffen SS): born 15 August 1905, in Rathenow/Brandenburg, Germany; studied medicine (1925–31) and biology/botany (1926–30) at the University of Halle; 1930, entered the NSDAP; 1931, joined the SS Sicherheitsdienst; 1931, received his M.D. and medical license; 1937, obtained his *Habilitation* also at the University of Halle, with a dissertation on hygiene problems in mining towns (Mansfeldischen Bergmannsdorfes); 1939, became a lecturer at the University of Berlin; professor in 1944. From 1937 until the end of the war, Mrugowsky was active as a medical officer in the SS, active in several branches of the SS bureaucracy; 1937, charged with building up the Hygiene-Institut der Verfügungstruppe der SS (Hygiene Institute of the Waffen SS Reserve), which became the Hygiene Institute of the Waffen SS on 1 September 1943; 1937, also appointed Standartenarzt der Leibstandarte Adolf Hitler.

At Nuremberg, Mrugowsky specifically testified that in the Waffen SS, he served as chief of the Hygiene Institute of the Waffen SS and of Office XVI, "Hygiene", in the SS Führungshauptamt (SS Administrative Headquarters); that between 1940 and 1943, his immediate supervisor was Dr. Karl Genzken. As director of the Hygiene Institute, Mrugowsky oversaw several publications, among them a collection of Christoph Wilhelm Hufeland's works on medical ethics entitled *Das arztliche Ethos* (München, Berlin: Lehmann, 1939) and a set of work instructions related to racial hygiene for medical clinics and laboratories entitled *Arbeitsanweisungen des Hygienes-Instituts der Waffen SS für Klinik und Laboratorium* (Berlin, usw.: Urban & Schwarzenberg, 1941). Sometime in 1941–42, Mrugowsky was named to Himmler's Command Staff (Komandostab des Reichführer's SS und Polizei). On 1 September 1943, Himmler reorganized the SS Medical Service and had the Hygiene Institute placed directly under Reichsarzt SS- und Polizei Dr. Ernst Grawitz. Mrugowsky retained directorship of the Hygiene Institute with the rank SS Oberführer. In the Health Department (Sanitätsamt) of the SS Führungshauptamt, he supervised four departments in Department D: XIII: Organization and Group Service; XIV: Dental Service; XV: Chemical and Pharmaceutical Service; XVI: Hygiene. All these positions involved Mrugowsky directly in the planning and implementation of the Nazi racial hygiene programs, and thus with the experiments on human subjects at the concentration camps.

He is known to have shot prisoners at Sachsenhausen with aconite-poisoned bullets to observe the effects of such munitions. In the Nuremberg Doctors' Trial, Mrugowsky

119 Interrogation Summary No. 322 of Karl Gebhardt, 17 October 1946, YVA, JM/5979, p. 1.
120 Klee, *Auschwitz*, p. 259.

was found guilty of war crimes in connection with his roles in the following experiments: high altitude tests, freezing, malaria, sulfanilamide, seawater, epidemic jaundice (hepatitis), sterilization, spotted fever (typhus), poisons, and incendiary bombs. He was sentenced on 20 August 1947, to death by hanging and executed on 2 June 1948 at Landsberg Prison.[121]

MUELLER, DR. HANS: pathologist for research at Buchenwald.[122]

MUENCH (MÜNCH), DR. HANS: born 1911 in Freiburg/Breisgau; member of the SS; worked at the Rajsko Hygiene Institute in Auschwitz from the summer of 1943 until the evacuation in January 1945; organized malaria testing in the vicinity of Zator, a village in swampy terrain not far from Auschwitz; acquitted of any wrongdoing in the Cracow Auschwitz Trial on 22 December 1947. Reported to reside in the Füssen/Allgäu region.[123]

MÜLLMERSTÄDT, DR. HELMUT (MUERMELSTAEDT): conducted typhoid experiments at Dachau.[124]

NACHTSHEIM, DR. HANS: 1943, experimented on the hereditary and non-hereditary nature of epilepsy and on the effects of low pressure on these patients; 1944, published the results (with Dr. Gerhard Ruhenstroth-Bauer) as "The Implications of the Lack of Oxygen for the Triggering of Epileptic Attacks".[125]

NAUL, DR.: conducted malaria research.[126]

NEFF, "DR." WALTER: although trained in agriculture (Landwirt), Neff carried out some medical procedures at Dachau, among them, at least one finger amputation. Neff was born in Westheim bei Augsburg; went to Austria to work and became involved in political resistance movements; was arrested by the Nazis after the Austrian *Anschluss* and sent to Dachau as a political prisoner; assumed responsibilities over prisoners first as a

121 Interrogation of Joachim Mrugowsky, 27 August 1946, YVA, JM/6006, p. 2; Affidavit of Joachim Mrugowsky, 17 October 1946, Translation of Document No-423, in RG-30.001M, pp. 1–2; Affidavit of Fritz Ernst Fischer, 19 November 1945, Document No-228, in RG-30.001M, p. 2; IAC, *Inhuman Medicine*, vol. 1, pt. 1, p. 39; "Nazi Doctors and Other Perpetrators of Nazi Crimes"; see also "Joachim Mrugowsky-Biography", at www.catalogues-professorum-halensis.de/mrugowskyjoachim.html, a German-language website on the professors at University of Halle. The StaBiKat; i.e., online catalogue of the Staatsbibliothek in Berlin, at www.StaBiKat.staatsbibliothek-berlin.de, lists Mrugowsky's publications.

122 Klee, *Auschwitz*, p. 55.

123 Correspondence with former SS physician Dr. Hans Muench, in Shelley, ed., *Criminal Experiments on Human Beings*, pp. 288–302, 305, 332; Klee, *Auschwitz*, p. 55.

124 Klee, *Auschwitz*, pp. 33; Nazi Doctor Database.

125 Klee, *Auschwitz*, pp. 228–230.

126 Interrogation Summary No. 39 of Wolfram Sievers, 16 August 1946, YVA, JM/6027, p. 3.

Stubenälteste, eventually became the Blockführer of Block 5, the TB ward; former prisoner-testimony indicated that Neff worked to prevent the extermination of several prisoners afflicted with TB who had been "selected" on account of their illness; in 1941, was appointed Oberpfleger of the Block and charged with setting up a research station on the Block so that homeopathic remedies could be tested; September 1942, was released from imprisonment but made a Zivilangestellter der Waffen SS (civilian member of the Waffen SS) and assigned to continue working at Dachau with Sigmund Rascher; assisted Rascher with the experiments on the effects of high altitude and freezing; recorded the deaths in an experiment log; is alleged to have been the source of the report that brought the arrests and executions of Rascher and his wife. After Rascher's death, Neff remained in the SS service and was returned to Dachau; he helped to organize an unsuccessful rebellion at the camp; was arrested by the Americans after the liberation of the camp on account of his participation in Rascher's medical experiments and taken to Nuremberg for the tribunal hearings, but then returned to Dachau for hearings on the rebellion; eventually released by the Americans but re-arrested by German authorities, again for participation in the medical experiments. Neff's case became a sort of "cause célèbre" in Munich, pitting those who believed he should be convicted for participating in the experiments against those who noted his efforts on behalf of prisoners.

Eventually a court in Munich convicted him for "Beihilfe zur Körperverletzung" and sentenced him (30 December 1948) to one month in prison. The sentence was never carried out and the conviction satisfied neither side in the controversy over his just fate. Neff died 31 August 1960 in Munich. No copies of his book on his Dachau experience, *Arzt des Todes* (Miesbach: Zwei-Brücken Verlag, 1949) can be located, but the manuscript has survived.[127]

NETTER, PROF. HANS: participated in various experiments at Dachau.[128]

NEUMANN, DR. ROBERT: pathologist; Lagerarzt at Buchenwald and Auschwitz; developed an instrument called a histotom for use in liver biopsies; tested the instrument on inmates at Buchenwald; many deaths occurred from the procedure.[129]

NONNEBRUCH (NOUNENBRÜCH), PROF. DR. WILHELM: Professor Nonnenbruch, was 1939–45 Professor of Internal Medicine, University of Frankfurt am Main; taught liver biopsy techniques; one of his students was Dr. Rudolf Brachtel; at Nuremberg, Blaha testified that Nonnenbruch participated in experiments with "Malaria-Milzen".[130]

127 Interrogation Summary No. 370 of Dr. Hans Romberg, 29 October 1946, YVA, JM/6018, p. 1. See also the German language article "Walter Neff" at http://members.aol.com/zbdachau/fates/ger/neff.htm; Klee, *Auschwitz*, pp. 32–33.

128 Klee, *Auschwitz*, p. 55.

129 Ibid., pp. 36, 48, 55.

130 Ibid., pp. 36, 36 n. 90, 184, 297.

OBERHEUSER (OBERHAUSER), DR. HERTA: born 1911 in Cologne; attended the Municipal Luisenschule in Düsseldorf; 1931–33, studied medicine in Bonn; 1933–37, continued medical studies in Düsseldorf; 1937, joined the NSDAP; after earning her medical degree, employed in the Medizinische Klinik in Düsseldorf; worked as a medical specialist and camp doctor at Ravensbrück; then as assistant physician at Hohenlychen, with Prof. Karl Gebhardt; participated in gangrene and bone transplantation experiments at Ravensbrück; also reportedly conducted brain experiments with Gebhardt on hospitalized prisoners.

Dr. Rolf Rosenthal claimed that he saw Oberheuser giving petroleum injections to patients that caused death within five minutes. She also killed patients by means of Evipan injection, incised inmates' limbs, and rubbed glass and sawdust into their wounds to produce infection. The only female defendant in the Nuremberg Doctors' Trial, she was convicted for war crimes in connection with the sulfanilamide, sterilization, and bone, nerve and muscle experiments; sentenced to twenty years imprisonment but released in 1952; became a family doctor in Stocksee, Germany; license revoked in 1960.[131]

PANNING, DR. GERHARD: before 1942, was a lecturer (Dozent) at the Institut für Wehrgerichtliche Medizin Institute for Defense-Forensic Medicine) in Berlin, one of the ten research institutes of the Military Academy of the Heeres-Sanitätsinspektion; was the Beratender Gerichstmediziner (forensic medicine advisor) for the Military Academy; was entrusted with the testing of new explosives and, in August 1941, allowed at least six Russian prisoners at Shitomir to be shot in tests; published photographs of the resulting injuries in the journal *Der Deutsche Militärarzt.*[132]

PAPE, DR. HERMANN: a doctor at Dachau, supervised by Dr. Heinrich Schütz; worked on phlegmone experiments beginning in November 1942; disappeared after the war.[133]

PETERS, DR. GERD: cooperated with Dr. Gerhard Rose in testing the efficacy of new synthetic remedies against malaria.[134]

PLAZA, DR. HEINRICH: the second camp doctor at Buchenwald from 1941 to January 1944; was involved in administering phenol injections and carrying out typhus experiments; also served in Dachau, Natzwelier and Auschwitz.[135]

131 Interrogation of Herta Oberhauser, 31 October 1946, YVA, JM/6009, pp. 4, 8–9; Klee, *Auschwitz,* pp. 156, 158; Aziz, *Doctors of Death,* vol. 3, p. 154; "DOCTORS OF THE HOLOCAUST", Internet website.
132 Klee, *Auschwitz,* pp. 196–198.
133 Ibid, pp. 56, 147–149.
134 Extracts from Report of Professor Dr. E. Gildemeister Concerning the Activities of the Robert Koch Institute – Reich Institute for the Fight Against Infectious Diseases, Partial Translation of Rose Document II, Rose Defense Exhibit 27, published in *Trial IMT,* vol. 1, p. 298.
135 Declaration of Dr. Erwin [Ding-]Schuler, 20 July 1945, Document No-257, in RG-30.001M; Declaration of Gerhard Schiedlausky, 7 August 1945, Translation of Document No-508, in RG-30.001M, p. 29; Klee, *Auschwitz,* p. 56.

PLOETNER (PLÖTNER), DR. KURT (SS-Sturmbannführer): assistant professor at the University of Leipzig; 1933, joined the NSDAP and SS; worked for the Ahnenerbe; involved initially with Pectin research; developed Styptoral; conducted experiments at Schlacters, near Lake Constance; sent to Dachau to work with Prof. Dr. Schilling and Dr. Rascher, assisting in Schilling's malaria experiments and Rascher's blood coagulation experiments; however, he "broke away from them when Dr. Rascher was arrested". Ploetner took over Rascher's Ahnenerbe-sponsored research station (at which time the institute's name in the Ahnenerbe was changed from "R", for Rascher, to "P", for Ploetner) after the latter's arrest; was assigned to the experiments with N-Stoff, a poisonous chemical (chlortrifluorid or C_3 Stoff) that was being investigated secretly for its warfare potential; experiments were carried out on camp prisoners.[136]

POHL, OSWALD: (SS Obergruppenführer) born 30 May 1892 in Duisburg; professionally trained as a Navy purser; 1926, joined the NSDAP; amassed considerable power by concurrent appointments in the SS administration; thus 1934, appointed chief of the SS-Hauptamt, which became the Wirtschaftverwaltungshaupamt (Economic Administration Head Office, or WVHA) in 1942; 1935, also appointed chief of three additional main offices in the SS administration: the SS Sicherheitshauptamt (security), the Rasse- und Siedlungshauptamt (Race and Settlement Main Office), and the Hauptamt Haushalt und Bauten (budget and buildings).

The WVHA administered the concentration camps through its Department D (see the entries for Richard Glücks and Enno Lolling), and thus Pohl, though not a doctor, was heavily involved with camp activities, including the medical experiments on inmates; he reportedly made some of the selections of prisoners for Hirt's skeleton collection and was involved in the nutritional experiments at Dachau. Pohl was arrested in May 1945; tried by the International Military Tribunal in Nuremberg; sentenced to death; imprisoned at Landsberg until June 1951 when the death sentence was finally executed.[137]

POKORNY, DR. ADOLF: a retired military doctor; specialist on skin and venereal diseases; a letter from Pokorny to Himmler, dated October 1941, reports that Madaus's research on dumb-cane might prove useful as a means of conquering the enemy (through sterilization); supported Clauberg's work on sterilization; acquitted after the war.[138]

136 Interrogation of Wolfram Sievers, Evaluation Report No. 98, Combined Intelligence Objectives Subcommittee, 13 June 1945, YVA, JM/10046, p. 2; Interrogation Summary of Wolfram Sievers, 16 August 1946, YVA, JM/6027, pp. 2–3; Letter to Himmler, 22 November 1944, writer illegible, Translation of Document No-005, in RG-30.001M, p. 1; *Trial IMT*, vol. 1, pp. 280, 282; Hoedeman, *Hitler or Hippocrates*, p. 23; Klee, *Auschwitz*, pp. 83–87, 121, 354ff). Quotations are from Sievers's Interrogation.

137 Interrogation of Wolfram Sievers, 28 October 1946, YVA, JM/6027, p. 6; Klee, *Auschwitz*, p. 183. For Pohl and the WVHA, see www.deathcamps.org/reinhard/wvha.html.

138 "Nazi Doctors and Other Perpetrators of Nazi Crimes". For the letter from Pokorny to Himmler, see on the internet "A Teacher's Guide to the Holocaust: Sterilzation", at http://fcit.coedu.usf.edu/holocaust/timeline/Doc/Steri.htm, which offers a collection of sources on the sterilization experiments from the archives of Shamash, The Jewish Internet Consortium.

Poppendick, Dr. Helmut (Oberst, Waffen SS): December 1926, passed the state medical exams; 1932, joined the NSDAP and the SS (July); 1935, appointed as a physician in the SS Rasse- und Siedlungshauptamt (Race and Settlement Main Office) under Oswald Pohl; 1941, made Chief Physician; 1943 to the war's end, served as Chief of the Personal Office of Dr. Ernst Grawitz; ordered Dr. Rudolph Brandt to conduct seawater experiments on camp inmates. At the Nuremberg Doctors' Trial, Poppendick was convicted of war crimes in connection with the experiments on high altitude, freezing, malaria, sulfanilamides, seawater, hepatitis (epidemic jaundice), sterilization, typhus (spotted fever), poison, and incendiary bombs. He was sentenced on 20 August 1947 to ten years imprisonment; released on January 31, 1951; became a specialist in internal medicine in Oldenburg.[139]

Prachtol, Dr. (probably Rudolf Brachtel): conducted malaria experiments at Dachau.[140]

Rascher, Dr. Sigmund (SS Hauptsturmführer and Stabsarzt, Luftwaffe Medical Corps): born 1909 in Munich; third child of Hanns-August Rascher, a medical doctor; 1930, Abitur (secondary school diploma) in Konstanz; 1933, began medical studies at Freiburg, also joined the NSDAP; 1933–34, worked in Switzerland, in part for his father; October 1934, returned to Munich for more medical studies; 1936, passed the state medical examination and joined the SA; 1936–38, worked in Munich for Prof. Trumpp on cancer research; 1936–39, also assistant in surgery at the University Hospital in Munich; 1939, moved over into the SS; 1 May 1939, taken into the Ahnenerbe as a cancer researcher; involved with the Ahnenerbe's Institut für wehrwissenschaftliche Zweckforschung (Institute for Military Scientific Research, or for Research for Military Purposes), which received its funding from the Wehrmacht; proposed medical experiments in the concentration camps and was sent to Dachau; his Dachau research station was dubbed Institute R ("R" for Rascher); carried out the high altitude and hypothermia experiments at Dachau. Despite personal connections to Himmler (Rascher's wife, Karoline Diehl, was a Himmler friend), Rascher and his wife eventually fell into disfavor after they presented an adopted child as their own offspring. Both were imprisoned and Frau Rascher executed at Buchenwald; Dr. Rascher himself was sent back to Dachau and shot on 26 April 1945 in Cell 73, the so-called Dachau bunker, though this fact was not verified until after the Nuremberg trials; at the Doctors' Trial, General Telford Taylor noted that "Rascher was thought to be dead". In 1957, "barely ten years after [the Dachau trial] verdict, Roypan-Diätetik SP2 in Munich, cited Rascher's findings in an advertisement of its ginseng tablets, noting that their efficacy had been demonstrated in experiments on frozen people by former SS physician

139 Burman, ed., *The First German War Crimes Trial*, p. 237; Klee, *Auschwitz*, pp. 178–179.
140 Testimony of Father Leo Miechalowski, Nuremberg Military Tribunal, undated, National Archives Record Group 238, M887, National Holocaust Museum, Internet website, pp. 878–881.

Dr. Rascher, and that SS Führer Himmler held a very high opinion of their value and recommended them to his SS-men as a means of raising their physical fitness (*Frankfurter Allgemeine Zeitung* and *Der Spiegel*, Oct. 1957)."[141]

REICHMAN, DR.: was involved with Mengele's experiments using eyes taken from twins at Auschwitz.[142]

REITER, DR. HANS CONRAD: born 1881 in Leipzig, Germany, the son of an industrialist; 1906, obtained his M.D. after studies at Leipzig, Breslau and Tübingen; thesis entitled "Nephritis and Tuberculosis"; postgraduate training at the Pasteur Institute in Paris, St. Mary's Hospital in London (under Sir Almroth Wright) and in 1913, at the University of Berlin's Institute of Hygiene; worked at the Hygiene Institutes of the Universities of Berlin and Königsberg; became an avid proponent of eugenics; attracted to the NSDAP because of its endorsement of racial hygienics as an answer to socio-economic and health problems in Germany (was among the first group of professors to swear allegiance to Hitler, joined the party in 1932 and served as its delegate in the Mecklenburg state parliament); one of the leaders in Nazi Germany of research in eugenics-related matters; appointed honorary professor of hygiene at the University of Berlin in 1933, director of the Federation of Scientific Societies in 1934, and president of the Robert Koch Institute for Infectious Diseases in 1935; president of the Reichsgesundheitsamt (Reich Health Office); represented Germany at the International Health Organization in Paris until 1945.

During the war, Reiter was instrumental in the institution of medical experiments in concentration camps, especially Prof. Gerhard Rose's experiments at Buchenwald with typhus; arrested and detained for two years by the Americans; then released and returned to private life, practicing medicine at a clinic in Kassel/Hessen, 1949–52; awarded the Great Medal of Honor of the Red Cross and affiliate membership in the Royal Society of London; died 25 November 1969, at his country home in Kassel-Wilhelmshöhe.[143]

141 Interrogation of Wolfram Sievers, 28 October 1946, YVA, JM/6027, p. 3; Wadyslaw Fejkiel, *Przeglad Lekarski*, p. 1962; *The Second World War: A Day by Day Account*, (http://www/angelfire.com/my/rememberww2/index.html); Paul Berben, *Dachau 1933–1945: The Official History*, Eng. trans. Capt. Bernhard R. Hanauer (Bruxelles: Comité International de Dachau: 1968, 1975); Wolfgang Benz, "Sigmund Rascher, M. D.: A Career", *Dachau Review 2: History of Nazi Concentration Camps Studies*, Vol. 2, 1990, ed. W. Benz and Barbara Distel (Bruxelles: Comité International de Dachau, 1990); Hackett, *Buchenwald Report*, pp. 68–81, 228–230, 369–371. See also the German language biography at http://lexikon.freenet.de/SigmundRascher, and the Wikipedia.de website. For General Telford Taylor's remark at Nuremberg, see "[Gen.] Telford Taylor Opening Statement", on the U.S. Holocaust Memorial Museum website at ushmm.org/research/doctors/summary2.htm; also printed in *Trials NMT*, vol. 1. See also Klee, *Auschwitz*, passim.

142 Declaration of Dr. Jancu Vexler, undated, YVA, 0.33/4334, p. 2.

143 Daniel J. Wallace and Michael Weisman, "Should a War Criminal Be Rewarded with Eponymous Distinction? The Double Life of Hans Reiter (1881–1969)", *Journal of Clinical Rheumatology*, 6: 1 (February 2000), pp. 49–54; Document No-265, in RG-30.001M.

Ritter, Dr. Robert: 1927, received doctorate in psychology at the University of Munich; 1930, M.D., Heidelberg, licensed to practice medicine; specialty was antisocial youth. 1936, appointed to direct a new institute, the Rassenhygienische und Bevölkerungsbiologische Forschungstelle (Eugenic and Population Biology Research Station) in the Reichsgesundheitsamt (Reich Health Office). Ritter specialized in research on Gypsies, and in 1941 this research took a practical turn, with his appointment as chief of the new Kriminalbiologisches Institut der Sicherheitspolizei (Institute of Criminal Biology of the Security Police), located in the detective headquarters (RKPA, Office V) of the SS Reichsicherheitshauptamt. For example, he undertook an "anthropological" investigation of Gypsies at Auschwitz. Ritter died in 1950, in the course of an investigation by a Frankfurt court. He argued that he had actually tried to help the Gypsies. The courts were convinced, and consequently, none of his numerous collaborators in the research were convicted of crimes against Gypsies.[144]

Roeder, Dr. Fritz: researched the chemical behavior of a part of the brain in conditions of oxygen deficiency, as part of the Dachau high altitude experiments conducted by Rascher.[145]

Rohde, Dr. Werner: born 1904 in Marburg am Lahn; worked as a camp physician at Buchenwald and Auschwitz and as physician-in-chief at Natzweiler; conducted experiments in conjunction with Dr. Bruno Weber on brain-altering chemicals; tried by a British military court at Wuppertal on charges of having killed prisoners (Allied nationals interned at the camp) by means of lethal injections; hanged on 11 October 1946.[146]

Romberg, Dr. Hans Wolfgang: conducted high altitude experiments at Dachau with Rascher; was an assistant to Dr. Siegfried Ruff at the German Research Institute for Aviation (Deutsche Versuchsanstalt für Luftfahrt, or DVL). Romberg was acquitted at the Nuremberg Doctors' Trial of the charge of war crimes in connection with these experiments.[147]

Rose, Prof. Dr. Gerhard August Heinrich: born 30 November 1896 in Danzig; studied at the Kaiser-Wilhelm-Akademie für das militärärztliche Bildungswesen in Berlin; 1921, began practicing medicine; 1922 joined the NSDAP; 1926–29, assistant at the surgical clinic of the University of Heidelberg; 1929–36, worked in China as a medical adviser to the Chinese government; 1936, succeeded Klaus Schilling as professor and

144 Müller-Hill, *Murderous Science*, pp. 70–71; Müller-Hill, "Genetics After Auschwitz", *Holocaust Genocide Studies*, 2: 1 (1987), p. 8. See also, Friedlander, *The Origins of Nazi Genocide*, passim.

145 Klee, *Auschwitz*, p. 223.

146 Shelley, ed., *Criminal Experiments on Human Beings*, p. 333; Klee, *Auschwitz*, p. 57; UNWCC, p. 535.

147 Interrogation of Dr. Hans Romberg, 29 October 1946, YVA, JM/6018, p. 1; Interrogation Summary No. 202 of Dr. Siegfried Ruff, 28 September 1946, YVA, JM/6020, p. 2; Klee, *Auschwitz*, p. 254.

head of the department of tropical medicine of the Robert Koch Institute; 1939, joined the Luftwaffe as a Lieutenant in the Medical Corp; rose to the rank of Generalarzt (Brigadier General) and served as Tropical Medicine Adviser to the two wartime directors of the Luftwaffe Medical Service, Erich Hippke and Oskar Schroeder.

Rose directed an institute at Pfafferode b. Mühlhausen in Thuringia, which was part of the larger Institut für Wehrhygiene (Institute for Military Hygiene) of the Luftwaffe; observed typhus experiments at Buchenwald; although initially opposed to conducting experiments on human beings, he nevertheless provided several experimental typhus vaccines to the camp researchers and participated in malaria and hepatitis experiments at Dachau; Rose was indicted at the Nuremberg Doctors' Trial for war crimes in connection with the typhus and hepatitis experiments and sentenced to life imprisonment on August 20, 1947; served fifteen years.[148]

ROSENTHAL, DR. ROLF: a camp doctor at Ravensbrück; assisted Dr. Karl Gebhardt in conducting both sulfanilamide and bone transplantation experiments; gave lethal Evipan injections to patients; sentenced to death by hanging by a British court in Hamburg on 3 February 1947 and hanged on 5 May 1947.[149]

RUFF, DR. MED. HABIL. SIEGFRIED (Flugkapitän): born 1907 in Frimersheim (possibly Friemersheim)/Niederrhein; educated in Aachen, Bonn and Berlin, graduating in 1926; medical studies at Bonn University; took an internship and then worked as an assistant at Bonn University Hospital; 1928, joined the NSDAP; 1934, began working at the Deutsche Versuchsanstalt für Luftfahrt in Berlin-Adlershof (German Aviation Research Institute); Drs. Romberg and Freitag worked under Ruff's direction; established the organization's Institut für Flugmedizin (Institute for Flight Medicine); remained at the institute until the end of the war, with the title Chief of Medical Research for Aviation; specialized in accident prevention and high altitude; 1942, initiated high altitude experiments at Dachau.

Ruff was charged at the Nuremberg Doctors' Trial with war crimes in connection with the high altitude experiments but acquitted on 20 August 1947, because the evidence against him was deemed circumstantial and insufficient. He was one of several German Nazi experts in military medicine whose services were sought by the U.S. military and CIA after the war. In Ruff's case, a threat by reporter Drew Pearson to reveal the efforts to President Truman ended the recruitment efforts; Truman had just issued an executive order banning former NSDAP members from entering the country; Ruff

148 "Diary of the Division for Research for Spotted Fever and Virus at the Institute of Hygiene of the Waffen SS", Translation of Document No-265, RG-30.001M, p. 2; in *Trial IMT,* vol. 1, p. 281; Burman, ed., *The First German War Crimes Trial,* pp. 241–241; Wallace and Weisman, "Should a War Criminal be Rewarded with Eponymous Distinction?", p. 51; Aziz, *Doctors of Death.*

149 Statement of Dr. Herta Oberhauser, Translation of Document No-487, in RG-30.001M, p. 4; Deposition of Gustawa Winnowska, in RG-30.001M, p. 1; Klee, *Auschwitz,* pp. 119, 126ff., 153, 212, 215, 287–288, 292, 324f., 326, 337, 343; UNWCC, p. 535. Quote is from the Winnowska deposition.

had been a party member. Ruff remained in Germany, working as chief doctor for Lufthansa and as professor and director of the Institut für Flugmedizin at the University of Bonn; 1978, received the Strughold-Preis of the Deutschen Gesellschaft für Luft- und Raumfahrtmedizin (Strughold Prize of the German Association for Aviation and Space Medicine).[150]

Rühl, Dr. Helmut: assistant to Dr. Bickenbach in the experiments with *Lost* (mustard gas) at Natzweiler, June–August 1944. Rühl disappears from official records 1948–60; after 1960, appears as an Amtarzt (bureau physician); retired in 1983 as a leading medical director with a pension; an indictment was filed against him on 29 June 1983.[151]

Rühl, Marrianne: assisted Prof. Dr. Eduard May in conducting malaria experiments.[152]

Sachs, Prof. Dr. Hans (SS Hauptsturmführer): a leading pathologist who was assigned to observe experiments with N-substance on prisoners.[153]

Sagel, Dr. Wilhelm: director of a mental institution in Arnsdor[f?]/Saxony; cooperated with Prof. Gerhard Rose in testing the efficacy of new synthetic remedies against malaria.[154]

Samestrang, Dr. (SS-Hauptsturmführer): conducted early (1938) freezing (hypothermia) experiments on prisoners in Sachsenhausen.[155]

Schenk, Prof. Dr. Ernst-Günther: physician and chemist; specialist in Ernährung (diet, nutrition) and natural cures; born 3 August 1904; 1930–31, served as an assistant at the Ludolf-Krehl-Klinik (Eiweiss-Chemie und Heilpflanzen) in Heidelberg; 1931–34, Oberassistent in the pathology section of the Kaiser-Wilhelm-Institut für medizinische Forschung; 1933, joined the SA and in 1934, the NS-Lehrerbund; 1934, returned to his former place of employment in Heidelberg as Oberarzt; did independent research on Fastenkuren (fasting as a means of healing); 1937, joined the NSDAP and NS-Ärztebund; 1938, became the Referent für Ernährung (Diet Expert) at the NSDAP Hauptamt für Volksgesundheit (Bureau for the Health of the People) in Munich; 1940, appointed

150 Interrogation of Dr. Siegfried Ruff, 22 September 1946, YVA, JM/6020, p. 1; Interrogation of Dr. Siegfried Ruff, 28 September 1946, YVA, JM/6020, pp. 1–2; Klee, *Auschwitz*, pp. 254, 515; "The CIA-Nazi Connection". Quotes are from "The CIA-Nazi Connection".

151 Klee, *Auschwitz*, pp. 382–383, 388.

152 Declaration of Wolfram Sievers, Evaluation Report No. 98, Combined Intelligence Objectives Subcommittee, 13 June 1945, YVA, JM/10046, p. 1.

153 Letter to Himmler, 22 November 1944, writer illegible, Translation of Document No-005, in RG-30.001M, p. 1.

154 Extracts from Report of Professor Dr. E. Gildemeister Concerning the Activities of the Robert Koch Institute – Reich Institute for the Fight Against Infectious Diseases, Partial Translation of Rose Document II, Rose Defense Exhibit 27, published in *Trial IMT*, vol. 1, p. 298.

155 Letter of S. Rascher, 23 April 1944, Translation of Document No-322, in RG-30.001M, p. 1.

Ernährungsinspekteur for the Waffen SS and Reserve SS Untersturmführer; 1944, given the rank SS Standartenführer and made inspector of diet and nutrition for the Waffen SS and the Wehrmacht; spent the last days of the war in the Reichs Chancellery in Berlin.

Schenk advised the Wirtschaftsverwaltungshauptamt (WVHA) on concentration camp nutrition problems; sought to situate Europe's largest institute for medicinal plants at Dachau. He suggested adding brewer's yeast and Pervitingaben – an indigestible mixture of sawdust and tree bark – to concentration camp diets Pervitin, a product of Pharma-Firma Temmler, is a stimulant. The Nazis used it to increase performance; had tried it with German troops and discontinued its use because of problems with addiction, but authorized further trials in the camps; thus the camp nutrition supplements also contained a stimulant drug. Schenk was taken prisoner by the Russians at the close of the war and only returned to Germany in 1955, with the last transport of unpardoned Nazis; he published books capitalizing on his experiences.

In 1960, the Bavarian State Ministry for Education (Unterricht) and Cultural Affairs (Kultus) discharged him from its civil service ranks; 1963, the personnel board recommended opening a formal "service penalty procedure" (Dienststrafverfahrens) against him on the grounds that he had participated in "frivolous experiments that demonstrate a view of humans as objects and as medical test rabbits". Two legal investigations followed, in 1963 and 1968, but formal charges were not filed and the investigation was closed; Schenk described his occupation in the years 1963–77 as "scientific work in the pharmaceutical industry".[156]

SCHIEDLAUSKY, DR. GERHARD: SS doctor; March–September 1941, stationed at Mauthausen; then at Flossenbürg as troop and prison doctor; December 1941, was transferred to Ravensbrück as senior doctor of the camp (Standortarzt); conducted gangrene experiments; supervised Dr. Herta Oberheuser; August–October 1943, transferred to Natzweiler; October 1943 to 11 April 1945, was at Buchenwald where he succeeded Dr. Waldemar Hoven as Standortarzt; sentenced on 3 February 1947 to death by hanging by a British war crimes court in Hamburg; hanged 3 May 1947.[157]

SCHILLING, PROF. DR. KARL KLAUS (in documents appears also as Klaus Schilling, Claus Schilling, and Karl Claus Schilling): 1894, physicians degree received from the University of Munich; did research in Africa on malaria and tsetse-fly diseases such as sleeping sickness; 1911, received a Rockefeller Foundation grant for research; 1941, in

156 Declaration of Wolfram Sievers, Evaluation Report No. 98, Combined Intelligence Objectives Subcommittee, 13 June 1945, YVA, JM/10046, p. 2; Klee, *Auschwitz*, pp. 179–189. On Pervitin, see Klee, Ibid., p. 225 and the website "DFG MedTagung".

157 Declaration of Gerhard Schiedlausky, 7 August 1945, Translation of Document No-508, in RG-30.001M, pp. 1–2, 6; Affidavit of Ferdinand Roemhild, Translation of Document No-434, in RG-30.001M, p. 1; Interrogation of Herta Oberhauser, 31 October 1946, YVA, JM/6009, pp. 4–5; Deposition of Janina Iwanska, Translation of Document No-877, in RG-30.001M, p. 4; Klee, *Auschwitz*, p. 153; UNWCC, p. 535. Quote is from Iwanska's deposition.

Rome, he was invited by Leonardo Conti to meet with Himmler who asked him to leave retirement in order to do research on malaria drugs; 1942, sent to Dachau to carry out this research on camp prisoners whom he deliberately infected with the disease. Schilling also infected patients with other tropical diseases to study the stages of illness and compare the effects of the diseases in patients from different blood groups.

After the war, the General Military Court at Dachau brought Schilling to trial in the case "United States vs. Weiss, Ruppert, et al." Schilling was condemned to death by hanging; sentence carried out at Dachau on 29 May 1946. Schilling tried to defend himself with the argument that he was working for the good of humanity. He appealed for leniency unsuccessfully to the President of the United States on the grounds that he should be allowed to continue this research.[158]

SCHLINK, PROF.: was involved with malaria experiments.[159]

SCHMICK, DR. HUGO: worked at Hohenlychen and Sachsenhausen on experiments with burns caused by gasses and *Marfanilpuder,* the latter a product of I. G. Farben. Schmick developed the method by which *Marfanilpuder* was applied to deliberately inflicted wounds in experimental subjects; he is known also to have conducted experiments at Sachsenhausen with *Lost* (mustard gas).[160]

SCHMITZ, DR. EMIL CHRISTIAN: 1941–42, Erster Lagerarzt at Sachsenhausen; conducted experiments with gas-induced burns. After the war, worked as a scientist at the pharmaceutical company Boehringer.[161]

SCHMITZ, HEINRICH: Vertragsarzt (consulting physician) at Flossenbürg, 1944–45, was hanged in Landsberg Prison on 26 November 1948, having been condemned for his senseless operations, amputations, and injections.[162]

SCHOLZ, PROF. DR. WILLIBALD: brain pathologist at the Kaiser-Wilhelm-Institut für Psychiatrie; in the high altitude experiments at Dachau, investigated the effects of oxygen deprivation on the brain.[163]

158 See Document No-856, in *Trials NMT,* vol. 1, pp. 291–292, on the web at www.mazal.org/archives/nmt/01/NMT289 ff., which presents the evidence and findings at Nuremberg related to the malaria experiments at Dachau. It includes Dr. Schilling's sworn and unsworn testimony before the American Military Tribunal at Dachau. See also, the Interrogation Summary No. 39 of Wolfram Sievers, 16 August 1946, YVA, JM/6027, p. 3; "Nazi Doctors and Other Perpetrators of Nazi Crimes".

159 Memorandum of Wolfram Sievers, 3 April 1942, Translation of Document No-721, in RG-30.001M, p. 1.

160 Klee, *Auschwitz,* p. 153, 270.

161 Ibid., p. 57 and 153–154 n. 42.

162 Ibid., p. 57 n. 204

163 Ibid., pp. 76, 223.

SCHREIBER, PROF. WALTER (Generalarzt): 1 September 1943, appointed commander of Lehrgruppe C of the Militärärztliche Akademie der Heeres-Sanitätsinspektion (Military Academy of the Armed Forces Medical Services Inspectorate) in Berlin. The ten medical research institutes of the Military Academy were combined in Lehrgruppe C under his oversight. Schreiber was also the authority on epidemic control (Bevollmächtigter für Seuchenbekämpfung) on the Reich Research Council (Reichsforschungsrat). He had knowledge of many of the camp experiments and testimony at Nuremberg revealed that he was in charge of hepatitis experiments at Sachsenhausen.

He was captured by the Soviets 29 April 1945; imprisoned until September 1948 when he was released in the Soviet sector of Berlin; a few months later fled to the American sector and was taken by the Americans to the intelligence center called Camp King; 11 September 1951, arrived at the U.S. Air Force Medical School at Randolph Field in Texas; the *Boston Globe* published information about his Nazi past in December 1951, triggering an outcry and in February 1952, he left the United States for Rio Negro, Argentina.[164]

SCHROEDER (SCHRÖDER), PROF. DR. OSKAR (Generaloberstabsarzt): born 1889; served as a medical officer during World War I; after the war continued as a medical officer and consultant in the medical inspectorate; rose through the ranks of the Luftwaffe medical services and on 1 January 1944, replaced Erich Hippke as Chef des Sanitätswesens des Luftwaffe (Chief of the Medical Service of the Luftwaffe); in this position, Schröder's many duties included direct oversight of the Physicians' Academy of the Luftwaffe (Ärtzliche Akademie der Luftwaffe), especially its department for Wissenschaft und Forschung (Science and Research) and of Dr. Strughold's Luftfahrtmedizinisches Forschungsinstitut (Flight Medicine Research Institute); also supervised Gerhard Rose's Institut für Wehrhygiene (Institute for Military Hygiene); played a central role in the seawater experiments at Dachau, which were funded by the Luftwaffe; at the Nuremberg Doctors' Trial, was charged with and convicted of war crimes in connection with the experiments on high altitude, freezing, sulfanilamide, seawater, hepatitis (epidemic jaundice) and typhus (spotted fever); sentenced to life imprisonment on 20 August 1947; served 15 years.[165]

SCHULER, DR. ERWIN (see the entry on Ding-Schuler): conducted typhus and phenol-injection experiments at Buchenwald.[166]

164 *Trial IMT,* vol. 1, pp. 495–96; Klee, *Auschwitz,* pp. 195, 88ff, 151, 159, 199, 203, 237, 288 n. 28, 311, 328 n. 151.

165 Interrogation Summary of Dr. Siegfried Ruff, 28 September 1946, YVA, JM/6020, p. 2; Statement of Rudolph Brandt, 14 October 1946, Translation of Document No-370, in RG-30.001M, p. 2; Burman, ed., *The First German War Crimes Trial,* pp. 222–223; Klee, *Auschwitz,* pp. 210–216, 254.

166 "Nazi Doctor Database".

SCHULZE, DR. RICHARD: an orthopedic surgeon at Hohenlychen who worked with Dr. Franz Stumpfegger on bone transplantation experiments; the transplanted bone tissue was taken from mentally disturbed female inmates in Ravensbrück.[167]

SCHUMANN, DR. HORST (SS Sturmbannführer): born 1906 in Halle; the son of a physician; joined the NSDAP in 1930, the SA in 1932; 1933, employed as a doctor in the Public Health Office in Halle; recruited as an Air Force physician after Germany invaded Poland. January 1940, joined the T4 euthanasia program at Viktor Brack's suggestion; headed the Gräfeneck euthanasia institute in Württemberg and the Sonnenstein asylum in Pirna, Sachsen, both of which served as killing centers; belonged to a commission of doctors who personally supervised the transfer of weak and sick prisoners in Auschwitz, Buchenwald, Dachau, Flossenbürg, Gross-Rosen, Mauthausen, Neuengamme and Niederhagen concentration camps to the euthanasia centers; 28 July 1941, arrived at Auschwitz; participated in sterilization research, which was another component of the Nazi project to rid the Third Reich of unwanted populations; specifically carried out procedures to sterilize both men and women by means of X-ray; 1944, left Auschwitz; October 1945–1951, under the assumed name "Gladbeck", openly practiced medicine; 1949, set up a private consulting practice with refugee credits; 1951, recognized as a war criminal; fled, worked as a ship doctor, then settled in 1955 in the Sudan; 1959, fled again through Nigeria and Libya to Ghana; 1966, was extradited to the German Federal Republic; September 1970, placed on trial; proceedings delayed April 1971, because of the defendant's high blood pressure; defendant released 29 July 1972 and lived in Frankfurt until he died 5 May 1983.[168]

SCHÜTZ, DR. HEINRICH (SS Sturmbannführer): born 12 April 1906 in Bad Schmiedeberg/Halle; his father was a doctor at a health spa; 1936, took a position as an assistant at a city hospital in Chemnitz (Stadtkrankenhaus); joined the SS in 1936 and the NSDAP in 1937; at first did background investigations for the SS; sent in 1940 to the G. und V. Prufstelle in Dachau, directed by Stabsarzt Dr. Karl Fahrenkamp; 1941, assigned to the Panzer division "Leibstande Adolf Hitler", then in March 1942, returned to Dachau; June, 1942, appointed head of the Biochemische Versuchsstationen (Biochemical Research Station) in the Dachau sick-bay, where homeopathic remedies were being tested in the treatment of sepsis; beginning November 1942, worked on phlegmone experiments; continued working as a physician after the war until charges

167 Interrogation Summary No. 54 of Joachim Mrugowsky, 27 August 1946, YVA, JM/6006, p. 5; Klee, *Auschwitz*, p. 154.

168 Declaration of Jakov Freimark, undated, YVA, 0.33/4334, pp. 1–2; Testimony of Dr. Viktor Brack, 19 May 1947, in "Nuremberg Trials Transcript of the Proceedings, USA vs. Karl Brandt et al.", p. 7733; Viktor Brack's Organizational Chart on "Euthanasia Program", undated, Document No-2758, p. 2; both Brack documents in Mendelsohn, ed., *The Holocaust, Selected Documents*, Vol. 9, pp. 108, 133; Joseph Bogusz, in IAC, *Inhuman Medicine*; Shelley, ed., *Criminal Experiments on Human Beings*, p. 335; "Jewish Virtual Library".

against him were filed in December 1972; sentenced to ten years imprisonment by a Munich court but immediately released on account of critical illness.[169]

Sievers, Wolfram (SS-Standartenführer): 1929, joined the NSDAP; 1935, also joined the SS with the rank of Standartenführer; from July 1935 until the end of the war served as Reichsgeschäftsführer (Reich Business Manager) of the Ahnenerbe Society (Ancestral Heritage Society) and director of the Ahnenerbe's Institut für Wehrwissenschaftliche Zweckforschung (Institute for Military Scientific Research); 1935 became Deputy Chairman of the Managing Board of Directors of the Reich Research Council. Sievers was tried at Nuremberg in the Doctors' Trial and found guilty of war crimes in connection with the experiments on high altitude, freezing (hypothermia), malaria, mustard gas, seawater, hepatitis (epidemic jaundice) and typhus (spotted fever); also with ordering and planning the murder of 112 Jews "for the purpose of completing a skeleton collection for the Reich University of Strasbourg"; sentenced to death by hanging and executed on 2 June 1948.[170]

Simona, Prof.: conducted post mortem examinations; later sent the corpses to Hirt's Anatomical Institute in Strasbourg for his skeleton collection.[171]

Sonntag (Sontag), Dr. Walter: worked at Ravensbrück; was the immediate superior of Dr. Herta Oberheuser in bone transplantation and gangrene experiments; Sonntag also worked at Sachsenhausen, Dachau and Natzweiler.[172]

Stein, Dr. Johannes: participated in the research of "race biologist" Wolfgang Lehmann; conducted experiments on POWs.[173]

Stieve, Dr. Hermann: director of the Institute of Anatomy at Berlin University; conducted experiments on women prisoners at Ravensbrück; studied the effects of stress on menstrual cycles, including irregular bleeding in women who had been told they were to be executed.[174]

Strughold, Prof. Hubertus: born 1898; chief of the Luftfarhtmedizinisches Forschungsinstitut (Aviation Medicine Research Institute) in the Reich Air Ministry;

169 Affidavit of Dr. Franz Blaha, Document 3249-PS, Exhibit No. USA-663, in *Trial IMT,* vol. 5, p. 171; Klee, *Auschwitz,* pp. 57, 144–145, 144 n. 12, 145 n. 16, 147–148, 150.

170 UNWCC, p. 534; Burman, ed., *The First German War Crimes Trial,* pp. 129–135, 162.

171 Testimony of Henri Henripierre, Nuremberg Trial Transcript USA vs. Karl Brandt et al., 18 December 1946, p. 716; reprinted in Mendelsohn, ed., *The Holocaust, Selected Documents,* Vol. 9, p. 196.

172 Interrogation of Herta Oberhauser, 31 October 1946, YVA, JM/6009, p. 4; Deposition of Zofia Sokulska, Translation of Document No-873, in RG-30.001M, p. 4; Klee, *Auschwitz,* p. 58.

173 Klee, *Auschwitz,* p. 58.

174 Annas and Grodin, eds., *The Nazi Doctors and the Nuremberg Code,* pp. 32–52.

reported to Oskar Schroeder and Erich Hippke; worked with Rascher and Romberg on the Dachau high altitude experiments; disappeared immediately after the war; one of twenty-one Nazi doctors whom U.S. Air Force surgeon Colonel Harry Armstrong wanted to recruit for the American military; 1947, entered the United States, placed under government protection by the Joint Chiefs of Staff and sent to Randolph Air Force Base in San Antonio, Texas; assisted the military with recruiting other Nazis from Germany and Austria; 1949, appointed director of the Department of Space Medicine at the School of Space Aviation; supervised experiments with weightlessness, decompression, and oxygen deprivation; called "Father of Space Medicine"; honorary member of the Air and Space Medicine Society in Munich; received by Pope Paul VI in conjunction with professional conventions in Paris and Rome; 1970s, investigated by the Immigration and Naturalization Service; case was closed at the request of a Texas congressman; retire in 1968 and died, 1986.[175]

STUMPFEGGER (STUMPFAECKER), DR. FRANZ: born 1906(?); Himmler's attending physician; 1942, along with Dr. Richard Schulze worked on bone transplantation experiments at Hohenlychen, taking transplant tissue from female inmates at Ravensbrück; 1966, tried, convicted and sentenced to life imprisonment; 1967, died in Bautzen Prison, in East Germany.[176]

TREITE, DR. PERCY (PERCIVAL) (SS-Obersturmführer): 1943 to the end of the war, a camp doctor at Ravensbrück; Nuremberg tribunal testimonies name him repeatedly; convicted by a British tribunal in Hamburg of war crimes: specifically the performance of sterilizations and abortions, and tests of clysters of urine of pregnant women in the treatment of typhus; sentenced 3 February 1947; on the night of 8–9 April 1947, committed suicide.[177]

TROMMER, DR. RICHARD: an SS doctor at Ravensbrück associated with the surgical experiments at that camp; August 1943, became Standortarzt (senior camp doctor) when Gerhard Scheidlausky was transferred to Natzweiler; also served at Flossenbürg and Neuengamme.[178]

175 Interrogation of Dr. Siegfried Ruff, 22 October 1946, YVA, JM/6020, pp. 1, 22; Klee, *Auschwitz*, pp. 196, 212–216, 253–255; "The CIA-Nazi Connection". Quotes are from "The CIA-Nazi Connection".

176 Interrogation of Herta Oberhauser, 31 October 1946, YVA, JM/6009, p. 8; Interrogation Summary No. 322 of Karl Gebhardt, 17 October 1946, YVA, JM/5979, p. 3; Klee, *Auschwitz*, p. 154.

177 Deposition of Helena Piasecka, Translation of Document No-864, in RG-30.001M, p. 1; UNWCC, p. 536; Klee, *Auschwitz*, pp. 58 and 58 n. 208. See Weindling, *Nazi Medicine and the Nuremberg Trials*, pp. 48, 177, 177; and Dörner, ed. *The Nuremberg Medical Trial*, p. 147, for some of the complications that arose in the case against Treite.

178 Deposition of Helena Piasecka, Translation of Document No-864, in RG-30.001M, p. 1; Declaration of Gerhard Schiedlausky, 7 August 1945, Translation of Document No-508, in RG-30.001M, pp. 2, 5; Klee, *Auschwitz*, p. 58.

TRZEBINSKY, DR. ALFRED: in Fall 1943, SS senior doctor (Standortarzt) at Neuengamme; oversaw tuberculosis experiments and was involved with killing the children who had served as experimental subjects; also served at Auschwitz and Lublin; was executed in fall 1946 at Hameln.[179]

VAERNET, DR. CARL (see the entry on JENSEN, DR. CARL PETER): Vaernet is a pseudonym used by Jensen in Germany.

VERSCHUER, PROF. OTMAR FREIHERR VON: 1942, director of the Kaiser Wilhelm Institute of Human Genetics and Eugenics in Berlin-Dahlem; teacher and mentor of Joseph Mengele. Having received a set of heterochromatic eyes taken by Mengele from twins (victims in his Auschwitz experiments), Verschuer decided to investigate the phenomenon, using additional specimens of twins' eyes supplied by Mengele from Auschwitz; thus linked the Dahlem Institute directly to the deadly experiments at Auschwitz. After the war, von Verschuer became a full professor at the University of Münster.[180]

VETTER, DR. HELMUT (SS Obersturmführer): born 1910 in Rastenburg; 1933, joined the SS; 17 February 1938, began working on experimental drugs at I. G. Farbenindustrie in Leverkusen; 1941, moved over to the Waffen SS; camp physician at Oranienburg, Dachau, Auschwitz and Mauthausen; carried out experiments with Ruthenol, Preparation B-1034 and Praeparat-3582 as treatments for tuberculosis; sentenced to death by an American Military Tribunal and executed on 2 February 1949.[181]

VILLMAN, DR.: conducted experimental operations on the legs of females imprisoned at Ravensbrück.[182]

VOEGT, DR. HANS: carried out hepatitis experiments; also experimented on mentally ill people; assisted Dr. Kurt Gutzeit with vaccine experiments on English POWs interned on the island of Crete.[183]

WAGNER, DR. ERICH (SS Untersturmführer): from Komotau/Sudetengau; a junior doctor (Assistenzarzt) in 1940 at Buchenwald; carried out research on tattooing practices for his doctoral dissertation (*Ein Beitrag zur Tätowierungsfrage*); he records that his tattoo samples (skin with tattoos) came from a large concentration camp.[184]

179 Klodzinski, in IAC, *Inhuman Medicine*, vol. 1, pt. 2, pp. 165, 171; Schwarzberg, *Children of Bullenhuser Damm*, pp. 35–46; Klee, *Auschwitz*, pp. 58 58 n. 210.

180 Astor, *The Last Nazi*, pp. 91, 98–98; Müller-Hill, *Murderous Science*, p. 70, and "Genetics After Auschwitz", *Holocaust Genocide Studies*, 2: 1 (1987), p. 8.

181 Klodzinski, in IAC, *Inhuman Medicine*, vol. 1, pt. 2, p. 177; Shelley, ed., *Criminal Experiments on Human Beings*, p. 336; "Doctors of the Holocaust", Pasternak, Personal Notes.

182 Deposition of Helena Piasecka, Translation of Document No-864, in RG-30.001M, p. 1.

183 *Trial IMT*, vol. 1, p. 499; Klee, *Auschwitz*, pp. 259–260.

184 Klee, *Auschwitz*, pp. 43, 48.

WEBER, DR. BRUNO NIKOLAUS (SS Hauptsturmführer): born 1915 in Koblenz; assigned to the Rajsko Institute to test blood sera groups; investigated interactions between human blood types by injecting patients with blood of various types and observing the effects; also injected patients with phenol; experimented with hallucinogens, barbiturates and morphine derivatives as mind control agents; accused of having cut flesh from human corpses for use in bacteriologic cultures; died in Homburg an der Saar on September 23, 1956.[185]

WEHRER, DR.: participated in experiments to test the effectiveness of the drugs R 17, Echinacine and Echinacine Extra in the treatment of wounds from phosphorous burns, on inmates given burns for the purpose.[186]

WIDMAN[N], DR. ING. ALBERT GOTTLOB (SS Sturmbannführer): not a medical doctor but did conduct experiments with human subjects in the camps; born 1912; associated as a consultant in chemistry with the Kriminaltechnisches Institut (KTI) of Department V (RKPA) in the Reichsicherheitshauptamt (RSHA) of the SS; conducted the first experimental gassing in an unused prison in Brandenburg; worked on poisoned weapons and tested them on psychiatric patients and prisoners: for example, 1944, accompanied his superior, SS Gruppenführer Nebe, to the Kriminalmedizinischen Institut in Vienna (supported by the KTI) and there tested poison munitions on human subjects, and 11 September 1944, tested poison bullets on five camp inmates who had been sentenced to death at Sachsenhausen. In September 1967, Widmann was found guilty by a court in Stuttgart for his part in the development and use of a gas van.[187]

WIMMER, DR. KARL: Luftwaffe medical officer; senior physician at the Strasbourg Anatomical Institute; first assistant of Dr. August Hirt; involved with Hirt in mustard gas experiments at Natzweiler and Strasbourg.[188]

WIRTHS (WIRTZ), DR. EDUARD (SS Sturmbannführer): born 1909 in Würzburg; brother of Helmut Wirths; SS physician in Dachau; from September 1942 until the evacuation, served as Standortarzt (chief doctor) at Auschwitz; experimented on dwarfs together with Mengele; also conducted experiments on the pre-cancerous conditions of the cervix; arrested by the British; committed suicide at the Neuengamme camp on 20 September 1945.[189]

185 Shelley, ed., *Criminal Experiments on Human Beings*, pp. 290, 315, 337; Lifton, *The Nazi Doctors*, pp. 269–302.

186 Affidavit of W. Hoven at Nuremberg Trial.

187 Klee, *Euthanasie*, pp. 207 and 502, and *Auschwitz*, pp. 173–174; Friedlander, *Index to NS-Justiz und Verbrechen*, p. 33; Testimony of SS Oberführer Dr. Mrugowsky, in *Trial IMT*, vol. 4, p. 208; Achim Thom and Genadiz Caregorodcev, *Medizin unterm Hakenkreuz* (Volk und Gesundheit, 1989), p. 503.

188 Interrogation Summary No. 48 of Wolfram Sievers, 20 August 1946, YVA, JM/6027, p. 3; Letter of Wolfram Sievers, 22 April 1943, Translation of Document No-193, in RG-30.001M, p. 1; Mitscherlich and Mielke, eds., *Doctors of Infamy*, p. 214.

189 Shelley, ed., *Criminal Experiments on Human Beings*, pp. 291, 337; Declaration of Elisabeth Ovitz-Moskovitz, undated, YVA, 0.33/4334, p. 2; Klee, *Auschwitz*, p. 59.

WIRTHS, DR. HELMUT: gynecologist, brother of SS doctor Eduard Wirths; in 1943, was working at the Stadtischen Frauenklinik (City Women's Clinic) in Hamburg-Altona; visited his brother at Auschwitz and inspected Block 10, where his brother was experimenting on female prisoners. He arranged to have specimens sent to his Altona clinic for research on pre-cancerous conditions of the cervix.[190]

WITTELER, DR. WILHELM: Erster Lagerarzt at Dachau; stated at the Dachau trials that no prisoner hanging could occur in the absence of a doctor; involved in Schilling's malaria experiments by falsifying death certificates to conceal the cause of death; was condemned to death by the American Military Tribunal sitting at Dachau, but the sentence was commuted in 1946 to twenty years imprisonment.[191]

WOLTER, DR. WALDEMAR: Erster Lagerarzt (camp doctor) at Dachau; also served as a camp doctor at Sachsenhausen and Mauthausen; participated in sepsis therapy experiments beginning in November 1942; was tried by a U.S. military court in Dachau at the trial of Mauthausen staff (U.S. vs. Hans Altfuldisch et al.) and condemned to death; executed (beheaded) 28 May 1947 at Landsberg Prison, along with four other SS doctors who had worked at Mauthausen.[192]

ZABEL (SS Hauptsturmführer): worked at Auschwitz's Institute of Hygiene (Rajsko Institute) under Dr. Hans Muench; participated in malaria research.[193]

ZAJITSCHEK, DR.: participated in typhus experiments in Buchenwald, using the drugs Rutenol and Nitroacridin 3582.[194]

190 Klee, *Auschwitz*, pp. 411–412; Nazi Doctor Database.
191 Klee, *Auschwitz*, pp. 21, 58, 58 n. 213, 122.
192 Klee, *Auschwitz*, pp. 34, 59, 59 n. 214, 145, 149, 361. See also "Dachau Scrapbook: Mauthausen".
193 Correspondence with Former SS Physician Dr. Hans Muench, in Shelley, ed., *Criminal Experiments on Human Beings*, p. 305.
194 Dr. Erwin Ding [-Schuler], "On Treatment of Typhus with Acridin Derivatives", Translation of Document No-582, in RG-30.001M, pp. 2, 8–11.

Bibliography

ABBREVIATIONS

BDC A3340-RAK-005: Berlin Documentation Center

BDC A3340-RAK-010: Berlin Documentation Center

BDC SS Officer Files A3343 SSO-096: Berlin Documentation Center

IAC: International Auschwitz Committee

RG-30.001M: (Microform) Records of the United States Nuernberg War Crimes Trials, United States vs. Karl Brandt et al., The "Medical Case" (Case I), 21 November 1946–20 August 1947, U.S. National Archives, mss. archives RG-30.001M

Trial IMT: *Trial of German Major War Criminals: Proceedings of the International Military Tribunal Sitting at Nuremberg Germany,* 22 vols

Trials NMT: *Trials of War Criminals before the Nuremberg Military Tribunals Under Control Council Law No. 10,* 15 vols (Washington, D.C., 1949–52). Volumes 1–2 of this publication contain materials from "The Medical case", i.e., United States vs. Karl Brandt et al., also known as The Doctors' Trial, The Medical Trial, or The Medical Case

UNWCC: United Nations, War Crimes Commission, *History of the United Nations War Crimes Commission and the Development of the Laws of War* (London: HMSO, 1948)

YVA: Yad Vashem Archives

SOURCES

Biographische Enzyklopedie deutschsprachiger Mediziner, 2 vols. (K. G. Saur, 2002).

Documented Report of the Sachsenhausen Trial (Berlin: SWA Verlag, 1948).

Experimental Operations on Prisoners of Ravensbrück Concentration Camp (Poznan and Warsaw: Wydawicho Zachodnie, 1960).

Nazi Conspiracy and Aggression (Washington: U.S. Government Printing Office, 1946 and Supp. A, 1947).

Report of the Atrocities Committed at the Dachau Concentration Camp, Vol. 1, Yad Vashem Archives, JM/10046.

The Trial of Major German War Criminals Proceedings of the International Military Tribunal Sitting at Nuremberg, Germany, Part 8, 27 February 1946–11 March 1946, Official Transcription (London: His Majesty's Stationery Officer, 1947).

Alexander, Major Leo, "The Treatment of Shock from Prolonged Exposure to Cold, Especially in Water", Combined Intelligence Objectives Subcommittee, Target No. 24, Report No. 250 (Washington, D.C.: Office of Publications Board, Dept of Commerce, 1946).

Altman, Lawrence K., "Nazi Data on Hypothermia Termed Unscientifc", *New York Times* (17 May 1990), p. B-11; recovered through the website *ProQuest Historical Newspapers.*

Aly, Götz, Peter Chroust and Christian Pross, *Cleansing the Fatherland* (Baltimore and London, 1994).

American Medical Association, "Letters", *Journal of the American Medical Association,* 276: 20 (27 November 1996), p. 1633.

Annas, G. J., and M. A. Grodin, eds., *The Nazi Doctors and the Nuremberg Code: Human Rights in Human Experiments* (New York and Oxford: Oxford University Press, 1995).

Astor, Gerald, *The Last Nazi: The Life and Times of Dr. Josef Mengele (*New York: Donald I. Fine Books, 1985).

Atlas, Michel C., "Ethics and Access to Teaching Materials in the Medical Library: The Case of the Pernkopf Atlas", *Bulletin of the Medical Librarians' Association,* 89: 1 (January 2001), pp. 51–58.

Aziz, Philippe, *Doctors of Death,* 3 vols. (Geneva, Switzerland: Ferni Publishers, 1976).

Beecher, Henry K., "Ethics and Clinical Research", *New England Journal of Medicine,* 274 (1966), pp. 1354–1360.

Belmont Report: "Ethical Principles and Guidelines for the Protection of Human Subjects of Research", Department of Health, Education, and Welfare Publication no. (05), 78–0012, vol. 1 (Washington, D.C.: U.S. Government Printing Office, 18 April 1979).

Ben, Abraham, *The Angel of Death: The Mengele Dossier* (Paris: France-Empire, 1967).

Benz, Wolfgang, "Sigmund Rascher, M.D.: A Career", *Dachau Review 2: History of Nazi Concentration Camps Studies,* ed. by W. Benz and Barbara Distel, vol. 2, (Brussels: Comité International de Dachau, 1990).

Berben, Paul, *Dachau 1933–1945: The Official History,* transl. by Capt. Bernhard R. Hanauer, Comité International de Dachau (Brussels: 1968, 1975).

Berger, Robert L., "Nazi Science: The Dachau Hypothermia Experiments", *New England Journal of Medicine,* 322: 20 (17 May 1990), pp. 1438–1439.

Bernadac, Christian, *Devil's Doctors: Medical Experiments on Human Subjects in the Concentration Camps* (Geneva: Ferni Publishing House, 1978).

Burman, W. Paul, ed., *The First German War Crimes Trial: Chief Judge Walter B. Beals' Desk Notebook of the Doctors' Trial, Held in Nuremberg, Germany, December 1945 to August 1947* (Chapel Hill, North Carolina: Documentary Publications, 1985).

Caplan, Arthur L., ed., *When Medicine Went Mad: Bioethics and the Holocaust,* (Towota, New Jersey: Humana Press, 1992).

Cohen, Baruch C., "The Ethics of Using Medical Data from Nazi Experiments", on the website *Jewish Law Articles,* http://www.jlaw.com/Articles/NaziMedEx.html, April 28, 2004. Cohen's article appeared originally in *Midstream* (June/July 1989).

Desoille, H., and Lafitte, M. M., *Psychologie criminelle des Hitleriens* (Paris, 1972).

Dörner, Klaus, ed., *The Nuremberg Medical Trial, 1946/47* (München: K. G. Saur, 2001).

Edzard, Ernst, "Killing in the Name of Healing: The Active Role of the German Medical Profession during the Third Reich", *American Journal of Medicine,* 100 (May 1996).

Eule, Karsten, and Marco Siegert, *Kriminalistik im System der Kriminalwissenschaften,* on the web at www.marco-siegert.de/projektarbeit/KAP-03.htm.

Fejkiel, Wladyslaw, *Przeglad Lekarski*, p. 1962; *The Second World War: A Day by Day Account*, at http://www.angelfire.com/my/rememberww2/index.html.

Fischer, Klaus P., *Nazi Germany: A New History* (New York: Continuum Books, 1995).

Franzblau, Michael, MD, "Nazi Medical Crimes Go Unpunished", *Dermatopathology: Practical and Conceptual*, 2: 2 (April–June 1996), pp. 83–86.

Freedman, Monroe H., "Letter from Monroe H. Freedman", *The Hastings Center Report* (August 1985), p. 31.

Friedlander, Henry, *Index to NS-Justiz und Verbrechen* (USHMM, unpublished).

Friedlander, Henry, *The Origins of Nazi Genocide: From Euthansia to the Final Solution* (Chapel Hill and London: University of North Carolina Press, 1995).

Friedman, Steven G., "Terrorists in Hamburg Redux", *Midstream: A Monthly Jewish Journal* (April 2002), on the website www.midstreamhf.com/200204/feature.html.

Greene, Vevl W., "Can Scientists Use Information Derived from the Concentration Camps? Ancient Answers to New Questions", in Caplan, ed., *When Medicine Went Mad*, pp. 155–170.

Grunfeld, Gerson B., "Letter to the Editor", *Journal of Medical Ethics*, 17 (1991), p. 162.

Hackett, David A., *The Buchenwald Report* (Boulder, Colorado: Westview Press, 1995).

Hoedeman, Paul, *Hitler or Hippocrates: Medical Experiments and Euthanasia in the Third Reich*, transl. by Ralph de Rijke, forew. by E. A. Cohen (Sussex, England: Book Guild, 1991).

Kater, Michael H., *Das Ahnenerbe der SS, 1935–1945* (Stuttgart: Deutsche-Verlags Anstalt, 1974).

Kater, Michael H., "The Burden of the Past: Problems of a Modern Historiography of Physicians and Medicine in Nazi Germany", *German Studies Review*, 10: 1 (February 1987).

Kater, Michael H., *Doctors under Hitler* (Chapel Hill and London: University of North Carolina Press, 1989).

Katz, Jay, "Abuse of Human Beings for the Sake of Science", in Caplan, ed., *When Medicine Went Mad*: pp. 233–270.

Katz, Jay, "Development of Codes of Ethics", Ch. 2 in *A History of Experimentation*, pp. 37–39.

Katz, Jay, *Experimentation with Human Beings* (New York: Russell Sage Foundation, 1972).

Klee, Ernst, *Auschwitz: Die NS-Medizin und Ihre Opfer* (Frankfurt am Main: S Fischer, 1997).

Klee, Ernst, *Deutsche Medizin im Dritten Reich* (Frankfurt am Main: Fischer, 2001).

Klee, Ernst, *"Euthanasie" im NS-Staat: Die Vernichtung lebensunwerten Lebens* (Frankfurt am Main: Fischer Taschenbuch Verlag, 1994).

Klodzinski, Stanislaw, *Inhuman Medicine.* International Auschwitz Committee.

Kogon, Eugen, *Der SS-Staat, das System der deutschen Konzentrationslager* (Frankfurt am Main: Verlag der Frankfurter Hefte; and München: K. Alber, 1946).

Kogon, Eugen, *The Theory and Practice of Hell* (New York: Berkeley Books, 1998).

Kor, Eva Mozes, "Nazi Experiments as Viewed by a Survivor of Mengele's Experiments", in Caplan, ed., *When Medicine Went Mad.* (1992).

Lagnado, Lucette Matalon, and Sheila Cohn Dekel, *Children of the Flames: Dr. Josef Mengele and the Untold Story of the Twins of Auschwitz* (New York: William Morrow & Company, Inc., 1991).

Leake, C. D., ed., *Percival's Medical Ethics* (Baltimore, 1927).

Lerner, Barren H., and David J. Rothman, "Medicine and the Holocaust: Learning More of the Lessons", *Annals of Internal Medicine,* 122: 10 (1995).

Lifton, Robert Jay, *The Nazi Doctors: Medical Killing and the Psychology of Genocide* (New York: Basic Books, 1986).

MacLean, French, *The Camp Men: The SS Officers Who Ran the Nazi Concentration Camp System* (Atglen, PA: Schiffer Military History, 1999).

Mendelsohn, John, ed., *The Holocaust: Selected Documents in Eighteen Volumes* (New York: Garland Pub., 1982).

Mitscherlich, Alexander, and Fred Mielke, eds., *The Death Doctors,* transl. by James Clengh, (London: Elek Books, 1962), a translation of Mitscherlich and Mielke, eds., *Medizin ohne Menschlichkeit: Dokumente des Nürnberger Ärztlicheprozesses,* 1949 ed. reprint (Frankfurt am Main, 1978). This 1949 ed. (German) is the 2nd edition of the publication; the 1st edition appeared in 1947, as *Das Diktat der Menschenverachtung* (Heidelberg: Schneider, 1947), and was translated into English as *The Doctors of Infamy: The Story of Nazi Medical Crimes* (New York: Henry Schuman, 1949). There is also a paperback edition, *Medizin ohne Menschlichkeit: Dokumente des Nürnberger Prozesses,* (Frankfurt am Main: Fischer Taschenbuch Verlag, 1960).

Moe, Kristine, "Should the Nazi Research Data Be Cited", *The Hastings Center Report* (December 1984), pp. 5–7.

Müller-Hill, Benno, "Genetics After Auschwitz", *Holocaust Genocide Studies,* 2: 1 (1987).

Müller-Hill, Benno, *Murderous Science* (Oxford: Oxford University Press, 1998).

Neuhaus, The Rev. John, "The Use of Metaphors and Analogies Concerning the Holocaust in Contemporary Bioethical Debates", typescript of a lecture given at the conference "The Meaning of the Holocaust for Bioethics", 1993, in Minnesota.

Nixon, Alan C., "Opinion: If the Data's Good, Use It – Regardless of the Source", *The Scientist,* 2: 21 (14 November 1988).

Percival, Thomas, *Medical Ethics* (1803; reprinted by R. E. Krieger Publ., 1975, 1976).

Ploetz, Alfred, "Die Tüchtigkeit unserer Rasse und der Schutz der Schwachen" [The Competence of our Race and the Protection of the Weak], vol. 1, in Alfred Ploetz, *Grundlinien einer Rassenhygiene* [The Fundamentals of Racial Hygiene (Berlin, 1895).

Posner, Gerald L., *Mengele: The Complete Story* (New York: McGraw-Hill, 1986).

Post, Steven G., "The Echo of Nuremberg: Nazi Data and Ethics", *Journal of Medical Ethics* 17 (1991), pp. 42–44.

Proctor, Robert N., "Nazi Biomedical Policies", in Caplan, ed., *When Medicine went Mad* (Towota, New Jersey: Humana Press, 1992).

Proctor, Robert N., *Racial Hygiene: Medicine under the Nazis* (Cambridge, Mass. and London, England: Harvard University Press, 1988).

Rosenbaum, Alan S., "The Use of Nazi Medical Experimentation Data: Memorial or Betrayal?", *Journal of Applied Philosophy,* 4 (1989), pp. 59–67.

Scharsach, Hans-Henning, *Die Ärzte der Nazis* (Wien, München and Zürich: Orac, 2000).

Shelley, Lore, ed., *Criminal Experiments on Human Beings in Auschwitz and War Research Laboratories: Twenty Women Prisonier's Accounts* (San Francisco: Mellen Research University Press, 1991).

Schwarzberg, Günther, *The Murders at Bullenhuser Damm: The SS Doctor and the Children* (Indiana Univ. Press, 1984).

Schuster, Evelyn E., "Fifty Years Later: The Significance of the Nuremberg Code", N*ew England Journal of Medicine,* 337: 20 (13 November 1997), pp. 1436–1440.

Shabecoff, Philip, "Head of E.P.A. Bars Nazi Data in Study on Gas", *The New York Times* (23 March 1988).

Siegel, Barry, "Can Evil Beget Good? Nazi Data: A Dilemma for Science", *The Los Angeles Times* (30 October 1988), Front Section. Recovered through the *ProQuest Newspapers* website at http://proquest.umi.com.

Snyder, Louis L., *Encyclopedia of the Third Reich* (New York: McGraw-Hill Book Company, 1976).

Sun, Marjorie, "EPA Bars Use of Nazi Data", *Science,* 240: 4848 (1 April 1988), p. 21.

Thom, Achim, and Genadiz Caregorodcev, *Ärzte unterm Hakenkreuz* (VEB Verlag Volk und Gesundheit, 1989).

Timmermann, Carsten, "Rationalizing 'Folk Medicine' in Interwar Germany: Faith, Business and Science at Dr. Madaus & Co.", *Social History of Medicine,* 14 (2001), pp. 459–482.

Wade, Nicholas, "The Editorial Notebook: The Errors of Nazi Science", *The New York Times* (27 May 1990), Section 4, p. 12; courtesy of the website *LexisNexis,* http://web.lexis-nexis.com.

Waitz, Robert, "Experimental Typhus in the Buchenwald Camp", IAC, *Inhuman Medicine,* vol. 1, pt. 2, pp. 120–130.

Wall Street Journal, " 'Nazi Hypothermia Data is Useless,' Surgeon Says: A Wall Street Journal News Roundup", *Wall Street Journal* (17 May 1990), p. A-1; courtesy of the website *ProQuest Newspapers,* http://proquest.umi.com/pqdweb?index.

Wallace, Daniel J., and Michael Weisman, "Should a War Criminal Be Rewarded with Eponymous Distinction? The Double Life of Hans Reiter (1881–1969)", *Journal of Clinical Rheumatology* 6: 1 (February 2000), pp. 49–54.

Waltrich, Hans, *Zur Geschichte der Heilstalten vom Roten Kreuz in Hohenlychen* (http://www.oekostadt-online.de/oen/walt.1.htm and http://www.oekostadt-online.de/oen/walt.2.htm.

Weindling, Paul, *Health, Race, and German Politics between National Unification and Nazism, 1870–1945* (New York: Cambridge University Press, 1989).

Weindling, Paul, *Nazi Medicine and the Nuremberg Trials: From Medical War Crimes to Informed Consent* (Houndmills: Palgrave MacMillan, 2004).

Weisskopf, Michael, "EPA Bars Use of Nazi's Human Test Data After Scientists Object", *The Washington Post* (24 March 1988), First Section, p. A17.

Yad Vashem-YIVO The Holocaust, *The Nuremberg Evidence* (unpublished, USHMM Library).

Ziporyn, Terra, "What the Nazis called 'Medical Research' Haunts the Scientific Community to This Day", *Journal of the American Medical Association,* 263: 6 (9 February 1990).

INTERNET SOURCES

Avalon Project at Yale Law School, www.yale.edu/lawweb/avalon/imt, documents of the International Military Tribunal.

Bioprofiles, http://www.ess.uew.ac.uk/genocide/bioprofiles.htm

CIA-Nazi Connection,
http://www.angelfire.com/ca3/jphuck/Book14Ch.3.html

Dachau Scrapbook,
www.scrapbookpages.com/DachauScrapbook/DachauTrial.html

Dachau Scrapbook: Buchenwald Trial,
www.scrapbookpages.com/DachauScrapbook/DachauTrial/BuchenwaldTrial.html

Dachau Scrapbook: Mauthausen,
www.scrapbookpages.com/DachauScrapbook/Mauthausen01.html

Doctors of the Holocaust,
www.remember.org/imagine/doctors.html

Erich Hippke,
http://www.geocities.com/~onion47/WEHRMACHT/LUFTWAFFE/Sanitäts Offizier/HIPPKE Erich.html

Eule, Karsten and Marco Siegert, Kriminalistik im System der Kriminalwissenschaften,
www.marco-siegert.de/projektarbeit/KAP-03.htm

Inspektion der SS-Totenkopf-Standarten-Lexikon der Wehrmacht,
http://www.lexikon-der-wehrmacht.de/Gliederungen/SSTotenkopfStandarten-R.htm

Jewish Virtual Library, at www.jewishvirtuallibrary.org

The Mazal Archives,
www.mazal.org/archive/nmt/02/NMT02-t0875.html.
Texts and indices of the IMT and NMT publications listed above.

Nizkor, www.nizkor.org/hweb/imt, documents from the *International Military Tribunal.*

Nazi Doctors and Other Perpetrators of Nazi Crimes, at
www.webster.edu/~woolflm/nazidocsandothers.htm

United States Holocaust Memorial Museum,
http://www.ushmm.org/research/doctors/medical.htm

Die Zeit, 40/2003, "Von deutschen Ruhm", at http://zeus.zeit.de/text/2003/40 A-DBE, citing the entry on Kurt Gutzeit in *Biographische Enzyklopedie deutschsprachiger Mediziner,* 2 vols. (K. G. Saur, 2002).

Thou shalt not be a victim!

Thou shalt not be a perpetrator!

Thou shalt not be a bystander!

YEHUDA BAUER
Historian

List of illustrations

Photos of the doctors tried at the Nuremberg "Doctors' Trial", plus a photo of Mengle who was never taken to court.

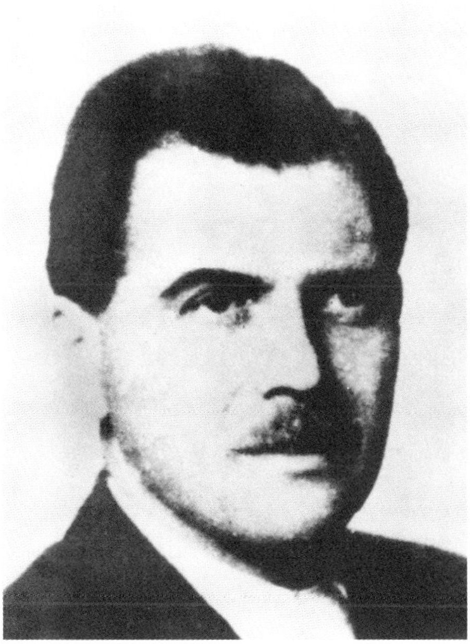

Josef Mengele

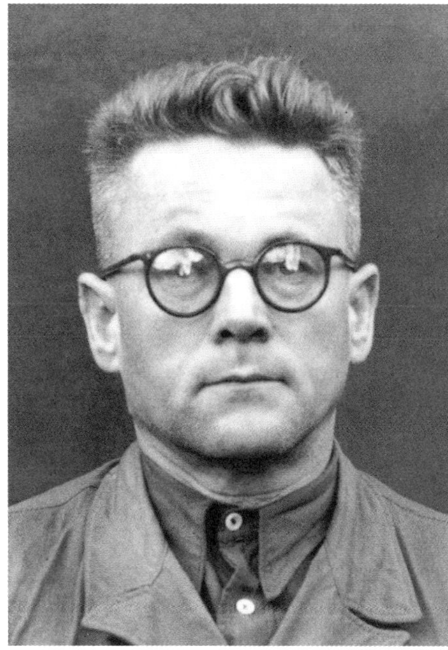

Karl Gebhardt

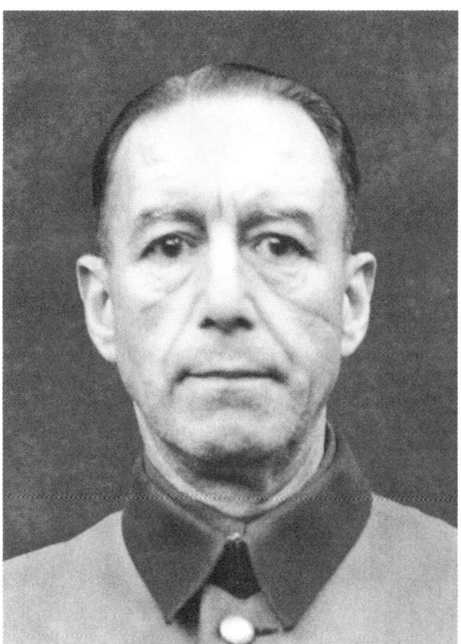

Siegfried Handloser

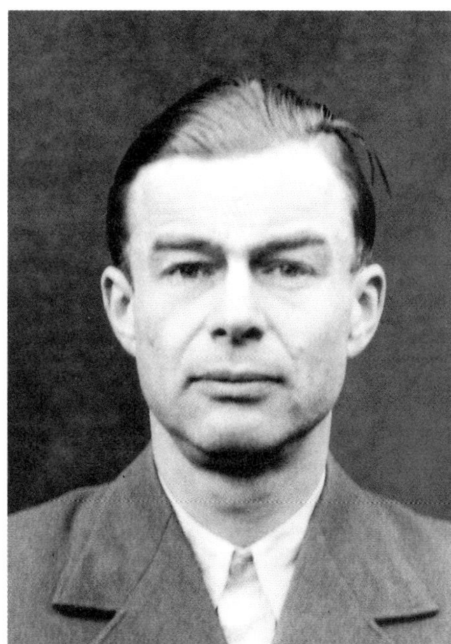

Siegfried Ruff

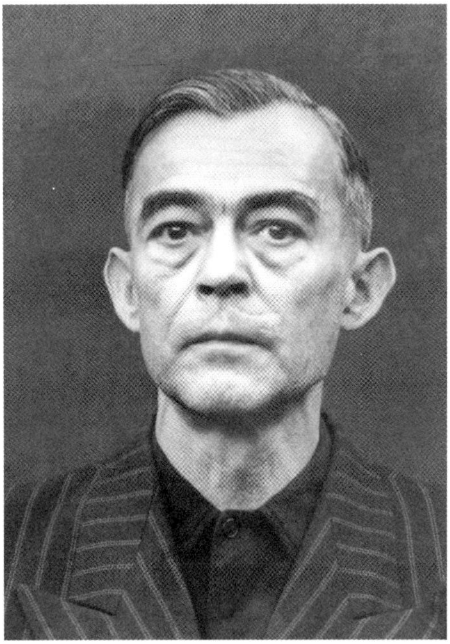

Kurt Blome

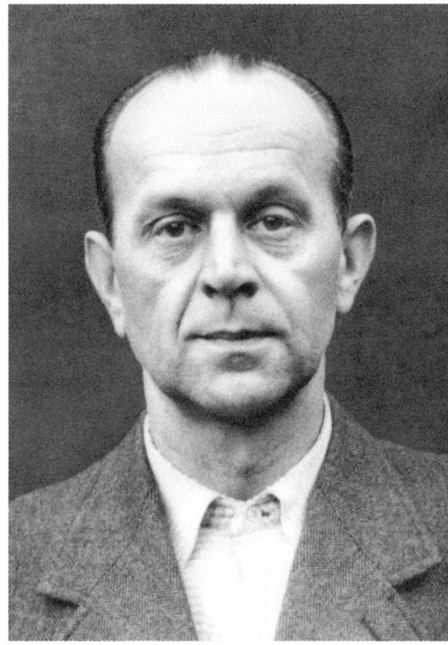

Adolf Pokorny

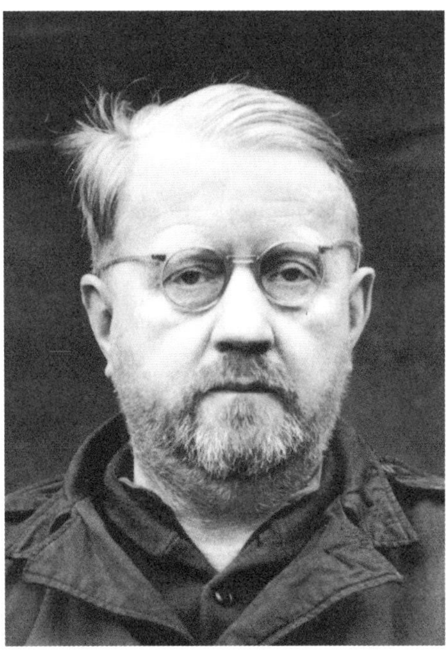

Gerhard Rose

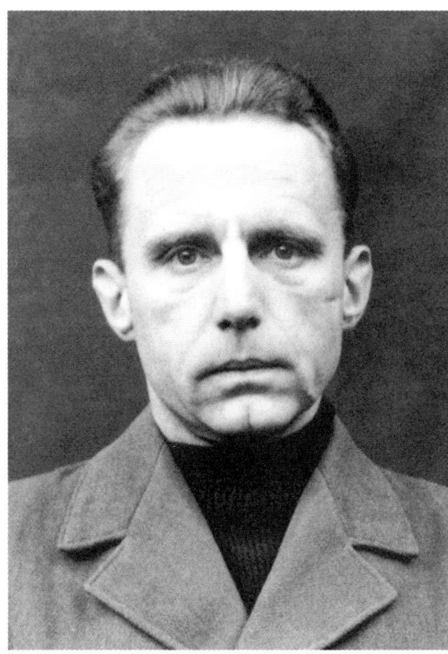

Wilhelm Beiglböck

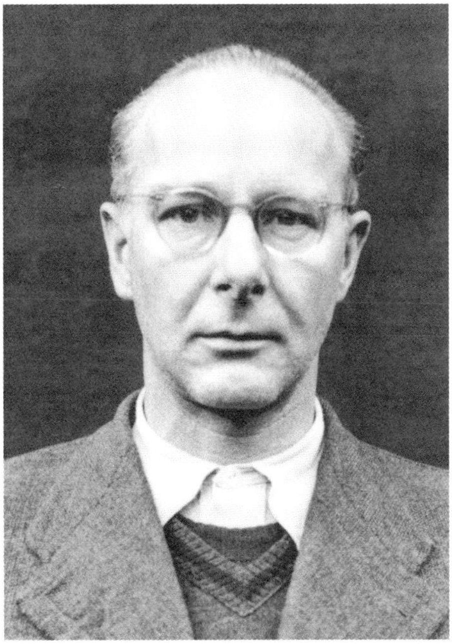

Viktor Brack

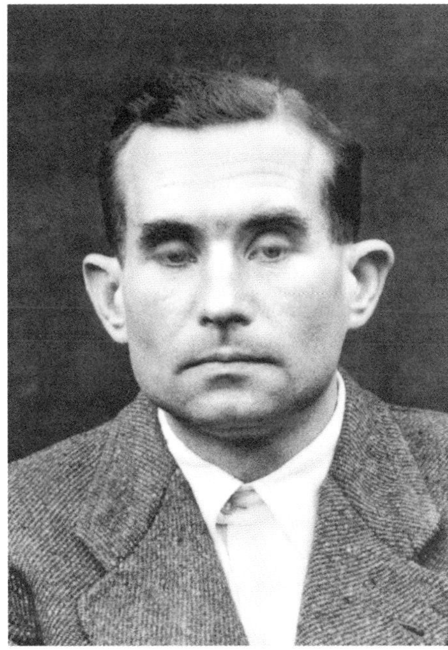

Hermann Becker-Freyseng

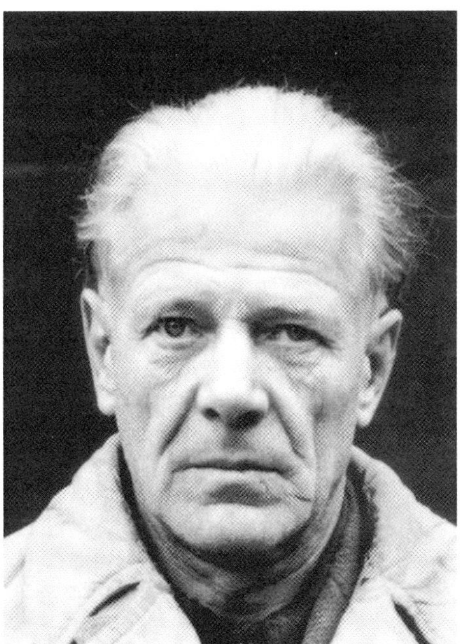

Georg August Weltz

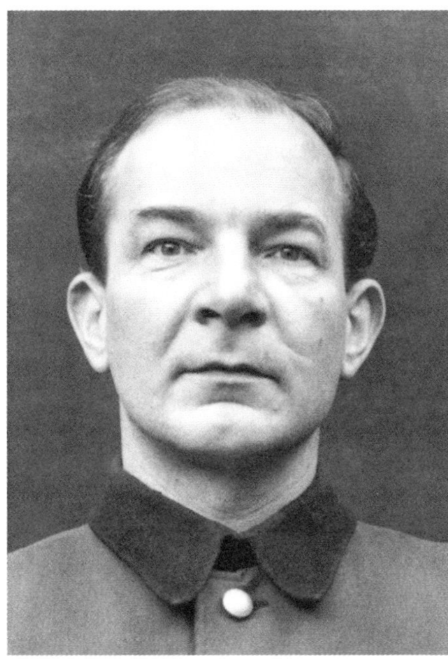

Joachim Mrugowsky

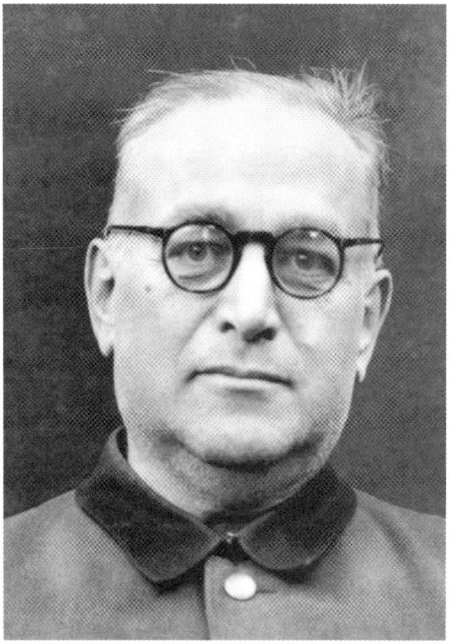

Paul Rostock

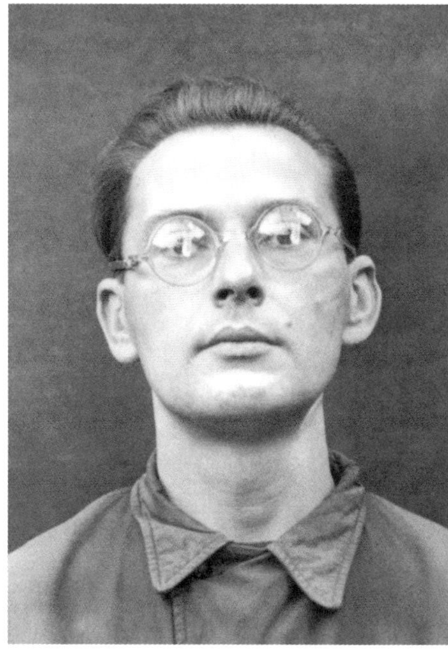

Rudolf Brandt

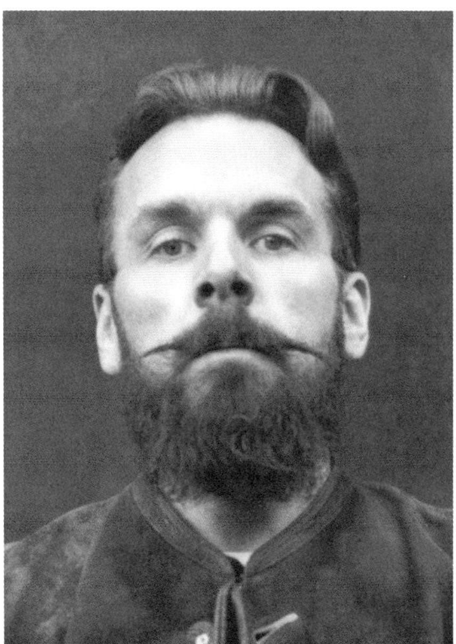

Wolfram Sievers

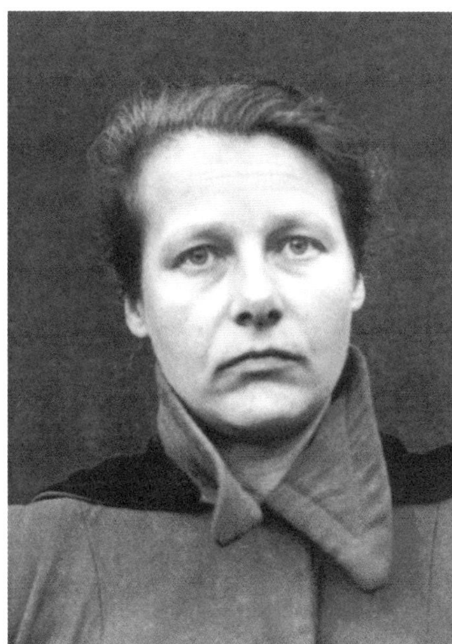

Herta Oberhauser

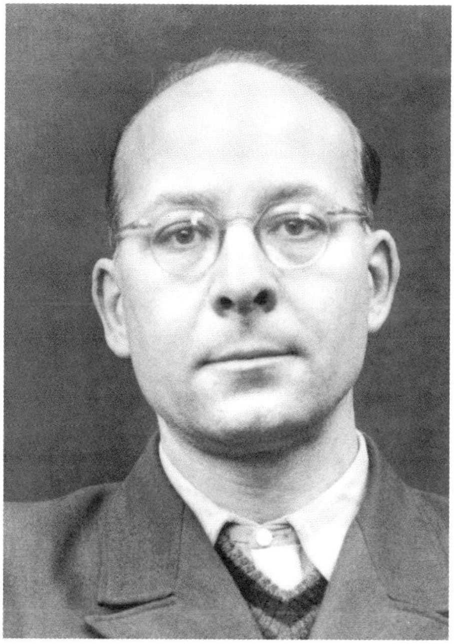

Helmut Poppendick

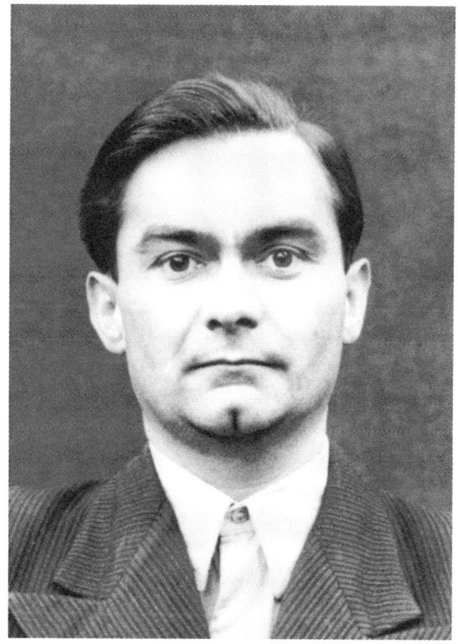

Hans Wolfgang Romberg

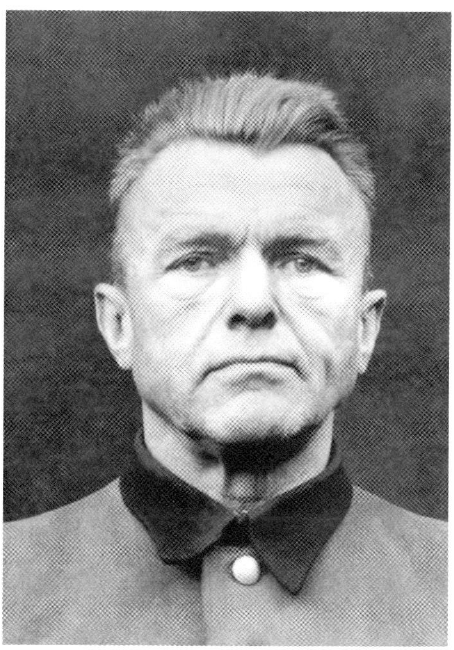

Karl Genzken

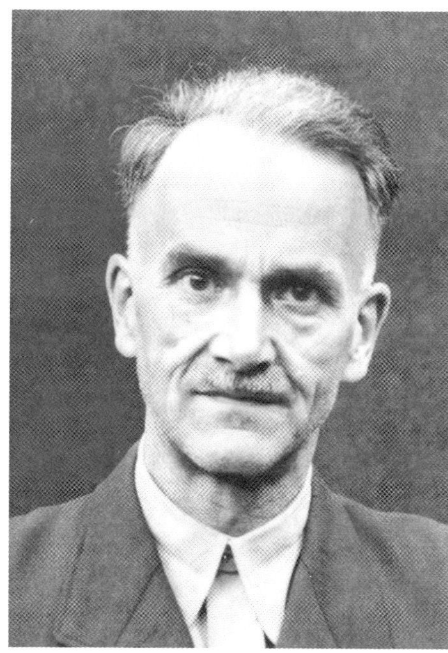

Oskar Schroeder

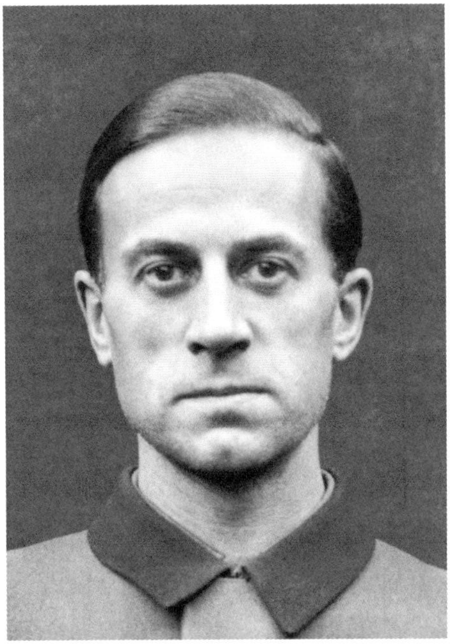

Karl Brandt

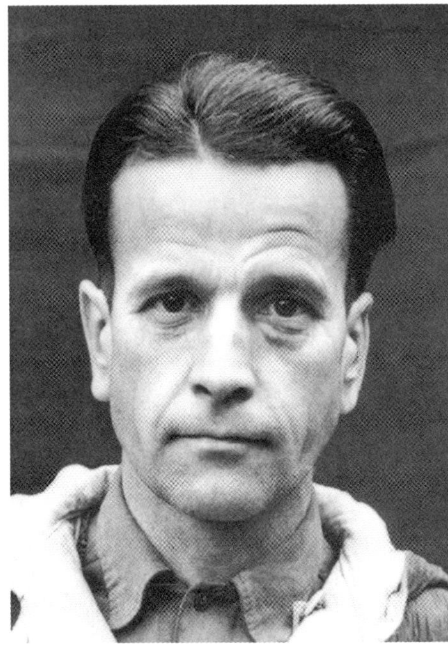

Waldemar Hoven

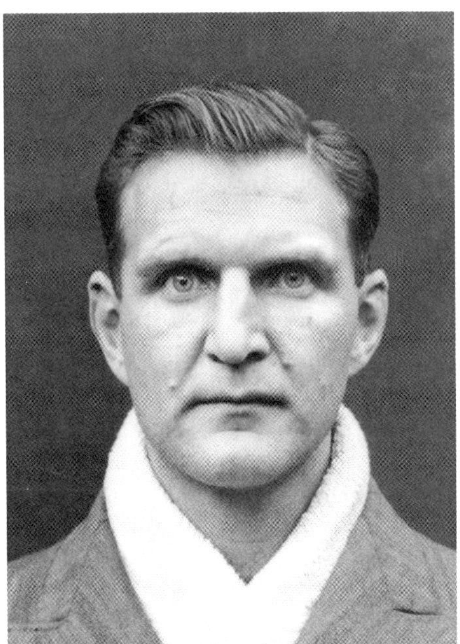

Fritz Fischer

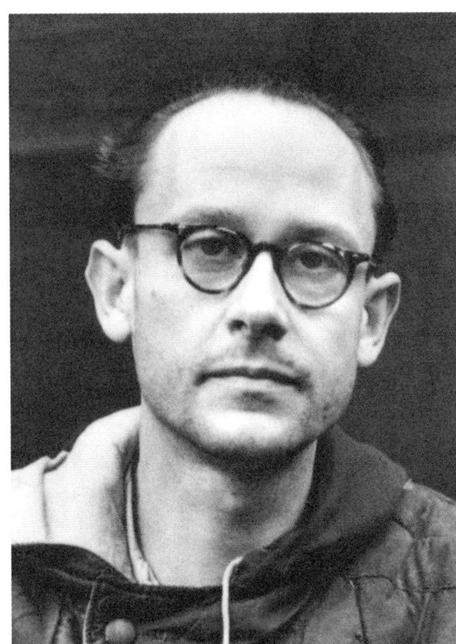

Konrad Schaeffer